W9-AVI-367

American Cancer Society's

Complete Guide to

PROSTATE
CANCER

Books published by the American Cancer Society

A Breast Cancer Journey: Your Personal Guidebook, Second Edition

American Cancer Society Consumers Guide to Cancer Drugs, Second Edition, Wilkes, Ades, and Krakoff

American Cancer Society's Complementary and Alternative Cancer Methods Handbook

American Cancer Society's Guide to Complementary and Alternative Cancer Methods

American Cancer Society's Guide to Pain Control, Revised Edition

Angels & Monsters: A child's eye view of cancer, Murray and Howard

Because Someone I Love Has Cancer: Kids' Activity Book

Cancer in the Family: Helping Children Cope with a Parent's Illness, Heiney et al.

Cancer: What Causes It, What Doesn't

Caregiving: A Step-By-Step Resource for Caring for the Person with Cancer at Home, Revised Edition, Houts and Bucher

Coming to Terms with Cancer: A Glossary of Cancer-Related Terms, Laughlin

Couples Confronting Cancer: Keeping Your Relationship Strong, Fincannon and Bruss

Crossing Divides: A Couple's Story of Cancer, Hope, and Hiking Montana's Continental Divide, Bischke

Eating Well, Staying Well During and After Cancer, Bloch et al.

Good for You! Reducing Your Risk of Developing Cancer

Healthy Me: A Read-along Coloring & Activity Book, Hawthorne (illustrated by Blyth)

Informed Decisions: The Complete Book of Cancer Diagnosis, Treatment, and Recovery, Second Edition, Eyre, Lange, and Morris

Kicking Butts: Your Path to Quitting Smoking

Our Mom Has Cancer, Ackermann and Ackermann

When the Focus Is on Care: Palliative Care and Cancer, Foley et al.

Also by the American Cancer Society

American Cancer Society's Healthy Eating Cookbook: A celebration of food, friends, and healthy living, Second Edition

Celebrate! Healthy Entertaining for Any Occasion

Kids' First Cookbook: Delicious-Nutritious Treats to Make Yourself!

American Cancer Society's

Complete Guide to

PROSTATE CANCER

Edited by
David G. Bostwick, MD, MBA
E. David Crawford, MD
Celestia S. Higano, MD
Mack Roach III, MD

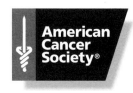

Published by
American Cancer Society
Health Promotions
1599 Clifton Road NE
Atlanta, Georgia 30329, USA

Copyright © 2005 American Cancer Society
All rights reserved. Without limiting the rights under copyright reserved above, no part of this publication may be reproduced, stored in or introduced into a retrieval system, or transmitted, in any form or by any means (electronic, mechanical, photocopying, recording, or otherwise), without the prior written permission of the publisher.

Printed in the United States of America
Cover designed by Jill Dible, Atlanta, Georgia

5 4 3 2 1   04 05 06 07 08

Library of Congress Cataloging-in-Publication Data

American Cancer Society's complete guide to prostate cancer / edited by David G. Bostwick ... [et al.].
    p. cm.
  Includes index.
  ISBN 0-944235-54-9 (pbk. : alk. paper)
  1. Prostate—Cancer—Popular works. I. Title: Complete guide to prostate cancer. II. Bostwick, David G. III. American Cancer Society.

RC280.P7A47 2004
616.99'463—dc22

                2004015407

A NOTE TO THE READER

The information contained in this book is not intended as medical advice and should not be relied upon as a substitute for talking with your doctor. This information may not address all possible actions, treatments, medications, precautions, side effects, or interactions. All matters regarding your health require the supervision of a medical doctor or appropriate health care professional who is familiar with your medical needs. For more information, contact your American Cancer Society at 800-ACS-2345 or http://www.cancer.org.

EDITORIAL BOARD

LEAD EDITOR:

David G. Bostwick, MD, MBA

clinical professor of pathology, University of Virginia,
  Charlottesville, VA
medical director, Bostwick Laboratories, Richmond, VA

Bostwick is an internationally renowned expert in prostate cancer, bladder cancer, and urologic diseases, with more than two decades of experience. He was formerly a professor of pathology and urology at the Mayo Clinic (1991–1999). He has authored 10 books, more than 25 book chapters, and over 400 papers. His textbook, *Urologic Surgical Pathology*, coauthored with John Eble, MD, is the best-selling book in uropathology. Bostwick published more papers with the keywords "prostate cancer" in the past decade (1990–2000) than any other investigator. He is also the most sought-after pathologist for second opinions in prostate pathology. Bostwick is on the editorial board of 10 journals and is past president of the International Society of Urological Pathology.

EDITORIAL BOARD MEMBERS:

E. David Crawford, MD

associate director, University of Colorado
  Comprehensive Cancer Center, Aurora, CO
professor of surgery and radiation oncology,
  head, Urologic Oncology, University of Colorado
  Health Sciences Center, Aurora, CO

Crawford is a nationally recognized expert in prostate cancer. The recipient of more than 69 research grants, he has conducted research in the treatment of advanced bladder cancer, metastatic adenocarcinoma of the prostate, hormone-refractory prostate cancer, and other areas of urological infections and malignancies. He has authored or coauthored over 400 articles and five textbooks. He is also an editorial reviewer or consultant for a large number of publications, including *Urology*, *Journal of Urology*, *The New England Journal of Medicine*, *Cancer*, and the *Journal of Clinical Oncology*.

Celestia S. Higano, MD

oncology specialist, Seattle Cancer Care Alliance
associate professor, Department of Medicine and
  Department of Urology, School of Medicine,
  University of Washington, Seattle, WA

Higano subspecializes in genitourinary oncology and heads the clinical research program in that area for the University of Washington. She runs the monthly Genitourinary Tumor Board. In addition to numerous clinical trials with investigational agents, her areas of ongoing research include intermittent androgen suppression and the effects of androgen deprivation on the male mind and body.

Mack Roach III, MD

professor of radiation oncology and urology,
director, Clinical Research, Department of Radiation
  Oncology, University of California at San Francisco,
  San Francisco, CA

Roach is president of the John Hale Medical Society. He was the lead author for the *American College of Radiology Guidelines for Treatment Planning* (1996; 2000). He is associate editor for *CA: A Cancer Journal for Clinicians* and is on the editorial boards of: *The Prostate Journal*; *International Journal of Radiation Oncology, Biology, and Physics*; and *Clinical Prostate Cancer*. Research interests include: defining methods of predicting outcome following treatment for prostate cancer, improving the delivery of and defining the role of radiation for treating prostate cancer, implementing PEREGRINE into routine clinical practice, and examining prostate cancer and race.

Editorial Review

Rick Alteri, MD,
associate medical editor,
American Cancer Society,
Atlanta, GA

Durado Brooks, MD, MPH,
director, Prostate and Colorectal Cancer,
American Cancer Society,
Atlanta, GA

Ted Gansler, MD,
director of medical content,
American Cancer Society,
Atlanta, GA

Tom Morris, MS,
prostate cancer survivor,
Richmond, VA

Patricia A. Parker, PhD,
assistant professor, Department of
Behavioral Science, the University of
Texas MD Anderson Cancer Center,
Houston, TX

Stan Rosenfeld,
prostate cancer survivor; *leader,*
American Cancer Society Man to Man
support group, Fairfax, CA

Carmen Rodriguez, MD, MPH,
senior epidemiologist; *director*,
Biospecimen Repository,
American Cancer Society,
Atlanta, GA

Leslie R. Schover, PhD,
professor, Department of Behavioral
Science, University of Texas MD
Anderson Cancer Center, Houston, TX

Editor
Amy Brittain

Managing Editor
Gianna Marsella, MA

Book Publishing Manager
Candace Magee

Director, Publishing
Diane Scott-Lichter, MA

Direct Channels Managing Director
Chuck Westbrook

CONTRIBUTING AUTHORS

Christopher L. Amling, MD, *assistant professor*, Department of Urology, Naval Medical Center, San Diego, CA

Rekha N. Attigere, MBBS, *special fellow*, University of Colorado Health Sciences Center, Denver, CO

Sylvie Aubin, PhD, *acting clinical instructor*, Department of Psychiatry and Behavioral Sciences, University of Washington School of Medicine; Seattle Cancer Care Alliance, Seattle, WA

Charles L. Bennett, MD, PhD, *professor of medicine*, Department of General Medicine/Division of Hematology/Oncology, Northwestern University; *director,* Health Service Research and Development, Lakeside, Chicago VA Health Care System, Chicago, IL

Jonathan C. Berger, *medical student*, Pritzker School of Medicine, the University of Chicago, Chicago, IL

David G. Bostwick, MD, MBA, *medical director*, Bostwick Laboratories, Richmond, VA; *clinical professor of pathology*, University of Virginia, Charlottesville, VA

Michael K. Brawer, MD, *director*, Northwest Prostate Institute, Northwest Hospital, Seattle, WA

Harry B. Burke, MD, PhD, *associate professor of medicine*, George Washington University School of Medicine, Washington, DC

Peter R. Carroll, MD, *professor*, Department of Urology, University of California, San Francisco, San Francisco, CA

Jenevie D. Clark-Dorsey, MS HED, *project manager*, Division of Population Sciences, Fox Chase Cancer Center, Philadelphia, PA

E. David Crawford, MD, *associate director*, University of Colorado Comprehensive Cancer Center; *professor of surgery and radiation oncology, head*, Urologic Oncology, University of Colorado Health Sciences Center, Aurora, CO

Nancy A. Dawson, MD, *director*, Genitourinary Oncology Program, Greenebaum Cancer Center, University of Maryland, Baltimore, MD

Michael A. Diefenbach, PhD, *associate member*, Division of Population Science, Fox Chase Cancer Center, Philadelphia, PA

Bob Djavan, MD, PhD, *vice chairman*, Department of Urology; *director*, Prostate Disease Center, University of Vienna, Vienna, Austria

L. Michael Glode, MD, *Robert Rifkin Chair for Prostate Cancer Research*, University of Colorado Health Sciences Center, Denver, CO

Ciril J. Godec, MD, PhD, *chairman*, Department of Urology, Long Island College Hospital, Brooklyn, NY

Nicolle S. Gorby, *project coordinator*, Institute for Health Service Research, Northwestern University, Chicago, IL

Michelle H. Gurel, *director*, Research and Education, Chicago Prostate Cancer Center, Westmont, IL

Shuk-Mei Ho, PhD, *professor of surgery and cell biology*, University of Massachusetts Medical School, Worcester, MA

Jeffrey M. Holzbeierlein, MD, *assistant professor of urology*, University of Kansas Medical Center, Kansas City, KS

Hedvig Hricak, MD, PhD, *chairman*, Department of Radiology, Memorial Sloan-Kettering Cancer Center, New York, NY

Brian D. Kavanagh, MD, MPH,
associate professor and vice-chair, Department of
Radiation Oncology, University of Colorado
Cancer Center, Aurora, CO

Naveen Kella, MD, *fellow*, the Baylor Prostate
Center, Baylor College of Medicine, Houston, TX

Arnon Krongrad, MD, *president*,
The Krongrad Clinic, Aventura, FL

Paul H. Lange, MD, *professor and chairman*,
Department of Urology, University of
Washington, Seattle, WA

John H. Lynch, MD, *professor and chairman*,
Department of Urology, Georgetown University
Hospital, Washington, DC

E. Allison Lyons, *project coordinator*,
Institute for Health Service Research,
Northwestern University, Chicago, IL

Paul D. Maroni, MD, *resident*, Division of
Urology, University of Colorado Health Sciences
Center, Aurora, CO

Viraj A. Master, MD, PhD, *clinical instructor*,
Department of Urology, University of California,
San Francisco Comprehensive Cancer Center at
Mt. Zion Medical Center, San Francisco, CA

Katherine C. Meade, *vice chairman*,
Virginia Prostate Cancer Coalition,
Mason Neck, VA

Maxwell V. Meng, MD, *assistant professor*,
Department of Urology, University of California,
San Francisco, San Francisco, CA

Rafael V. Miguel, MD, *professor and chairman*,
Department of Anesthesiology;
director, Pain Medicine Program,
University of South Florida, Tampa, FL

Bruce Montgomery, MD, *associate professor*,
University of Washington;
Seattle Cancer Care Alliance, Seattle, WA

Brian J. Moran, MD, *medical director*,
Chicago Prostate Cancer Center, Westmont, IL

Judd W. Moul, MD, *director*, Department of
Defense Center for Prostate Disease Research;
professor of surgery/urology, Uniformed Services
University of the Health Sciences, Rockville, MD

Mark A. Moyad, MD, MPH, *Phil F. Jenkins
Director of Complementary/Preventive Medicine*,
Department of Urology, University of Michigan
Medical Center, Ann Arbor, MI

Christian J. Nelson, PhD, *research fellow*,
Department of Psychiatry and Behavioral
Sciences, Memorial Sloan-Kettering Cancer
Center, New York, NY

William K. Oh, MD,
assistant professor of medicine and clinical director,
Multidisciplinary Care Team,
Dana-Farber Cancer Institute, Boston, MA

David K. Ornstein, MD, *assistant professor*,
Department of Urology, University of California,
Irvine, Orange, CA

Sangtae Park, MD, *resident*, Department of
Urology, University of California, San Francisco,
San Francisco, CA

Daniel P. Petrylak, MD,
associate professor of medicine, College of
Physicians and Surgeons, New York, NY

Darko Pucar, MD, PhD, *research fellow*,
Departments of Radiology and Medical Physics,
Memorial Sloan-Kettering Cancer Center,
New York, NY

Junqi Qian, MD, *director of molecular diagnostics*,
Bostwick Laboratories, Richmond, VA

Adam Raben, MD, *director of clinical research*,
Department of Radiation Oncology,
Helen F. Graham Cancer Center, Newark, DE

David Raben, MD, *associate professor*,
University of Colorado Health Sciences Center,
Aurora, CA

Nadeem U. Rahman, MD, *resident,*
Department of Urology, University of California,
San Francisco, San Francisco, CA

Mesut Remzi, MD, *resident,* Department of
Urology, University of Vienna, Vienna, Austria

Carrie W. Rinker-Schaeffer, PhD,
associate professor of surgery and medicine;
director of urologic research, University of Chicago,
Chicago, IL

Stan Rosenfeld, *American Cancer Society Man to*
Man group leader, Fairfax, CA

Andrew J. Roth, MD,
associate attending psychiatrist, Department of
Psychiatry snd Behavioral Sciences, Memorial
Sloan-Kettering Cancer Center, New York, NY

Fred Saad, MD, FRCSC, *director of urologic*
oncology, professor of surgery/urology,
Centre Hospitalier de l'Université de Montréal,
Montréal, Canada

Christian Seitz, MD, *resident,* Department of
Urology, University of Vienna, Vienna, Austria

Kevin M. Slawin, MD, *professor,* Department of
Urology; *director,* the Baylor Prostate Center,
Baylor College of Medicine, Houston, TX

Anthony Y. Smith, MD,
professor of surgery/urology, Division of Urology,
University of New Mexico School of Medicine,
Albuquerque, NM

Samira Syed, MD, *clinical assistant professor,*
University of Texas Health Science Center San
Antonio; *clinical investigator,* Institute for Drug
Development, Cancer Therapy & Research
Center, San Antonio, TX

James A. Talcott, MD, SM, *assistant professor,*
Center for Outcomes Research,
Massachusetts General Hospital, Boston, MA

Miah-Hiang Tay, MD, *clinical fellow,*
Dana-Farber Cancer Institute, Boston, MA

Ian M. Thompson, MD, *professor and chief,*
Division of Urology, University of Texas Health
Science Center San Antonio, San Antonio, TX

J. Brantley Thrasher, MD, *professor and William*
L. Valk Chair of Urology, University of Kansas
Medical Center, Kansas City, KS

Barry G. Timms, PhD, *professor,* Division of
Basic Biomedical Sciences, University of South
Dakota School of Medicine, Vermillion, SD

Anthony W. Tolcher, MD,
clinical associate professor, University of Texas
Health Science Center San Antonio;
director of clinical research, Institute for Drug
Development, Cancer Therapy & Research
Center, San Antonio, TX

James Clifton Vestal, MD,
director of urologic oncology, Urology Associates
of North Texas, Arlington, TX

BRIEF CONTENTS

CONTENTS

CHAPTER 13

BUILDING YOUR SUPPORT NETWORK 107

Jenevie D. Clark-Dorsey, MS HED;
Michael A. Diefenbach, PhD; James A. Talcott, MD, SM

SPECIAL SECTION: SUPPORTING THE PERSON WITH CANCER: A GUIDE FOR FAMILY, FRIENDS, AND CAREGIVERS 113

CHAPTER 14

TAKING CARE OF PRACTICAL MATTERS: WORK, INSURANCE, AND MONEY 117

Charles L. Bennett, MD, PhD; Nicolle S. Gorby;
E. Allison Lyons

SECTION V: STAGING AND PROGNOSIS

CHAPTER 15

STAGING 133

Peter R. Carroll, MD; Hedvig Hricak, MD, PhD;
Maxwell V. Meng, MD; Sangtae Park, MD;
Darko Pucar, MD, PhD

CHAPTER 16

LYMPH NODE BIOPSY 143

Peter R. Carroll, MD; Viraj A. Master, MD, PhD;
Maxwell V. Meng, MD; Nadeem U. Rahman, MD

CHAPTER 17

WHAT COMBINATION OF FACTORS PREDICT MY OUTCOME? 149

Harry B. Burke, MD, PhD

CHAPTER 30
QUALITY OF LIFE AND RELATIONSHIPS AFTER TREATMENT   293

Sylvie Aubin, PhD

SECTION VIII: RESEARCH IN PROSTATE CANCER

CHAPTER 31
MOLECULAR BIOLOGY   321

Jonathan C. Berger; Carrie W. Rinker-Schaeffer, PhD

CHAPTER 32
OTHER PROSTATE CANCER RESEARCH   329

Samira Syed, MD; Ian M. Thompson, MD; Anthony W. Tolcher, MD

PREFACE

David G. Bostwick, MD, MBA
Clinical Professor of Pathology, University of Virginia, Charlottesville
Medical Director, Bostwick Laboratories

THE QUIET PROSTATE, A WALNUT-SIZED ORGAN buried deep in the male pelvis, has the potential to break its silence—especially late in a man's life—in a dramatic way. It may enlarge and block urine flow or generate multiple precancers and cancers. Benign prostatic hyperplasia (noncancerous enlargement of the prostate) and prostate cancer are enormous public health issues, accounting for more than 1 million surgical procedures in the United States each year. The incidence of prostate cancer has tripled during the past decade; more cancers are being found chiefly because of early detection efforts such as PSA tests and digital rectal examinations (DREs).

This prostate cancer book was written as a practical aid for men and their loved ones who are concerned about prostate cancer or who are facing prostate cancer's many challenges. A knowledgeable and empowered man may be more likely to improve his outcome and feel more positively about it. It is hoped that this text will help you understand and cope with prostate cancer and the issues that accompany it.

This project brought together a remarkable group of dedicated volunteer physicians and health care providers who donated their time and expertise to create a guide to prostate cancer from the American Cancer Society. Unlike single-author books on this subject, we chose to include numerous individual contributors with proven and focused expertise in each topic, ensuring the inclusion of the most thoughtful and contemporary specialist views.

I am personally indebted to many individuals who have been involved in the preparation of this book. My fellow editors, Drs. E. David Crawford, Mack Roach, and Tia Higano—all continuing their lifelong devotion to the care of prostate cancer patients—took precious time from their practices to contribute to this work. They deserve special thanks for molding the original idea into a final text and gathering the expert contributors to ensure success. American Cancer Society colleagues provided essential support and encouragement as well.

To our spouses and children, we owe a particular debt of gratitude for their understanding and patience.

We hope you find this book valuable and helpful. On behalf of my fellow editors and the devoted staff of the American Cancer Society, I earnestly solicit constructive criticism from you so that the utility of this text can be expanded and improved to its maximum potential.

INTRODUCTION

MORE IS KNOWN ABOUT PROSTATE CANCER and how best to find and treat it than ever before. Today, men have more opportunities than ever to monitor their prostate health, and more power to influence their care and recovery if diagnosed with prostate cancer.

There is no "right way" to make decisions about cancer. Each person's cancer is different, and the way cancer affects a person's body is unique. And each person faces diagnosis in an individual way. Some men with prostate cancer choose to play an active role in their treatment decisions; others rely more heavily on their cancer care team to guide them through the decision-making process. Whatever choices you make, the *American Cancer Society's Complete Guide to Prostate Cancer* will help you through your experience with prostate cancer.

Who This Book Is For

You may be reading this book as a man or a loved one concerned with prostate health, or you may be facing the challenges that accompany a prostate cancer diagnosis. This book is a step-by-step guide through the physical and emotional aspects of the prostate cancer experience, from testing for prostate cancer to diagnosis to thinking about the future. It explores the experiences and challenges you're likely to face, provides important information and practical advice, and offers emotional support.

The *American Cancer Society's Complete Guide to Prostate Cancer* will walk you through the issues and details most important to you at different phases of your experience. You'll discover how cancer and its treatment may affect your body, your feelings, and your life in general. You'll learn how to find valuable information, evaluate it, and determine what's best for you. In addition, you'll find:

- stories and insights from men with prostate cancer who have sorted through some of the questions you're facing and experienced many of the feelings you're having

- strategies for managing the emotions, reactions, and side effects associated with prostate cancer and its treatment

- detailed questions to ask your medical team

- current information on prostate cancer treatment options and potential side effects, including the latest developments in cancer therapy, genetics, and research

- an overview of the latest *Prostate Cancer Treatment Guidelines for Patients* developed by the National Comprehensive Cancer Network (NCCN) and the American Cancer Society, as well as where to find important information on treatment options from the National Cancer Institute (NCI) and the American Urological Association (AUA) and American Foundation for Urologic Disease (AFUD)
- chapters addressing common issues at each phase of the journey, including a guide to recovery and life after cancer
- a special section for family, friends, and caregivers to help those close to you understand and cope with changes and feelings related to your prostate cancer

How the Book Is Organized

You may find it most helpful to read the chapters in consecutive order, considering each phase from beginning to end and anticipating future issues. Or you may want to read only the chapter (or chapters) most applicable to your current experience.

The chapters in Sections I and II explore the nature of prostate cancer, diagnostic tests and what the test results mean, and the terminology and concepts used by medical professionals. Section III will help you understand your diagnosis of prostate cancer or a non-cancerous prostate condition, including pathology reports and other information. Section IV guides you through coping with your diagnosis, building a medical team, and dealing with practical issues like work and finances.

Section V explains what staging and prognosis mean to you, and Section VI provides a comprehensive overview of treatment options, including surgery, radiation, and hormonal therapy. It explores "watchful waiting" as well as chemotherapy, hyperthermia, cryosurgery, and investigational treatments. This section explores the process of choosing a treatment that is right for you and examines each treatment and its potential benefits, risks, and side effects. We also cover clinical trials and complementary and alternative methods to ensure that you'll be aware of all your options before deciding on a treatment plan.

The chapters in Section VII guide you through life after treatment, including maintaining your health and pursuing follow-up care as well as facing the possibility of recurrence. Adjusting to changes after treatment and methods of coping with intimacy and sexuality issues are also explored. Section VIII focuses on exciting research that may pave the way for new developments in prostate cancer prevention, screening, and care.

The Resources section in the back of the book lists resources that may be helpful to men with prostate cancer and their loved ones. It includes a directory of American Cancer Society resources, prostate cancer organizations, cancer information sources, patient and family services, treatment and side effect resources, Internet sources and information, and additional reading. The Glossary offers definitions of terms you are likely to encounter as you learn about prostate cancer.

Many cancer-related issues change over time. Some—such as communication with others about your cancer and collaboration with your medical team—will be present continuously, while others—like your initial diagnosis—will be crucial at one particular phase. Cross-references within the book will refer you to additional sections where a topic is addressed.

HOW TO USE THIS BOOK

This book will allow you to be as active a participant in your care as you choose to be. It provides information and issues to consider at each phase of your prostate cancer experience. You may also want to use this book as a guide to maintaining medical records, addressing financial issues, and making notes about your insurance coverage.

About the American Cancer Society

Represented in more than 3,400 communities throughout the country and Puerto Rico, the American Cancer Society is a nonprofit health organization dedicated to eliminating cancer as a major health problem. This book is just one example of the many ways the Society seeks to fulfill its mission: to save lives and diminish suffering from cancer through research, education, advocacy, and service.

The American Cancer Society is the largest private source of cancer research dollars in the United States. Founded in 1913 by 10 physicians and 5 concerned members of the community, the organization now has over 2 million volunteers. Most offer their time free of charge to the American Cancer Society to work to conquer cancer and improve the lives of those affected by it.

Looking Ahead

Let the *American Cancer Society's Complete Guide to Prostate Cancer* be a resource as you as you make your way through the prostate cancer experience. Take one step at a time and find what works best for you. The chapters in this book will help you explore the issues ahead and educate you about your options. Being informed and empowered to make knowledgeable decisions about your care will help you better understand and meet the challenge of prostate cancer.

ACKNOWLEDGMENTS

MANY MEN WITH PROSTATE CANCER and their loved ones shared their individual stories and wisdom for inclusion in this book in the hopes of helping others. We thank them for frankly and honestly sharing their prostate cancer experiences.

WHAT IS PROSTATE CANCER
AND WHO IS AT RISK?

ALL MEN ARE AT RISK OF DEVELOPING PROSTATE CANCER. But a *risk factor* for prostate cancer is not the same as a cause of prostate cancer. Many factors affect a man's risk of prostate cancer, and it is not possible to pinpoint why one man with certain risk factors develops prostate cancer while another does not. Changing the risk factors you can control (like diet) is one way to reduce prostate cancer risk. Being aware of risk factors and understanding more about the factors you can control is important to prostate health.

All Men Are at Risk for Prostate Cancer

It is not possible to pinpoint why one man develops prostate cancer while another does not.

CHAPTER 1

WHAT IS THE PROSTATE AND HOW DOES PROSTATE CANCER DEVELOP?

David G. Bostwick, MD, MBA

THE FUNCTION OF THE PROSTATE IS NOT FULLY UNDERSTOOD, but it appears to play two important roles in sex. First, the prostate produces some of the prostatic fluids for semen that nourish sperm during and after intercourse. Its second function is to push the prostatic fluid through the urethra, the tube that carries this fluid out of the body through the penis during ejaculation.

Where Is the Prostate?

The word prostate means, literally, to "stand before or in front of." The walnut-sized prostate is located in front of the bladder behind the muscular wall of the abdomen. It surrounds part of the urethra and is adjacent to the seminal vesicles (glands at the base of the bladder that release fluid into semen during orgasm). (See Figure 1.1; Figure 3.1 on page 28 of chapter 3 shows front and side views of the male urinary tract.)

What Makes Up the Prostate and Surrounding Area?

The prostate is made up of compressed tissue and an intricate series of channels and canals called ducts and ductules, which are lined by fluid-producing cells.

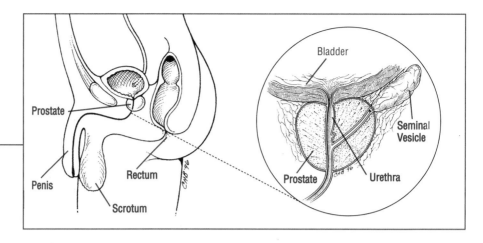

Figure 1.1.
The Prostate Gland
and Surrounding Area

These cells empty their secretions into the ducts and ductules and the prostate squeezes those fluids into the urethra to mix with sperm during ejaculation.

The outer surface of the prostate is known as the capsule. The capsule is not well defined and can be difficult to identify in areas; therefore it is sometimes not possible for doctors to determine whether cancer has grown beyond the edge of the prostate.

The prostate is supplied by large, paired groups of nerves and blood vessels called neurovascular bundles that run along the outside edge of the prostate. (Protecting these bundles during radical prostatectomy or cryosurgery through "nerve-sparing" procedures may preserve men's ability to have unassisted erections.)

The seminal vesicles are just behind the prostate. Because they are often felt during a digital rectal examination (DRE), they may be mistaken for benign prostatic hyperplasia (BPH, the non-cancerous enlargement of the prostate that occurs in many men as they get older) or cancer. In adult men, the seminal vesicles are approximately 4 inches long and 2 inches wide, although this varies.

The vas deferens is a tube that carries sperm from the testicles (also called the testes; the male reproductive glands found in the scrotum) to the urethra. The seminal vesicle ducts merge with the vas deferens and then enter the prostate and join before ending at the urethra.

The bladder is a hollow organ with flexible walls that stores urine. Urine is carried from the kidneys to the bladder by two tubes called ureters and is carried out of the bladder through the urethra.

What Is Cancer?

Cancer develops when cells in a part of the body begin to grow out of control. Although there are over a hundred kinds of cancer, they all start because of the out-of-control growth of abnormal cells.

Normal body cells grow, divide, and die in an orderly fashion. During the early years of a person's life, normal cells divide more rapidly until adulthood. After that, cells in most parts of the body divide only to replace worn-out or dying cells and to repair injuries. Because cancer cells continue to grow and divide, they are different from normal cells. Instead of dying, they outlive normal cells and continue to form new abnormal cells.

Cancer cells can enter the bloodstream or lymph vessels and travel to other parts of the body, where they begin to grow and replace normal tissue. This process is called metastasis. When cells from a cancer like prostate cancer spread to another organ like the lung, the cancer is still called prostate cancer, not lung cancer.

Some Men Don't Want to Know About Their Bodies

I counsel men who have been diagnosed with prostate cancer, and I'd say more than half of them don't know about their bodies, what the prostate is for, what the testicles do. Some men turn their backs and don't want to know what's going on or if they have prostate cancer.

— *Dave R.*

Many Men Will Face Prostate Cancer

We know from statistics that many of us are eventually going to live with prostate cancer whether we get treatment or not, and if we get treatment, the odds are that we are going to live with it, and we're going to die from something else.

— *Peter*

How Prostate Cancer Develops

The origin and development of prostate cancer is not completely understood, but the best available evidence indicates that a precancerous condition called high-grade prostatic intraepithelial neoplasia (PIN), which involves microscopic changes in the appearance of cells lining the prostate, leads to the development of invasive cancer. Invasive cancer occurs when cancer spreads beyond the initial layer of cells where it first developed to involve nearby tissues. For more information about PIN, see chapter 2.

Five unique characteristics contribute to the often unpredictable way prostate cancer develops and progresses. They are outlined here.

PROSTATE CANCER GROWS SLOWLY

Prostate cancer tends to grow slowly, typically taking 2 to 4 years to double in size. This is significantly longer than breast or colon cancer, for example. This slow growth rate is probably why prostate cancer can exist for so long without detection

TYPES OF PROSTATE CANCER

There are different types of prostate cancer. Doctors study where the cancer started and its appearance under a microscope to determine the type of prostate cancer a man has. A cancer is classified as carcinoma if it begins in the lining layer of an organ. More than 95 percent of prostate cancers are adenocarcinomas. When we talk about prostate cancer, usually we are referring to adenocarcinoma. Prostate cancer can be classified into the following types:

- **adenocarcinoma:** cancer that begins in the glandular cells that line the ducts in the prostate; the most common type of prostate cancer
- **small cell carcinoma:** cancer made up of small, round cells; this type of cancer develops from nerve-like cells and generally doesn't cause rises in PSA levels; it tends to be aggressive and is usually advanced when found
- **squamous cell carcinoma:** cancer that begins in non-glandular cells. Squamous cell carcinomas usually do not cause a rise in PSA levels; they are thought to be more aggressive than adenocarcinomas
- **transitional cell carcinoma:** transitional cell carcinomas in the prostate commonly develop from primary tumors in the bladder or urethra; they rarely develop in the prostate
- **other rare types of cancer:** other rare types of prostate cancers also exist, such as sarcomas and other epithelial tumors

and why 10 times more cases of prostate cancer exist than are diagnosed. (See chapter 4 for more information about screening for prostate cancer and the factors involved.)

PROSTATE CANCER IS AGE-RELATED

Prostate cancer rarely appears in a man younger than 40 years old. It is typically identified in men about 70 years old (although cancer is increasingly being detected in younger men because men without symptoms are more widely and effectively tested for prostate cancer). This extraordinary link with age suggests that prostate cancer results from the accumulation of damage to genes over time, perhaps from chemical reactions or other internal or external factors.

MEN OFTEN HAVE MULTIPLE PROSTATE CANCERS

Prostate cancer is usually multifocal (present in multiple locations in the prostate), so most men have prostate cancers, not just one cancer. Prostatic intraepithelial neoplasia (PIN), the likely precursor to cancer, is also usually multifocal.

PROSTATE CANCER MAY DEVELOP IN MULTIPLE WAYS

A gene is a specific sequence of DNA (deoxyribonucleic acid) that stores information telling a cell how to grow and function properly. DNA is organized into structures called chromosomes. Genes carried by chromosomes contain information about a person's inherited characteristics, including his or her likelihood of developing certain diseases. Virtually all chromosomes appear to participate in the development of prostate cancer. Experts have found very few unique "prostate cancer genes" (gene changes, or mutations, that may be responsible for a man's inherited tendency to develop prostate cancer; see chapter 2) such as those observed with some other cancers. Therefore, it seems that prostate cancer may develop in multiple ways.

PROSTATE CANCER WILL EVENTUALLY DEVELOP IN ALMOST ALL MEN

Prostate cancer is one of the most common types of cancer. Men around the world have a similar likelihood of having localized prostate cancer (tumors contained within the prostate gland) regardless of diet, occupation, lifestyle, or other factors. Nearly all men will develop prostate cancer if they live long enough, although it may never cause symptoms or be diagnosed.

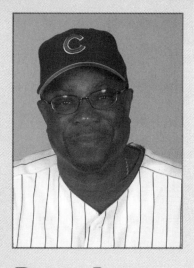

DUSTY BAKER,
MANAGER,
CHICAGO CUBS

I knew I had to attack prostate cancer instead of letting it attack me.

FAMILY HISTORY

I NEVER THOUGHT I HAD CANCER in my family. My grandfathers on both sides died in their 40s, and my uncle on my mom's side died in his mid-40s. But no one talked about why.

After my prostate cancer diagnosis my aunt sent me death certificates that showed the causes of death for my uncles and grandfather: prostate cancer. I had no idea—their cancers were never mentioned. My dad had been diagnosed with prostate cancer 8 years earlier, but I didn't know it affected my risk.

If I had known about my family history in my 20s, 30s, or even 40s, I could have improved my diet and made healthier lifestyle choices. I could have paid attention to my PSA to see if it went up. Now my brothers know they are prime candidates for prostate cancer, and they know about the importance of screening.

DIAGNOSIS AND SUPPORT

My diagnosis came when I was in my mid-50s. I happened to be at a crossroads in my career—I was in the last year of a contract and it was less than 2 months before spring training.

I didn't know what to do. At first I was in denial. But my wife was extremely supportive. She had just lost her mother to breast cancer and encouraged me to be proactive. I reminded myself that I had a lot to live for, and I set out to understand what I was dealing with. My son was 2 and my daughter was 20, and I wanted a long future with them. I knew I had to attack prostate cancer instead of letting it attack me.

Support is essential. After my diagnosis, I went home, hugged my son, daughter, and wife. I relied on my family support group throughout my prostate cancer experience. I also prayed a lot and had friends and teammates and family members who prayed for and with me.

TREATMENT DECISIONS

It was a challenge making a major decision in such a short time. A part of me wanted the doctor to make the treatment decision for me, but I knew every man's situation is different, and I had to make my own choice.

After learning about the therapies available to me and treatment side effects, I pursued a radical prostatectomy. I had learned enough to be confident that I was making the right decision for me and my life.

SIDE EFFECTS

After treatment, the psychological effects of incontinence and erectile dysfunction were tough to cope with. But things were also difficult physically. I had a lot of fatigue and wasn't able to pick up my 2-year-old son, and I was headed right to spring training.

Before treatment, I never got up in the night to go to the bathroom—but after treatment I was up 3 to 4 times a night, and I couldn't go to sleep for a couple of hours, so I had sleep deprivation.

Luckily I had a great coaching staff who realized what I was going through and looked out for me at work. They wouldn't let me overextend. Two to 3 months after treatment I was still weak and tired. One day at spring training we were playing a split double header, so we had a game at 1 o'clock and a game at 7 o'clock. Early in game 2, my staff was trying to talk me into going home and resting. I was exhausted, but I was trying to be tough. By early in the second inning, I was falling asleep. I had to understand my limitations and take care of myself while I was recovering.

CHANGES IN DIET AND LIFESTYLE

I had always taken vitamins, but after diagnosis I looked into information about diet and healthy changes I could make. Once you feel like you've beaten cancer, you don't want to die of something you could have prevented.

I eat a lot of tofu dishes and drink soy milk, especially in shakes with fruits, soy protein, and yogurt. I take vitamin E and selenium, eat stewed tomatoes, watch the fried food—I try to be healthful. My cholesterol and blood pressure have even gone down. I do have occasional treats, but not with the frequency I once would have. We know my son is at risk for developing prostate cancer, so we keep an eye on his diet as well.

FOLLOW UP AND OUTLOOK

I was diagnosed 2 years ago, and my checkups have now gone from every 3 months to every 6 months. I had a recent appointment and everything is great.

Before treatment, I had an older man tell me the experience would make me a better person. I didn't know what he meant. But now I do have a keener sense of what is important in life, and I am a better person— a better husband, father, a better man.

SCREENING

Awareness and early detection could have helped me. You can't be too proud or afraid to get checked for prostate cancer. If the doctors find something wrong, you can keep an eye on it or deal with it early. Don't wait to get screened—early detection is the key.

CHAPTER 2

WHY DO SOME MEN GET PROSTATE CANCER?

David G. Bostwick, MD, MBA
Shuk-Mei Ho, PhD
Barry G. Timms, PhD

F YOU ARE A MAN DIAGNOSED WITH PROSTATE CANCER, one of your first questions may have been "What did I do?" or "Why me?" Some men believe that if they had done something differently, they could have prevented cancer. Others wonder if they caused the cancer themselves.

Having prostate cancer is not your fault.

Prostate cancer is the most common cancer among men except for skin cancer. It accounts for nearly 1 of every 3 cancers diagnosed in men in the United States. Currently a man living in the United States has a 1 in 6 lifetime risk of being diagnosed with prostate cancer. In 2004, an estimated 230,110 new prostate cancer diagnoses and 29,900 deaths are expected. That's approximately 1 death every 15 minutes. These numbers include only men diagnosed with prostate cancer; many more men never know they have the disease. Most men die *with* prostate cancer rather than *from* it, yet doctors are unable to accurately predict which men will die from their cancer and which men will not.

Cancer is complex, and it is not possible to point to just one reason why a man develops prostate cancer. This chapter outlines risk factors for prostate cancer and explains how the disease is affected by circumstances both within and out of our control. It also discusses theories about how prostate cancer *may* be prevented. More study is needed into these potential preventive measures.

Table 2.1. RISK FACTORS FOR PROSTATE CANCER	
Factors That May Affect Risk	**Factors of Uncertain Risk Based on Current Evidence**
Older age	Vasectomy
Hormones	Smoking
Racial/ethnic background	Alcohol
Nationality	Sexual activity and marital status
Family history	Viruses and other infections
Diet	Social factors, including socioeconomic factors and education
Obesity	Other unidentified factors
Occupation	
Prostatic intraepithelial neoplasia (PIN)	
Physical inactivity	

Risk Factors Explained

We don't know what causes men to get prostate cancer, but we're learning more as scientists study potential causes and effects. Factors that appear to increase a man's chance of developing prostate cancer are referred to as risk factors.

Many men with one or more prostate cancer risk factors never develop the disease, and some men who develop it have no apparent risk factors. Even when a man with prostate cancer has a risk factor, there is no way to prove that it actually caused his cancer. Some factors, like a person's age or race, can't be changed. Others may be linked to cancer-causing elements in the environment or to personal choices such as diet and exercise. And a man's risk for developing prostate cancer can change over time. See Table 2.1 for some of the factors that are likely to increase risk—and those that have received attention but are not likely to affect risk.

Factors That May Affect Prostate Cancer Risk

Although we don't yet completely understand the causes of prostate cancer, researchers have found several factors that are linked to an increase in the risk of developing this disease.

Table 2.2. PROBABILITY OF DEVELOPING PROSTATE CANCER FOR UNITED STATES MEN, 1998–2000*

Age [in years]	
Birth to 39	1 in 12,833 (less than 1 percent)
40 to 59	1 in 44 (about 2 percent)
60 to 79	1 in 7 (about 14 percent)
Lifetime	1 in 6 (about 17 percent)

*for those free of cancer at beginning of age interval. Based on cancer cases diagnosed during 1998-2000. The "1 in" statistic and the inverse of the percentage may not be equivalent due to rounding.

Adapted from: DEVCAN: Probability of Developing or Dying of Cancer Software, Version 5.1. Statistical Research and Applications Branch, National Cancer Institute, 2003. http://srab.cancer.gov/devcan

American Cancer Society, Surveillance Research, 2004, *Cancer Facts and Figures 2004*.

OLDER AGE

Age is the most important risk factor for many cancers, including prostate cancer. The chance of having prostate cancer increases rapidly after age 50. More than 70 percent of all prostate cancers are diagnosed in men over the age of 65. It is still unclear exactly how an increase in age increases a man's risk for prostate cancer.

Most cells in young healthy individuals have defense mechanisms that protect against cell-damaging chemicals that are produced as part of normal body processes. As a person ages, these defenses weaken in most tissues. This may allow damage to accumulate in cells, which could eventually lead to cancer.

HORMONES

Androgens are male hormones that are required for the growth, maintenance, and function of the normal prostate. However, they also have the ability to speed prostate cancer growth. More studies are needed into the potential roles of androgens such as testosterone and dihydrotestosterone (DHT); leptin, a hormone related to fat concentration in the body; and the female hormone estrogen in the development of prostate cancer.

TESTOSTERONE REPLACEMENT THERAPY

The relationship between testosterone levels in the body and prostate cancer is controversial. We know that testosterone provides nourishment for prostate cancer cells and helps them grow and develop. However, the incidence (the number of new cases of a disease that occur in a population each year) of prostate cancer increases with age, while testosterone levels begin to decline with age. Therefore a paradox exists regarding the role of testosterone in prostate cancer.

About 15 percent of men have an extremely low level of testosterone and exhibit symptoms of decreased muscle mass, decreased sex drive, cognitive problems, and risk of bone fracture. Some of these men might benefit from testosterone replacement therapy. Perhaps the single greatest concern associated with any type of androgen replacement therapy is the possibility that it may significantly increase the risk for development of prostate cancer.

Although low levels of testosterone may protect against prostate cancer, no evidence exists that normal levels of testosterone promote the development of prostate cancer. However, administering testosterone may stimulate a pre-existing prostate cancer. Therefore careful screening for prostate cancer is recommended for men considering androgen therapy.

DHEA SUPPLEMENTS

Dehydroepiandrosterone (DHEA) is a steroid hormone produced by the adrenal gland (glands located on top of the kidneys) that is broken down into other important hormones, such as estrogen and testosterone. Advocates claim that DHEA supplements can slow the aging process and increase sex drive, and even prevent the growth and recurrence of some cancers. There is very little solid evidence at this time to support any of these claims.

Some researchers believe DHEA supplements might increase the risk of prostate cancer, as well as other conditions that respond to hormone levels. DHEA may stimulate tumor growth in men with prostate cancer. It may also increase the size of the prostate.

Further research is needed to better define the risks and benefits associated with DHEA and similar supplements. In the meantime, men considering taking DHEA, especially those known to be at risk for prostate cancer, should first discuss this with their doctors.

Table 2.3. PROSTATE CANCER INCIDENCE AND MORTALITY RATES* BY RACE AND ETHNICITY, US, 1996–2000

The incidence rate is the number of new prostate cancer cases diagnosed among 100,000 men each year, and the mortality rate is the rate of death from prostate cancer among 100,000 men each year.

	White	African American	Asian American and Pacific Islander	American Indian and Alaska Native	Hispanic/ Latino[†]
Incidence	164.3	272.1	100.0	53.6	137.2
Mortality	30.2	73.0	13.9	21.9	24.1

*Per 100,000, age-adjusted to the 2000 US standard population.

†Hispanic/Latinos are not mutually exclusive from whites, African Americans, Asian Americans and Pacific Islanders, and American Indians and Alaska Natives.

Ries LAG, Eisner MP, Kosary CL, Hankey BF, Miller BA, Clegg L, Mariotto A, Fay MP, Feuer EJ, Edwards BK (eds). Adapted from *SEER Cancer Statistics Review, 1975-2000,* National Cancer Institute, Bethesda, Maryland. Available at: http://seer.cancer.gov/csr/1975_2002,2003.

American Cancer Society, Surveillance Research, 2004, *Cancer Facts and Figures 2004*

RACIAL BACKGROUND

Prostate cancer occurs almost 70 percent more often in African-American men than in white American men, and African-American men are more likely to be diagnosed at an advanced stage than men of other races. African-American men are more than twice as likely to die of prostate cancer as white men.

The reasons for these racial disparities are not known, but may reflect differences in access to care, differences in the decision-making process of whether to seek medical attention and follow-up, different lifestyle choices, biologic differences, or a combination of these. For example, prostate cancer is not common in Africa, but as a group, African-American men in the United States have a higher intake of dietary fat, and this may contribute to their higher risk.

Studies have begun to focus on prostate-specific antigen (PSA; a protein made by the prostate that is often found in high levels in men with prostate cancer) screening and the answers it may hold for race-related differences in prostate cancer risk. PSA screening is more common among white Americans than among

African Americans, which should result in a higher incidence among whites, but higher cancer rates have been found in African Americans. One study found higher PSA levels in African Americans both with and without prostate cancer. The factors causing higher PSA levels in African Americans are not completely understood, but are believed to be a combination of biological, environmental, and socioeconomic causes.

Because of the increased risk for African-American men, it is recommended that they begin undergoing prostate cancer screening at age 45, earlier than the general population. However, men of all races are advised to be vigilant about prostate cancer screening and to follow screening guidelines (see chapter 4).

For more information about racial disparities and cancer, contact the American Cancer Society (800-ACS-2345 or http://www.cancer.org), the National Cancer Institute's Center to Reduce Cancer Health Disparities (301-496-8589 or http://crchd.nci.nih.gov/), or the Intercultural Cancer Council (713-798-4617 or http://iccnetwork.org/).

DIFFERENCES BETWEEN COUNTRIES

The incidence of prostate cancer varies greatly from country to country. Prostate cancer is most common in North America and northwestern Europe. It is less common in Asia, Africa, Central America, and South America.

In recent years, the number of prostate cancer cases has risen considerably in many countries, including those where prostate cancer risk is considered low. Some of this may be related to dietary factors. Japanese men, for example, traditionally consume a relatively low fat diet. As the fat content of the Japanese diet has increased, the incidence of prostate cancer has also increased. (See page 18 for more information about diet and risk.)

Several studies of immigrants have found that men's prostate cancer rates shift toward those of their host country. For example, the incidence rate of Japanese men who move to the United States rises above the low rate of Japanese men in Japan but does not match the high rate of white men in

Getting Information to the African-American Community

Based upon my observations, there's a stigma in the black community associated with cancer more than any other disease. Somehow you're considered a fallen angel or fallen soldier if you get cancer. The new attitudes, the new knowledge regarding treatment, and new longevities possible with cancer have not yet been communicated, or maybe accepted, in the black community, as they may have been in other communities.

— *Westley*

African-American Men Have a Higher Risk of Dying

The mortality rate from prostate cancer is 50 percent higher in African-American men. I think it's very important for African-American men to speak to their church groups and fraternities and spread the word about prostate cancer screening.

— *Bill*

the United States. This suggests that at least some of the difference in risk relates to environmental factors. Some of the differences may also to be related to varied levels of reporting and detection of cancer cases around the world.

FAMILY HISTORY AND GENETICS

In chapter 1 we mentioned that genes contain information about a person's inherited characteristics, including his or her likelihood of developing certain diseases. Prostate cancer seems to run in some families, suggesting that an inherited or genetic factor may affect risk. This risk appears to be even stronger than that for colon or breast cancer, two cancers with well-recognized genetic links.

Having a father or brother with prostate cancer doubles a man's risk of developing this disease. The risk is even higher for men with several affected relatives, particularly if their relatives were young at the time of diagnosis.

Scientists have identified some inherited genes such as RNASEL, ELAC2, and MSR1 that may be involved in hereditary prostate cancer, but they probably account for only a small fraction of cases. Genetic testing for these genes is not yet available and the identification of these "genetic markers" for prostate cancer appears to be more difficult than for other cancers.

Some inherited genes increase risk for more than one type of cancer. For example, mutated (damaged) BRCA1 or BRCA2 genes are the reason that breast and ovarian cancers are much more common in some families. The presence of these gene mutations may also increase prostate cancer risk. But they are believed to be responsible for only a small percentage of prostate cancer cases.

One concern about the reliability of family history studies in showing prostate cancer risk is that aggressively screening the families of men with prostate cancer may make it more likely to find others in the family with the disease, which may skew the results of the study.

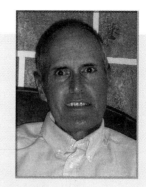

Prostate Cancer in the Family

Within 5 years, my father, 3 of my uncles, and 2 brothers were diagnosed with prostate cancer. I felt like I was on the railroad tracks with my foot stuck and I could see the train coming. Then I was diagnosed. Although I knew what my family members had been through, I knew I had to find out what course of treatment was right for me.

         – *Steven*

Younger Brother with Prostate Cancer

Two weeks after I was diagnosed with prostate cancer, my kid brother, age 48, was diagnosed with it as well. I'm very happy to say that he came through treatment with flying colors like I did. Misery loves company, I guess, and we kind of helped each other.

         – *Bill*

PROSTATIC INTRAEPITHELIAL NEOPLASIA (PIN)

Prostatic intraepithelial neoplasia (PIN) is a condition in which the microscopic appearance (e.g., size, shape) of prostate gland cells change. These changes have the potential to progress to prostate cancer. PIN begins to appear in men in their twenties. Almost 50 percent of men have PIN by the time they reach 50.

PIN is classified as either low grade, meaning the tissue appears almost normal, or high grade, meaning it looks abnormal. The significance of low-grade PIN is not known at this time. But men with high-grade PIN are more likely to develop prostate cancer. They should be watched carefully and should have repeat prostate biopsies.

DIET

Some studies have suggested that men who consume very high amounts of calcium (through food or supplements) have a higher risk of developing advanced prostate cancer. Most studies, however, have not found a prostate cancer link to the levels of calcium consumed in the average diet, and calcium is known to have other important health benefits.

Figure 2.1

Normal Prostate
Epithelial Cells and PIN

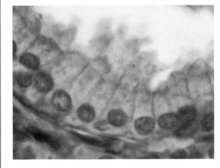

Normal prostate epithelial cells

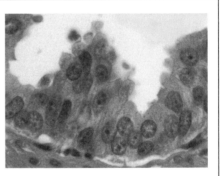

PIN

When a pathologist looks at a sample of prostate tissue under the microscope, normal epithelial cells (cells that line the prostate gland) look like those in the left picture. The presence of prostatic intraepithelial neoplasia (PIN), shown in the right picture, may be the first sign of cancer.

Left image used with permission of Dr. Barry Timms, Professor, Division of Basic Biomedical Sciences, University of South Dakota

Right image used with permission of Dr. Joel Ziebarth, Laboratory Medicine and Pathology, University of South Dakota School of Medicine, Sioux Falls, SD.

CAN WHAT YOU EAT AFFECT YOUR CANCER RISK?

This list shows some of the foods we eat and some of the vitamins and substances that have been studied in relationship to prostate cancer risk. Keep in mind that there's a crucial difference between getting nutrients through food and taking supplements. Also note that certain antioxidant supplements may interfere with the effectiveness of certain chemotherapy agents or with radiation therapy.

An arrow pointing up indicates that diets containing high levels of this dietary factor may increase your risk for developing prostate cancer. An arrow pointing down indicates that this dietary factor may protect you, and a question mark (?) means scientists haven't established the effect of this dietary factor on prostate cancer risk.

Table 2.4. DIET AND PROSTATE CANCER RISK

Food Type (examples)	Effect on Risk
Red meat	↑
Dairy products (high fat)	↑
Green vegetables (broccoli, peas)	↓
Fish (salmon, mackerel)	↓
Tomato products	↓
Fruits (pink grapefruit, watermelon)	↓
Soy products (tofu, soy milk)	↓
Supplements	**Effect on Risk**
Omega-3 fatty acids (flaxseed oil)	↓
Vitamin E*	↓
Selenium*	↓
Vitamins A, D, C	?

*A large study called the Selenium and Vitamin E Cancer Prevention Trial (SELECT) is exploring the idea that these supplements may lower prostate cancer risk (see chapter 32).

Lycopenes (antioxidants found in tomatoes and tomato products, pink grapefruit, and watermelon), vitamin E (found naturally in green, leafy vegetables and whole grains), and the mineral selenium (found naturally in seafood and whole grains) may lower prostate cancer risk. Studies are underway to assess whether supplements containing these substances may reduce risk as well.

Eating large amounts of red meat and high-fat dairy products may increase prostate cancer risk. Men in some countries with high prostate cancer risk, including the United States, eat more red meat and foods with a higher fat content than men in Asian countries, for example, who eat more vegetables, fish, and soy products and have low prostate cancer risk and prostate cancer deaths. Green vegetables and fish are good for our general health, but we know less about soy's effects on the body (see page 24).

Current evidence related to many dietary factors is inconsistent or unavailable. See the *Diet and Prostate Cancer Risk* table on page 19 for an indication of likely links between dietary factors and cancer risk.

Men who are in the age group that is most likely to develop prostate cancer have usually been eating the same type of diet for many years. We don't know how long it takes to see a benefit (or harm) because of diet, but changing a dietary habit for a short time will probably not affect your risk very much.

A well-balanced diet that includes many plant-based foods and lean meats and dairy products rather than high-fat options helps your health in many ways.

OCCUPATION

Some men's occupations may put them at increased risk for developing prostate cancer.

Men who have worked for a long time making batteries like those used in portable electronic products and have been exposed to cadmium may have a slightly higher risk for developing prostate cancer than other men. Welders and workers in the rubber manufacturing industry are also exposed to toxic chemicals that may put them at higher risk for prostate cancer.

Studies have shown that farmers may be at higher risk because of their exposure to high levels of pesticides.

PHYSICAL INACTIVITY AND BEING OVERWEIGHT OR OBESE

Physical inactivity may increase a man's risk of prostate cancer. Being overweight or obese may also increase a man's risk. This link is not clearly established; more research is needed.

Factors Not Likely to Affect Risk

There have been many attempts to establish links between various factors and the risk for prostate cancer. You may have heard about some of the following factors as potentially affecting prostate cancer risk. Most of these factors have shown little or no effect on the risk for developing prostate cancer.

VASECTOMY

A vasectomy is a surgical procedure performed to make a man infertile. Some studies have suggested that men who have had a vasectomy—especially those under 35 at the time of the procedure— may have a slightly increased risk for prostate cancer, but this link has not been consistently found. After a man undergoes a vasectomy for birth control, he is more likely to have thorough medical examinations at physician checkups. The more often men have a prostate examination, the more likely doctors are to find evidence of the disease. The mixed results are not strong enough to warrant recommendations that men wait to have this procedure or reverse the procedure.

SMOKING

Many multi-year studies have tried to identify a link between smoking and prostate cancer risk. Because cigarette smoke contains cancer-causing chemicals (also called carcinogens), some scientists thought smokers might be increasing their risk of not only lung cancer, but other cancers, such as prostate cancer. Evidence does not suggest a link between smoking and the development of prostate cancer, but men who smoke may have a higher mortality rate from prostate cancer than nonsmokers. And smoking has been clearly linked to other poor health outcomes, including cancers of the lung, mouth, throat, bladder, kidney, pancreas, and stomach, as well as heart disease, pneumonia, cataracts, and a serious form of gum disease called periodontitis.

SEXUAL ACTIVITY

The prostate is part of the male reproductive system, so an obvious question is whether a man's level of sexual activity has anything to do his risk for developing prostate cancer. Answering this question definitively is difficult, in part because sexual activity is a private topic. The following groups have been studied in an effort to establish some links between sexual activity and prostate cancer risk: married men with and without children, unmarried men with one or more sexual partners, men who abstain from sex, young men, older men, and men with sexually transmitted diseases. The results have been varied, but none of the studies provide any strong evidence of a relationship between sexual activity (or inactivity) and the risk for prostate cancer.

VIRUSES AND OTHER INFECTIONS

Many viruses can infect the prostate, just as they can infect any other tissue in the body. Viral infections can cause inflammation and problems with urination. However, there have been few reports of these infections resulting in higher risk for cancer of the prostate. (Men with infections will probably see their physicians and may end up getting prostate examinations, which might lead to earlier diagnosis of any prostate cancer that is present.)

Some viruses *are* related to cancer risk (for example, some types of human papillomavirus—HPV, a sexually transmitted infection—are strongly associated with the development of cervical cancer). Recent studies have looked at a potential relationship between HPV infections in men and the risk of prostate cancer. No conclusive evidence exists, but in the light of concern about sexual activity in younger men and increases in sexually transmitted diseases, there will likely be more studies over the next few years.

Current Theories About Prevention

The development of prostate cancer is a complex process affected by a combination of many factors, not all of which are known or controllable. It's not possible to identify a single reason why prostate cancer occurs.

While some lifestyle factors can be changed in an attempt to reduce prostate cancer risk, others are beyond a person's control. In this section, we outline measures that *may* help stop some cases of prostate cancer from forming, and we highlight ongoing developments in the area of prevention.

BLOCKING THE EFFECTS OF HORMONES

As noted earlier, hormones seem to play a role in the development of prostate cancer. Androgens are important in promoting the growth of both normal and cancerous prostate cells, and high levels of androgens may encourage the development of prostate cancers in some men.

Finasteride (Proscar) and dutasteride (Avodart) are drugs that lower the body's levels of a potent androgen called DHT. Both drugs are already used to treat benign prostatic hyperplasia (BPH). One large study found that finasteride reduced the risk of developing prostate cancer by about 25 percent, but those who did develop prostate cancer may have had a more aggressive form of cancer. More studies are needed to clearly establish the potential risks and benefits of using finasteride to prevent prostate cancer. (See chapter 32 for more information about the Prostate Cancer Prevention Trial and finasteride.) Meanwhile, men who have BPH and are currently being treated with finasteride should continue this therapy. Men at risk for prostate cancer who are interested in finasteride should talk to their doctor about what is appropriate for their situation.

EATING A HEALTHFUL DIET

Some cases of prostate cancer might be prevented by altering potential risk factors, such as diet. Many studies are examining dietary factors in the hope that men might be able to modify their diets to reduce the risk of developing cancers, including prostate cancer.

The American Cancer Society recommends eating a variety of healthful foods with an emphasis on plant sources and limiting your intake of red meats, especially those that are processed or high in fat. These nutrition guidelines may also lower the risk for some other types of cancer, as well as other serious diseases. Eating 5 or more servings of fruits and vegetables each day is also recommended. Beans, along with whole-grain bread, cereals, pasta, and rice are also healthful dietary choices.

LIMITING RED MEAT AND DAIRY PRODUCTS

Men who eat red meat and high-fat dairy products tend to eat fewer fruits and vegetables; doctors are not sure which of these factors may be responsible for increasing prostate cancer risk. Eating less red meat and fewer high-fat dairy products may reduce a man's risk of developing prostate cancer. Men who eat a lot of red meat or who consume a lot of dairy products appear to also have a greater chance of developing a more aggressive form of prostate cancer.

INCLUDING ANTIOXIDANTS IN MODERATION

Antioxidants are compounds that block the actions of activated oxygen molecules, known as free radicals, that can damage cells. Antioxidants may help lower prostate cancer risk. Current studies are assessing whether antioxidants such as lycopenes (antioxidants found in high levels in some fruits and vegetables, such as tomatoes, pink grapefruit, and watermelon), vitamin A, vitamin C, vitamin D, vitamin E, and the mineral selenium actually reduce risk. Talk to your doctor before taking any dietary supplements or high-dose vitamins.

Theories about the potential benefits of antioxidants, particularly vitamin E and dietary selenium, have inspired a large, ongoing chemoprevention trial studying their potential preventive effects on prostate cancer. Results of the study will not be available for several years.

SOY

Many scientists have begun to look at the possible benefits of adding more soy-based products to our diets. Dietary soy such as tofu, soybeans (edamame), or soy milk *may* lower prostate cancer risk. It may do so by inhibiting the growth of cancer cells. There is a good chance that the substances (possibly the estrogen-like substances) in the soybean may be beneficial. Studies are underway to more closely examine the possible effects of soy.

Until additional studies of dietary factors and prostate cancer are completed, the safest tactic for lowering prostate cancer risk is to pursue a generally healthful lifestyle, eating fewer red meats and high-fat dairy products and eating five or more servings of vegetables and fruits each day.

EXERCISE

Many studies indicate that regular exercise may help prevent disease. It may reduce a man's risk of prostate cancer, but this has not been clearly established. Keeping fit also helps maintain a healthy weight and a healthy heart. Any reduction in risk may be related to the benefits of reducing body fat and lowering male hormone levels.

FINDING OUT IF YOU HAVE
PROSTATE CANCER

UNLESS IT IS ADVANCED, PROSTATE CANCER USUALLY DOES not cause symptoms. More often it is found through screening (testing). Many symptoms that are linked to prostate cancer are more commonly due to benign (noncancerous) conditions, but they may cause men to consult their doctors and be screened for prostate cancer. The decision to screen for prostate cancer is between you and your doctor, and should take factors such as your age and health into account.

In this section we explore symptoms and screening, as well as what happens at a doctor's visit and what is involved with various tests that help doctors evaluate you for prostate cancer.

Consider Your Situation and Unique Factors

The decision to screen for prostate cancer is between you and your doctor.

CHAPTER 3

WHAT SYMPTOMS DO MEN WITH PROSTATE CANCER EXPERIENCE?

Anthony Y. Smith, MD

BECAUSE OF IMPROVED SCREENING METHODS, most men today are diagnosed when their prostate cancer is not causing symptoms. Some men may show symptoms of cancer before diagnosis, however. Here we'll explore potential symptoms men may experience that could indicate prostate cancer is present, as well as symptoms that may lead to diagnosis but are often not directly caused by prostate cancer.

What Symptoms May Indicate

Urinary symptoms are a common problem as men age. Because the prostate surrounds the urethra, changes in the prostate can affect urinary flow. Both benign prostatic hyperplasia (BPH, non-cancerous enlargement of the prostate) and prostate cancer may block the outlet of the bladder, causing various symptoms such as weak urination, difficulty urinating, or an inability to urinate, or even kidney failure. (In chapter 10 we discuss in more detail conditions such as BPH that are sometimes initially thought to be prostate cancer.)

A man with prostate cancer who has urinary symptoms doesn't necessarily have a more aggressive or harder-to-treat cancer than a man with prostate cancer experiencing no symptoms. At least one study has shown that men with prostate cancer who have obstructive symptoms seem to have similar outcomes to those who do not have symptoms.

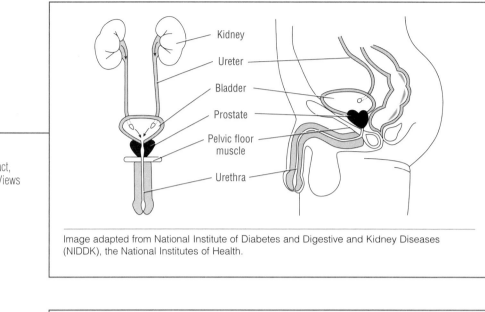

Image adapted from National Institute of Diabetes and Digestive and Kidney Diseases (NIDDK), the National Institutes of Health.

Figure 3.1.

Male Urinary Tract, Front and Side Views

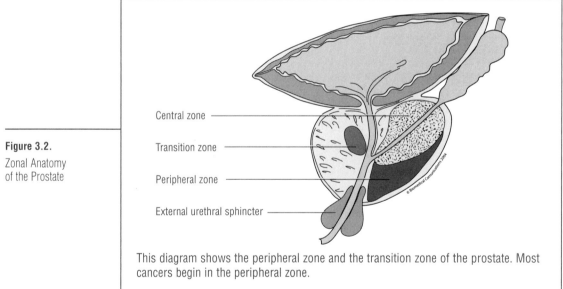

This diagram shows the peripheral zone and the transition zone of the prostate. Most cancers begin in the peripheral zone.

Figure 3.2.

Zonal Anatomy of the Prostate

Non-urinary symptoms do not always indicate that prostate cancer is present, but some of the symptoms listed below may be caused by prostate cancer and its spread. Many of them develop gradually. Men who notice a change in their health should consult their doctors.

URINARY SYMPTOMS

Men may have urinary symptoms that are not necessarily related to the cancer but that prompt them to go to the doctor for an evaluation. This examination may lead to a diagnosis of prostate cancer that is present but not causing symptoms.

WEAK URINATION OR INABILITY TO URINATE

Obstructive symptoms are those that men may be most likely to associate with prostate trouble. They include having a weak urinary stream, failing to empty the bladder, being unable to urinate, straining, waiting too long to start urinating, or having the urine stream stop and start during urination.

Obstructive symptoms may indicate that a man has prostate cancer, but more commonly they occur because of benign prostatic hyperplasia (the overgrowth of normal prostate cells), which is not cancerous. Benign prostatic hyperplasia (BPH) usually grows along the urethra (causing urinary symptoms) in what is called the transition zone, whereas more than 80 percent of prostate cancers grow in the outer part of the prostate (known as the peripheral zone) and do not cause urinary symptoms.

PAINFUL OR FREQUENT URINATION

Irritative symptoms, which may include frequent urination, an urgent need to urinate, and painful urination, may also be an indication of prostate cancer, but more likely indicate an infection of the prostate or urinary tract. Benign enlargement of the prostate, bladder cancer, or some other irritation in the bladder, such as a bladder stone, may also cause these symptoms.

INABILITY TO URINATE OR KIDNEY FAILURE

If severe symptoms such as an inability to urinate and kidney failure are due to prostate cancer and not to BPH, the prostate cancer is typically larger and more likely to have spread locally or elsewhere. Spread into the base of the bladder may have blocked the ureters, the tubes that carry urine from the kidneys to the bladder, or it may block the urethra where it courses through the prostate.

BLOOD IN URINE

Blood in the urine is often caused by conditions other than prostate cancer. However, in some cases prostate cancer may cause blood to appear in the urine, either microscopically or so it can be seen during urination. If prostate cancer is present, blood in the urine may signal that cancer has spread to the urethra or bladder, which generally indicates that the disease is relatively advanced.

SYMPTOM SCORE INDEX

The chart here, based upon the American Urological Association (AUA) BPH Symptoms Score Index, may be useful when a man is experiencing urinary symptoms. Because benign prostatic hyperplasia (BPH) and prostate cancer share some symptoms, it is important to talk to your doctor about your specific symptoms.

To complete this self-test, simply circle one number for each question. Mark your score from 0 (Not at all) to 5 (Almost always) on the right. Add all of the scores to reach your total. Total scores of less than 10 suggest mild symptoms, while 10 to 20 suggest moderate symptoms and scores above 20 suggests severe symptoms. Men with moderate to severe symptoms should consult their doctors.

	Not at all	Less than 1 time in 5	Less than half the time	About half the time	More than half the time	Almost always	Patient score
1. Incomplete emptying Over the past month, how often have you felt the sensation of not having emptied your bladder completely after you have finished urinating?	0	1	2	3	4	5	
2. Frequency Over the past month, how often have you had to urinate less than 2 hours after last urinating?	0	1	2	3	4	5	
3. Intermittency Over the past month, how often have you found that during urination you stopped and started urinating again several times?	0	1	2	3	4	5	
4. Urgency Over the past month, how often have you found it difficult to postpone urination?	0	1	2	3	4	5	
5. Weak Stream Over the past month, how often have you had a weak urinary stream?	0	1	2	3	4	5	
6. Straining Over the past month, how often have you had to push or strain to begin urinating?	0	1	2	3	4	5	
7. Nocturia Over the past month, how many times did you typically get up to urinate from when you went to bed at night until you got up in the morning?	0	1	2	3	4	5	
						Total score	

Based on the American Urological Association (AUA) BPH Symptoms Score Index, American Urological Association Education and Research, Inc.

URINARY SYMPTOMS IN YOUNG MEN

Younger men who have obstructive or irritative symptoms should be evaluated for prostate cancer, because BPH usually appears after age 60. Several studies have suggested that African-American men more often have obstructive symptoms at a younger age.

URINARY SYMPTOMS THAT APPEAR SUDDENLY

Symptoms due to prostate cancer may appear more suddenly over a matter of months, while urinary symptoms due to benign enlargement of the prostate tend to progress slowly over many years.

OTHER SYMPTOMS

ERECTILE DYSFUNCTION

Some men may have erectile dysfunction (the inability to have and maintain an erection). This may be unrelated to the cancer, but in evaluating the erectile dysfunction, a doctor will usually screen for prostate cancer. This is because prostate cancer may invade the nearby nerves that normally help a man achieve erections. (Rarely, aggressive local spread of prostate cancer can also cause a prolonged, painful erection known as priapism.)

BLOOD IN SEMEN

Blood in ejaculated semen is most commonly associated with inflammatory conditions of the prostate (known as prostatitis), but may occasionally indicate that prostate cancer is present, particularly in men over age 55.

ABDOMINAL PAIN OR DIGESTIVE SYMPTOMS

Locally advanced prostate cancer can invade or encircle the rectum and produce obstructive symptoms similar to colorectal cancer symptoms. This is rare. A tough tissue separates the prostate from the rectum and tends to serve as a barrier to prevent prostate cancer from invading the rectum directly. When it does happen, however, it may cause constipation, abdominal pain and cramping, bleeding, or intermittent diarrhea.

> ### Urinary Symptoms Didn't Seem Unusual
>
> I really wasn't having urinary symptoms before my diagnosis of cancer other than what you'd normally think would happen with age. I was getting up a couple of times at night to go to the bathroom. But I just thought, after you're 55, that's normal. I never connected it with cancer. It was not something that stood out like a sore thumb.
>
> – John D.

WEIGHT LOSS, FATIGUE, OR GENERALIZED WEAKNESS

As cancer advances, it metastasizes (spreads) to other sites in the body. Prostate cancer is occasionally diagnosed because of the symptoms of metastasis. But because of better tests and improved screening, fewer than 5 percent of men show symptoms of advanced prostate cancer at diagnosis.

General symptoms of an advanced cancer of any kind include loss of weight, loss of appetite, tiredness, and weakness, although in early stages of advanced disease, a person may not experience any of these symptoms.

BACK OR PELVIC PAIN

Back and pelvic pain are common symptoms that can be related to a host of different conditions more common than prostate cancer. But unrelenting pain in the back or pelvic region is a common symptom of advanced prostate cancer. This is because prostate cancer typically first spreads to the bones, specifically the pelvis and spine. Bone pain in other areas is also possible, as prostate cancer can also spread to the ribs and bones in the extremities.

In some cases, a broken bone is the first sign of bone metastasis. Fractures, especially in hip bones that have been weakened by cancer, cause pelvic pain.

Bone Pain Sent Me to the Doctor

From September or October until March, when I was diagnosed with advanced cancer, I was having back pain. My spine was hurting, hurting. I'd had some back problems in the past. Nothing significant, but enough that I thought at first, well this was just a little more of what I had before.

— *John D.*

PAIN, NUMBNESS, OR WEAKNESS IN THE LEGS

Extensive metastases in the spine can compress the nerves in or near the spinal cord and cause pain, numbness, or weakness in the lower extremities, problems with bowel or urinary control, or even paralysis. Nerves in or near the lower part of the spinal cord affect the legs, bladder, and intestines, which is why compression of the spinal cord can cause these problems.

Spinal cord compression should be treated as a medical emergency.

CLOTTING DISORDERS

On rare occasions, men with advanced prostate cancer experience severe bleeding, usually from multiple sites. Release of substances from the prostate cancer into the bloodstream is believed to cause both clotting in the body as well as destruction of a substance necessary for clotting. As a result, the normal clotting process (which routinely prevents excessive bleeding) is affected.

MENTAL CHANGES AND OTHER SYMPTOMS

Prostate cancer invading the bones can force large amounts of calcium out of the bones and into the bloodstream. Higher-than-normal levels of calcium in the blood (known as hypercalcemia) can cause mental changes, nausea, vomiting, and abdominal pain.

CHAPTER 4

HOW IMPORTANT IS FINDING PROSTATE CANCER EARLY?

Harry B. Burke, MD, PhD
Ciril J. Godec, MD, PhD

THE DEATH RATE FROM PROSTATE CANCER HAS DECREASED in the United States over the last ten years, probably because of the earlier detection, diagnosis, and treatment made possible by prostate cancer screening (testing), searching for prostate cancer in men without symptoms, or changes in the body caused by cancer.

Detecting Prostate Cancer Early

Screening for prostate cancer appears to trigger a chain reaction that may help save lives: early detection, early treatment, and fewer deaths from prostate cancer. See page 38 for more information about the American Cancer Society's recommended prostate cancer screening guidelines.

RECOMMENDED SCREENING TESTS

Getting screened for prostate cancer makes it more likely that any cancer present will be found at an early stage, and more likely that it will be curable. Since the early 1990s the American Cancer Society and the American Urological Association have recommended screening for prostate cancer through two methods: the digital rectal examination, a physical exam in which the doctor inserts his or her gloved finger into the rectum to detect any irregularity in the nearby prostate gland's surface, and the prostate-specific antigen test, a blood test that measures levels of a protein made by the prostate. (See chapters 5 and 6 for more information about these screening tests.) Prostate-specific antigen (PSA) testing uses chemical methods to provide a PSA number indicating how much of the protein is in the blood, while the digital rectal examination (DRE), depends upon a doctor's ability to physically detect an abnormality in the prostate. A combination of both the DRE and PSA is most effective in finding prostate cancer.

High PSA levels do not always mean that prostate cancer is present. Benign prostatic hyperplasia (enlargement of the prostate; BPH) and prostatitis (inflamed prostate) may also cause the PSA level to be increased. Only about 10 percent of men who are screened for prostate cancer will have an elevated PSA level, and only one third of those will have prostate cancer.

THE POSITIVE EFFECTS OF SCREENING

When a population is screened (tested) for prostate cancer, there is an immediate rise in prostate cancer incidence (the total number of new cases diagnosed in a year). Screening allows doctors to diagnose prostate cancer early, before it advances to more critical stages and makes itself known through symptoms. Screening also allows for diagnoses in younger men. According to the National Cancer Institute, men today are diagnosed with prostate cancer up to 5 years earlier than they were before screening was introduced.

Early study results support the clinical value of screening, but this issue has not been settled. Initial data from two major long-term and ongoing studies of prostate cancer screening show approximately a 20-percent reduction in death from prostate cancer due to screening. Both studies are being performed on thousands of patients and will provide extensive data on screening and mortality between 2005 and 2008.

SCREENING AND ADVANCED PROSTATE CANCER

Men whose cancer was detected by screening are diagnosed earlier than other men and therefore are less likely to have disease that has spread beyond the prostate. This is particularly important because currently available treatments are much less effective for men with prostate cancer that has spread.

Detect Cancer Earlier through PSA Testing

My father never went for a PSA check until, upon his retirement, I convinced him to have a PSA test. His PSA was extremely high. Despite hormonal therapy, he died of prostate cancer. I strongly urge all men to follow prostate cancer screening recommendations and undergo testing for prostate cancer.

— Ihor

Early Detection Was a Lucky Break

When I had the exam and finally confirmed that it was cancer, in the middle of panic and fear, I still felt lucky. It was detected early. If I had not had regular checkups, if I had waited until things got more serious and discovered it after cancer cells had spread, I would feel completely differently.

— Tieh Huei

Screening seems to have allowed cancers to be diagnosed at earlier stages. Since screening with the PSA test became common, metastatic prostate cancer accounts for a smaller percentage of all new cases of prostate cancer diagnosed (although there have been more cases diagnosed overall).

IS DETECTING PROSTATE CANCER EARLY ALWAYS IDEAL?

In the recent past a "normal" PSA level was considered from 0 to 4 nanograms per milliliter (ng/ml). Some doctors argue that lowering the cutoff point and further testing men with PSA levels of 2.5 ng/ml or more would help detect cancer earlier, especially in younger and African-American men. This might give patients a better chance of surviving prostate cancer.

Other doctors would like to lower the age at which screening begins or establish a "baseline" PSA value at an earlier age so a man's PSA level may be monitored for change. They feel that screening at a younger age will detect a higher number of patients likely to be treated successfully.

THE IMPACT OF EARLY DETECTION

Not all prostate cancers progress quickly, and some will never cause health problems. Some doctors note that screening younger men and lowering the PSA levels that lead to a biopsy (a procedure in which a sample of tissue is removed and then examined under a microscope) may result in "over-diagnosis"—that is, the detection of cases of prostate cancer that were not likely to grow and spread for many years (if at all).

> **Talking About Prostate Cancer Screening**
>
> Years ago when I was a youngster growing up in the 50s and early 60s, we never used the word breast. Obviously you didn't see mammograms on the evening news, and now they're being talked about daily. I think that we need to do that with prostate cancer: bring the topic out in the open, talk about screening, and face it head on.
>
> *— Bill*

Opponents of screening men who show no symptoms of prostate cancer argue that with screening, doctors may diagnose cancer that would never hurt a man if it were not diagnosed. They note that this could lead to unnecessary treatment that could harm men's sexual or reproductive health, and might even increase death rates.

A major problem is that scientists cannot determine with certainty which cancers will be harmful and which will not. Finding cancer early through screening allows doctors to inform patients about the possibilities and allows men with prostate cancer to make the best possible decisions.

WHAT EACH MAN SHOULD CONSIDER

Early detection of prostate cancer is a complex issue for doctors and patients. If you are considering being screened for prostate cancer, ask your doctor to provide available data and information about situations like yours. Being informed will enable you to make educated decisions about screening, detection, and treatment.

In chapter 2 we explored various risk factors for prostate cancer, and throughout section II of this book we discuss tests that allow doctors to detect prostate cancer. As you learn about risk factors for prostate cancer and consider undergoing screening tests, it's important to keep in perspective your likely risk of developing prostate cancer and the possible impact on your life of being diagnosed with prostate cancer. Putting your risk of prostate cancer into context requires understanding three things:

- your risk of having or developing prostate cancer
- your risk of prostate cancer as compared to the other risks you face in your life
- the potential consequences for your health and life if you did develop prostate cancer

ASSESSING RISK

A man's risk of prostate cancer refers to his chances of having detectable prostate cancer by the end of a defined time interval. For example, an average 60-year-old man may be said to have a 14 percent chance of developing detectable prostate cancer within 19 years. In other words, among 100 60-year-old men who do not have prostate cancer, 14 will have prostate cancer diagnosed (either by screening tests or because they developed symptoms) during the next 19 years. This number is based on the "average" outcomes of many men. However, no individual man is exactly average. Based on risk factors discussed in chapter 2, doctors can estimate that some men may have a higher-than-average risk and others may have a lower risk. Even when these factors are considered, it is important to realize that these predictions are quite accurate in predicting how many men out of 1,000 will develop prostate cancer, but are not at all accurate in predicting the outcome of any single man. One way to help understand the difference between predictions for groups and individuals is to think of coin tosses. If you flip a coin 1,000 times, you can confidently predict that the number of heads will be very close to 500. On the other hand, if you toss the coin only once, it's impossible to accurately predict how it will land.

Your doctor can't say for certain whether you will have prostate cancer or not, but he or she can help evaluate your risk factors and advise you about your likely risk.

COMPARATIVE RISK

Another factor to consider with screening is the probability of prostate cancer as compared to other risks in a man's life. In other words, if a man has severe heart disease and is not expected to live more than a couple of years because of it, his risk of death from prostate cancer is lower than his risk of death from heart disease. Therefore it is less necessary to assess his risk of prostate cancer. The issue of comparative risk becomes more difficult if a man has other illnesses but it is not clear that they are currently life threatening. In that situation, doctors can help evaluate the man's risk of prostate cancer and discuss his potential screening plan.

POTENTIAL CONSEQUENCES OF A PROSTATE CANCER DIAGNOSIS

As noted elsewhere in this chapter, the vast majority of men screened for prostate cancer are not found to have the disease (only about 3 percent of men screened are found to have prostate cancer). However, if men live long enough, they are likely to develop prostate cancer. One man in 6 will be diagnosed with prostate cancer during his lifetime, but only 1 in 33 will die from prostate cancer.

In many cases, prostate cancer grows slowly. Some men opt not to treat prostate cancer, especially if they are elderly and if treatment side effects are more likely to cause detriments to their health than the cancer itself. Younger men often want prostate cancer treated early when it can most easily be controlled. Screening is something for you and your doctor to decide about.

Early Detection Recommendations

The American Cancer Society, the American Urological Association, and the National Comprehensive Cancer Network believe that prostate cancer testing can save lives. The American Cancer Society and the American Urological Association recommend that health care professionals offer men 50 years or older who are at average risk of developing prostate cancer the option of annual testing for early detection of the disease. (The National Comprehensive Cancer Network recommends offering a baseline screening at age 40 and possibly again at age 45 before annual testing beginning at age 50). Testing for prostate cancer in men without symptoms can detect tumors at an earlier stage, allowing for earlier treatment and potentially more favorable results.

Most major medical organizations recommend that doctors discuss the benefits and potential risks of PSA screening, consider patient preferences, and individualize the decision to screen. Generally the most appropriate candidates are men over 50 or younger men at increased risk. Screening is not likely to benefit men with a life expectancy of less than 10 years.

American Cancer Society Recommendations for the Early Detection of Prostate Cancer

The American Cancer Society believes that health care professionals should offer the PSA blood test and digital rectal examination (DRE) yearly, beginning at age 50, to men who have at least a 10-year life expectancy. Men at high risk— such as African Americans and men who have a first-degree relative (father, brother, or son) diagnosed with prostate cancer at an early age (younger than 65)—should begin testing at age 45. Men at even higher risk (because they have several first-degree relatives who had prostate cancer at an early age) could begin testing at age 40. If the results of this initial test are less than 1 ng/ml, further testing might not be needed until age 45.

The American Cancer Society also recommends that men discuss with their doctors potential benefits, side effects, and questions regarding early prostate cancer detection and treatment so they can make informed decisions about testing. If you feel that you are at risk and would like to be tested for prostate cancer, work with a physician who will offer you screening.

If you elect to be tested, keep in mind the following:

- Digital rectal examination and PSA testing are most effective when used together to detect prostate cancer.

- A PSA of less than 4.0 ng/ml does not mean that you do not have prostate cancer, and a normal DRE does not mean that you do not have prostate cancer.

- An abnormal DRE or a high PSA level does not necessarily mean that you do have prostate cancer. Some elevations in PSA may be due to benign (not cancerous) conditions of the prostate. If you have a PSA result of 4.0 ng/ml or higher, your doctor will work to determine the cause of this elevated PSA level. (Some doctors use a cutoff point of 2.5 ng/ml.)

CHAPTER 5

WHAT HAPPENS WHEN I SEE THE DOCTOR?

Paul H. Lange, MD
Bruce Montgomery, MD

WHETHER YOU ARE PURSUING PROSTATE CANCER SCREENING based on recommendations from the American Cancer Society and other organizations or you have experienced worrisome symptoms and want to figure out what may be causing them, visiting your doctor is important in evaluating and preserving your health.

A physical examination and discussion of your personal history is the first step. If any potential for a prostate condition is found, you may visit the doctor again for additional tests in order to pinpoint the cause of any problems. In the next chapters, we'll continue to explore testing, such as biopsy and transrectal ultrasound, as well as the factors that help men decide if testing and diagnosis—potentially followed by treatment—are appropriate for them.

In this chapter we'll explore the likely progression of discussion and tests recommended when you consult the doctor to rule out or diagnose a prostate condition, especially cancer.

Being Informed and Involved

By providing your doctor with information about your health and situation, you ensure that together you determine the treatment decisions that are right for you. By reading this book and otherwise learning about prostate health as well as asking questions, you will make sure you understand the reasons for any suggested tests or treatments.

DOCTORS WHO EVALUATE PROSTATE CONDITIONS

You may see different doctors to evaluate and diagnose problems with your prostate, including:

- **a family doctor, general practitioner, or internist:** a doctor who treats many medical problems and is often a primary care provider
- **a specialist such as a urologist:** a doctor who specializes in the diagnosis and treatment of problems in the genitals, bladder, kidney, and prostate
- **a radiation oncologist or medical oncologist:** a doctor who specializes in the treatment of patients who have cancer

We explore the roles and specialties of the different members of a prostate cancer health care team in more depth in chapter 12.

An initial visit to your doctor will usually involve an interview and a discussion of your medical history. Along with a physical examination—and, potentially, studies of your prostate gland—this will help determine if you need additional testing.

Discussing Your Medical History and Condition

It is crucial that the members of your health care team have all relevant information about your health and the health of your family. It is important to tell your doctor about any symptoms that might be related to prostate cancer, especially symptoms that involve the urinary or genital tract. See chapter 3 for more information about potential symptoms of prostate cancer.

FAMILY HISTORY

Your family history is important. If your father or brother—or multiple relatives—had prostate cancer, particularly at an early age, your risk of developing the disease is increased. Prostate cancer can also run in families with histories of other cancers, and your doctor will ask you if anyone else in the family has had other types of cancer.

URINARY AND SEXUAL SYMPTOMS

You may feel uncomfortable providing some information that relates to personal issues such as urinary function or sexual functioning. These topics aren't always easy to talk about. Be assured that the doctor's questions are both important and standard. Try to share all the information you can about patterns, challenges, and

What Happens at a Doctor's Visit

When visiting the doctor for a checkup or because of troublesome urinary or sexual symptoms, you may undergo some of the following examinations and tests, explored further in the remainder of this chapter and in later chapters.

The interview: talking about history and condition

- family history
- urinary and sexual symptoms
- other symptoms
- medications and conditions

Physical examination

- general examination
- digital rectal examination (DRE)

Laboratory studies

- prostate-specific antigen (PSA) blood test, complete blood count (CBC), other studies

Imaging studies

- transrectal ultrasound
- computed tomography (CT) scan, magnetic resonance imaging (MRI) scan, bone scan

changes. Your doctor will use this confidential information to decide how to proceed and to guide any potential treatment.

Men's sexual function can vary a great deal depending on age and the presence of other medical problems that interfere with erections. It is essential that your doctor know if your prostate health has had an impact on your sexual function, for example, your ability to develop and maintain an erection, any discomfort during orgasm, or any blood in ejaculate.

MEDICAL CONDITIONS AND MEDICATIONS

Other medical conditions can be important factors in weighing the risks and benefits of testing for prostate cancer—and, if necessary, in determining which treatment might be right for you. It is also important that your doctor know what medications you are already receiving to treat symptoms or medical conditions and if you have allergies to any specific medications.

Tell the Doctor about Symptoms

In preparing for your doctor's visit, you may want to consider how you would answer the questions below. Provide any detail you can, and bring your answers to discuss at your consultation.

Urinary and sexual symptoms:

- Do you have urinary symptoms such as a need to urinate frequently during the day or at night?
- Do you have trouble beginning urination?
- Are you unable to stop or start urinating when you go to the bathroom?
- Do you feel as though you don't get rid of all of the urine in your bladder?
- Have you noticed that your urine stream is weaker than usual?
- Do you have to strain to go to the bathroom?
- Have you seen blood in your urine?
- Do you have pain or bleed when you have an orgasm?

Other symptoms:

- Do you have pain in your bones, lower back, muscles, chest, or pelvis?
- Have you experienced any weight loss in the past few months? How much did you lose, and how quickly? (Were you trying to lose weight?)
- Have you experienced excessive tiredness, fevers, or night sweats?

Physical Examination
GENERAL EXAMINATION

A complete physical examination is often performed to help determine your risk of having prostate cancer. Prostate conditions may involve more than just the prostate itself, and your doctor may also examine your skin, lymph nodes, chest, heart, and abdomen.

Your doctor might also suggest a digital rectal examination (DRE) and a prostate-specific antigen (PSA) blood test. As we noted in the last chapter, the American Cancer Society recommends offering these two prostate cancer screening tests—in conjunction with a discussion of the pros and cons of testing—for many men 50 and older and for men at high or very high risk who are 40 or 45 and older. Other tests may also be offered.

DIGITAL RECTAL EXAMINATION

A digital rectal exam allows a doctor or experienced health care professional to determine if the prostate is enlarged, hard, or if there are irregularities in it (see Figure 5.1). The digital examination also gives your doctor an idea of how extensive any abnormality of the prostate might be and helps the doctor plan and direct a potential biopsy, in which sample of tissue is removed and examined under a microscope. Additional testing can determine the cause of any abnormality.

The prostate gland is located just in front of the rectum, which means that part of it (fortunately, the part where cancers most often begin) can be felt through the rectum. The health care professional gently places a gloved, lubricated finger ("digit") into the rectum to feel the part of the prostate that is just under the skin of the rectum. A DRE should be performed as part of any screening process for prostate cancer and should be performed by a physician, physician's assistant, or nurse practitioner who is experienced in performing these examinations.

The digital examination can help detect both prostate and rectal cancer. It is sometimes a standard element of a thorough physical examination of an adult man. The DRE is also used after a man is diagnosed with prostate cancer to help determine if the cancer has spread beyond his prostate gland and is used to detect cancer that has returned after treatment.

WHAT IS INVOLVED?

The doctor may ask you to bend over the edge of the examination table or to lie on the table on your side with your knees held close to your chest for this examination. The examination itself may cause slight discomfort, but it is not painful and is usually very brief.

WHY IS IT NEEDED?

Digital rectal examination and PSA testing are paired because neither test alone provides adequate testing for prostate cancer. About one fifth of prostate cancers do not produce enough PSA to make the blood PSA level abnormal; as a result, the PSA test may not detect these cases. DRE alone does not provide adequate screening for prostate cancer. It is

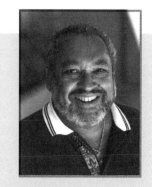

DRE Diagnosed Cancer When PSA Was Normal

I had a normal PSA and had been checked annually in my physical exam. I happened to notice on a bulletin board that males over 55 were needed for a prostate cancer screening research program. So I signed up. A urologist examined me and said, "Hey, your prostate feels like a rusty piece of metal. I'm going to send this report to your doctor, and you should really see a urologist." And I did, and I was diagnosed with prostate cancer.

— Freeman

Physical Exam Led to Diagnosis

I was diagnosed at age 50 through a physical examination. I was quite devastated, which goes without saying. Anyone would be. I was always sort of a macho-type pilot, you know, a Vietnam veteran, and of course I always thought that these things happened to other people.

— Fred

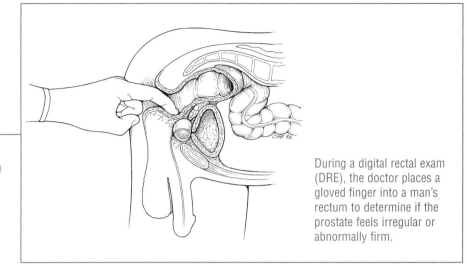

Figure 5.1.
The Digital Rectal Exam
(DRE)

During a digital rectal exam (DRE), the doctor places a gloved finger into a man's rectum to determine if the prostate feels irregular or abnormally firm.

difficult for a doctor's finger to reach all parts of the gland through the rectum—although it reaches the back part of the gland, where most prostate cancers begin. Small cancers may be difficult to feel and therefore difficult to detect through DRE.

Laboratory Tests

Other studies may help the doctor assess your prostate health. These may include blood tests, such as the prostate-specific antigen (PSA) test, the prostatic acid phosphatase, and complete blood count (CBC).

- **Prostate-specific antigen (PSA)** is a protein made by the prostate that liquefies semen so it can travel up the female reproductive tract. When prostate cancer develops, the PSA level in the blood usually rises. The PSA test directly measures these levels. An elevated PSA level suggests a higher risk of prostate conditions. PSA results alone do not provide enough information to diagnose or rule out cancer. They help doctors understand whether further testing may be helpful or necessary. PSA tests are explored in more detail in the next chapter.

- The **prostatic acid phosphatase** is a blood test that searches for a different protein, also secreted by prostate cancer. This test generally does not detect as many cancers as PSA testing. Most doctors no longer order it to screen for prostate cancer.

- The **complete blood count (CBC)** and coagulation studies provide information about blood cell counts and the risk of abnormal bleeding. They help determine if it is safe to perform other studies, such as biopsies of the prostate (see next section). Men who will undergo a prostate biopsy or have symptoms which could be related to low blood counts may have these tests performed.

- Your doctor may also ask to test a sample of your urine, known as a **urinalysis**, to look for blood or other abnormalities.

Biopsy

A biopsy is a procedure in which a sample of tissue is removed and examined under a microscope. A core needle biopsy is the main method used to diagnose prostate cancer. For a core needle biopsy, the doctor inserts a narrow needle through the wall of your rectum into several areas of your prostate gland, removing a cylinder of tissue and sending it to the laboratory to be examined and determine if cancer is present. See chapter 7 for more information about biopsies.

Imaging Studies

If your doctor feels that your physical exam, blood tests, or health history suggest the need for further tests, you may undergo an imaging study (a method used to produce a picture of internal body structures). Imaging studies, such as transrectal ultrasound (TRUS), allow doctors to better see and evaluate the prostate and surrounding area.

Transrectal ultrasound (see chapter 8 for more detail) uses sound waves to produce an image of the prostate gland that can help doctors identify areas that are suspicious and would be appropriate for biopsy. TRUS helps guide a precise biopsy, so the two tests are often performed together.

Other imaging studies are most often performed *after* a diagnosis of prostate cancer, to evaluate whether or not cancer has spread to other areas of the body. These include bone scans, computerized tomography (CT) scans (also sometimes called CAT scans), and magnetic resonance imaging (MRI). See chapter 15 for more information about these tests.

CHAPTER 6

WHAT DO PROSTATE-SPECIFIC ANTIGEN (PSA) LEVELS INDICATE?

Michael K. Brawer, MD

THE PROSTATE-SPECIFIC ANTIGEN (PSA) TEST has dramatically changed the detection of prostate cancer that may cause no outward symptoms. Using PSA tests to screen for prostate cancer has also changed prostate cancer care. In this chapter we will discuss what PSA is, how the PSA test may be used, and what a PSA level indicates.

What Is PSA?

Prostate-specific antigen is a protein made in the prostate gland. The function of PSA is to liquefy semen so sperm are better able to travel up the female reproductive tract.

When the prostate is healthy, very little PSA escapes into the bloodstream. However, if any of a variety of diseases is present—and sometimes if the prostate is simply enlarged—the walls between the prostate and the bloodstream may break down and allow more PSA into the blood. In these cases, PSA can be detected by a blood test.

Prostate-specific antigen is produced by both normal cells and cancer cells. PSA can be found in large amounts in the blood of some men with prostate cancer; less often, large amounts of PSA can also be found in the blood of men who do not have prostate cancer.

The PSA Test

Abnormal levels of prostate-specific antigen often indicate that a man has prostate cancer. Therefore testing for high PSA levels allows doctors to assess a man's prostate cancer risk. Generally, when cancer *is* present, the higher the PSA level is, the larger the prostate cancer is and the more likely it is to have spread beyond the prostate.

But the PSA test cannot determine the presence or absence of prostate cancer. PSA levels alone do not provide enough information to distinguish between benign prostate conditions and cancer. PSA testing serves only as a screening device that can indicate that a prostate problem might exist. The doctor takes the result of a PSA test into account, along with other factors, then decides whether to suggest additional testing.

ESTABLISHING A MAN'S PSA LEVEL

Prostate-specific antigen is detected in the bloodstream through a simple blood test. A blood sample is drawn from a vein in the arm and sent to a laboratory for testing. Different test kits provide slightly differing results; even within a laboratory, which uses one manufacturer of test kits, there can be variation in the PSA level found. There is also significant day-to-day variation in PSA in the body in all men. See Table 6.1 for other factors affecting the PSA level.

WHAT DOES A PSA LEVEL INDICATE?

PSA test results report the level of PSA detected in the blood. The higher a man's PSA level, the more likely it is that he has prostate cancer. PSA is measured in terms of nanograms per milliliter, or ng/ml; a nanogram is one billionth of a gram. A PSA level of 4 to 10 ng/ml is considered slightly elevated, 10 to 20 is moderately elevated, and above 20 is highly elevated. But because certain factors can cause PSA levels to rise or fall (see page 49), one high PSA reading does not necessarily mean more involved tests, such as a biopsy, are needed. Doctors may monitor PSA levels to determine if they continue to rise over time, especially if the values are only slightly elevated. If levels continue to rise, the doctor will suggest more extensive tests.

WHAT IS A "NORMAL" PSA LEVEL?

For many years, the "normal" PSA level was below 4 ng/ml. However, the number of men with cancer who have PSA levels between 3 and 4 is comparable to the number of men with cancer who have PSA levels between 4 and 5. Therefore many authorities in the field have encouraged lowering the PSA level at which biopsy is recommended from 4 to 3, and some have suggested lowering it

Table 6.1. FACTORS AFFECTING PROSTATE-SPECIFIC ANTIGEN (PSA) LEVEL

Various factors can affect the PSA level. Several medicines and herbal preparations may lower blood PSA levels as well; tell your doctor if you are taking finasteride (Proscar or Propecia) or dutasteride (Avodart) or any supplement marketed "for prostate health."

Factor	Effect on PSA
Bed rest	Decrease
Digital rectal exam	None
Exercise (excluding cycling)	None
Ejaculation	Increase
Cycling	Increase
Prostatic massage	Increase
Cystoscopy	Increase
Perineal or transrectal needle biopsy	Increase
Transrectal ultrasound	Increase

to 2.5. A man with a PSA below 2.5 has a very low likelihood of having prostate cancer. (If he did have cancer, the cancer would likely be identified—and cured—when the PSA exceeded a level of 3 ng/ml.) (For more information about screening and the arguments for and against identifying all cases of prostate cancer, see chapter 4.)

FACTORS AFFECTING THE PSA LEVEL

A number of factors may result in a temporary change in a PSA level (see above). A man's PSA level falls after a long period of rest and increases slightly with movement.

Factors that may cause the PSA level to rise include medical procedures such as cystoscopy (a test in which a slender tube with a lens and a light is used to see the bladder and urethra), prostate biopsy, vigorous prostatic massage (sometimes used to treat prostatitis), and transrectal ultrasound (TRUS; see chapter 8). A digital rectal examination (DRE) does not appear to have any significant effect on the PSA level. Therefore a blood sample may be collected for a PSA test after a DRE if an abnormality is felt. (See chapter 5 for more information about DRE.)

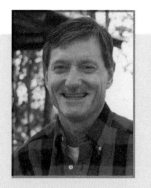

A Low PSA Can Accompany Prostate Cancer

Although my PSA was low, during a DRE my prostate felt firm to my doctor, so I underwent a biopsy. My urologist, my wife, and I were shocked when a biopsy showed cancer....It was the all-time lowest PSA the urologist had heard of accompanying cancer.

— *John B.*

High PSA Warning Allowed for Research

My PSA was over 20 when I was 55 years old. I highly suspected that I had cancer, but I was not ultimately diagnosed until about a year and a half later. Meanwhile I spent quite a bit of time researching my options.

— *Howard*

Until recently, the effect of sexual activity on PSA level was subject to debate. Now, however, investigators have demonstrated a slight elevation of PSA following sexual intercourse. The PSA level appears to peak approximately an hour after ejaculation and returns to its starting level within approximately 24 hours.

Before having a PSA test:

- Do not engage in sexual activity for 1 to 2 days.
- Schedule the test for several weeks after a cystoscopy.

PSA: NOT A PERFECT TEST

There are several reasons why some experts have mixed feelings about using PSA tests in screening for prostate cancer.

PSA LEVEL DOES NOT ALWAYS REFLECT WHETHER PROSTATE CANCER EXISTS

A perfect screening test for prostate cancer would give an abnormal result *only* in men who have cancer. Unfortunately, such a test does not exist. Most men with abnormal PSA levels are not diagnosed with cancer. Only 25 to 30 percent of men with "abnormal" PSA levels (levels higher than 4 ng/ml) will be biopsied and diagnosed with cancer. Abnormal PSA levels in men who do not have cancer are common. Older men have a greater chance this; 15 in 100 men over 50 will have elevated PSA levels but only 3 of these will have prostate cancer. Men may therefore be unnecessarily alarmed by PSA test results. When a man is told that he has an abnormal PSA, he and his family are likely to become anxious about what this might mean about his health and his future. The man may also face some invasive and costly testing that ultimately proves to be unnecessary (see the next section).

An ideal screening test would also detect every cancer. That is, if a man has cancer, the test result should be always be abnormal. But again, in reality there is no perfect test. Some men with prostate cancer have normal PSA levels. If the cancer is not detected by another means (such as a digital rectal exam), a normal PSA level could give a man a false sense of security.

PSA TESTING CAN LEAD TO COSTLIER (AND MORE INVASIVE) TESTS

Men with high PSA levels may be referred for a biopsy, even though cancer may not actually be present. There are many costs associated with prostate cancer biopsies: antibiotics (to prevent or treat infection), ultrasound charges (ultrasound is used to help guide doctors to the correct area of the prostate), biopsy fees, and the cost of examining and interpreting the biopsy specimen. Beyond copayments, these costs are typically covered by insurance or Medicare.

Because it is an invasive procedure, there is also a very small risk of problems during and after the biopsy, such as pain, infection, or excessive bleeding.

THE NEGATIVE SIDE OF FINDING PROSTATE CANCER EARLY

When considering testing for prostate cancer, it is important to consider whether a diagnosis of cancer would be likely to favorably impact a man's quality and length of life. Factors that complicate the issue include:

- Prostate cancer often grows slowly, and some very early-stage cancers detected by screening may never cause problems.
- Once some men find out they have cancer, they may become so focused on destroying the cancer that they decide to undergo treatment, even if the risks outweigh the likely benefits.
- Treatments often involve side effects, such as urinary and sexual problems, that negatively affect quality of life.
- Tests such as biopsies can cause bleeding and potential infection.

The issue of early testing for prostate cancer, including PSA testing, is complicated. For more information about this subject, see the chapter 4 section *Is Detecting Prostate Cancer Early Always Ideal?* on page 35.

RESEARCH INTO IMPROVING PSA TESTS

Some developments in PSA testing methods may provide doctors with more information and detail, allowing them to more accurately identify men who need biopsies. Not all doctors interpret these additional PSA tests in the same way, and most of these are still considered investigational. If your PSA test result is considered higher than normal, ask your doctor to discuss your cancer risk and your need for further tests.

AGE-SPECIFIC PSA RANGES

Age is an important factor in rising PSA levels. Therefore some doctors use age-specific PSA ranges (which are different for men in each decade of their lives) as guides when considering whether or not to pursue additional tests if a high PSA level is found.

But this strategy is not without its own problems. Lowering the PSA cutoff point for younger men could find more cancers that would likely need to be treated, but it would also increase the number of biopsies performed that show no cancer is present as well as the number of slow-growing cancers found early. Raising the PSA threshold recommended for biopsy in older men could have the effect of missing some significant cancers that otherwise would have been detected in that population. Some experts believe that a PSA cutoff of 3 ng/ml for all men may provide a larger benefit.

Because the usefulness of age-specific PSA ranges is not well proven, the manufacturers of the PSA tests, the American Cancer Society, the American Urological Association, and the National Comprehensive Cancer Network do not support their use at this time. You may want to ask your doctor if he or she relies on age-specific PSA ranges.

PSA DENSITY: CONSIDERING PROSTATE SIZE

Determining the size of the prostate (through transrectal ultrasound) and dividing the PSA number by the prostate volume provides PSA density. This number helps adjust for the fact that some men have bigger prostates than others and may therefore have higher "normal" PSA levels.

A higher PSA density indicates greater likelihood of cancer. PSA density may be useful, but the percent-free PSA test (see next page) has thus far been shown to be more accurate.

PSA VELOCITY: HOW QUICKLY PSA RISES OVER TIME

The PSA velocity is not a separate test. It is the change in PSA values over time. If a man has a slightly elevated PSA level, his doctor may want to follow the level over time by repeating the tests several months later. The theory behind this approach is that the PSA level in men with prostate cancer usually increases at a greater rate than in men without cancer.

A PSA that rises faster than 0.75 ng/ml per year (for example, if values went from 3 to 3.8 to 4.6 over the course of 3 years) is considered high, and a biopsy should be considered.

Most doctors believe that to be valid the PSA velocity should be measured over a minimum of 18 months. However, the interval of PSA tests that will correctly establish PSA velocity has not been determined. Another issue to remember is that a man's PSA level may change for a variety of reasons other than the development of prostate cancer. Nonetheless, it is important to watch the velocity of your PSA scores to help find out if a problem might exist.

MEASURING PERCENT-FREE PSA

PSA occurs in two major forms in the blood. Most PSA is bound (attached) to blood proteins and the other circulates free (unattached). The ratio of free PSA to total (bound plus free) PSA is called percent-free PSA. Percent-free PSA may help distinguish men with prostate cancer from those with benign conditions, since benign prostate conditions produce more free PSA, while cancer produces more of the attached form.

If your PSA results are in the borderline range (4–10 ng/ml), a low percent-free PSA (less than 10) means that your likelihood of having prostate cancer is about 50 percent, and you should pursue a biopsy. In fact, many doctors recommend biopsies for men whose percent-free PSA is 25 percent or less. A recent study found that if men with borderline PSA results had prostate biopsies only when their percent-free PSA was 25 percent or less, about 20 percent of unnecessary prostate biopsies could be avoided, and about 95 percent of cancers would still be detected. Although this test is widely used, not all doctors agree that 25 percent is the best value to use.

This test may decrease the number of abnormal PSA levels found in men without cancer. However, several concerns exist regarding the percent-free PSA. Handling specimens in the lab may affect results because free PSA is less stable than bound PSA. And different manufacturers' tests provide staggeringly different free-to-total ratios. Because of these factors, efforts to develop measurements for the bound form of PSA are underway.

WHEN TO TEST

A man and his doctor should talk about whether he should be screened for prostate cancer with a PSA test. Men should consider their individual situations and discuss the positive and negative aspects of testing with their primary care physicians.

If the patient and doctor agree that the early diagnosis of prostate cancer would be in the patient's best interest, then a PSA test along with a carefully performed digital rectal examination is recommended. Using both screening methods together may provide more information and is recommended.

Before testing, the doctor will likely discuss a man's situation with him and consider any factors that might affect the PSA level—for example, age, medications, recent sexual activity, and recent bedrest or resumed activity (see Table 6.1).

Some doctors may recommend biopsy for a man with a total PSA level over 3 ng/ml; others may more strictly adhere to the "normal" level of 4 and recommend biopsy for men with levels higher than that. If the DRE is abnormal or the PSA exceeds normal thresholds, the doctor will provide a referral to a urologist, a doctor who specializes in treating conditions and diseases of the genitals and urinary tract.

CHAPTER 7

WHAT IS A BIOPSY?

Bob Djavan, MD, PhD
Mesut Remzi, MD
Christian Seitz, MD

IF CERTAIN SYMPTOMS OR THE RESULTS OF EARLY DETECTION TESTS have raised the possibility of prostate cancer, your doctor will use other tests to find out if you have prostate cancer. A biopsy is the most reliable way of diagnosing or ruling out cancer. It involves removing a sample of tissue (usually surgically or with a needle) and examining it under a microscope to see whether cancer cells are present. There are several biopsy techniques that can be used in diagnosing prostate cancer.

What Is a Biopsy of the Prostate?

A prostate biopsy involves removing small pieces of tissue from the prostate for microscopic examination. A biopsy is most often done after a high prostate-specific antigen (PSA) level (see chapter 6) or a lump found during a digital rectal exam (DRE; see chapter 5) suggests cancer may be present. Several weeks may pass between a suspicious PSA or DRE is discovered and when a biopsy is performed. Because prostate cancers generally tend to grow very slowly, most men should not be concerned about a cancer growing or spreading during that period of time.

During a biopsy, several tissue samples are taken from different areas of the prostate. Anywhere from 6 to 13 samples are usually needed to determine if cancer is present and how much of the gland is affected, but as many as 24 samples may be taken from some patients. Transrectal ultrasound (TRUS) can be used to guide doctors to the area of the prostate they want to sample (see chapter 8 for more information).

A sextant biopsy is a procedure in which 6 core biopsy samples are taken, one each from the top, middle and bottom of each side of the prostate. Saturation biopsies (which involve taking more than 40 cores) are done only in cases in which there is a high suspicion of prostate cancer and a man has already had multiple biopsies that have been negative, or when a thorough mapping of the prostate is desired. This may require a hospital stay.

The biopsy samples are sent for study under the microscope by a pathologist, a doctor who specializes in diagnosing and classifying diseases, to determine if cancer is present. This analysis usually takes 1 to 3 days.

WHAT IS A CORE NEEDLE BIOPSY?

A core needle biopsy is the main method used to diagnose prostate cancer. A core needle biopsy involves using small needles to withdraw cylinders of tissue from the prostate. Each sample, or core, is usually about ½ inch long and ¹⁄₁₆ inch across. Though the procedure sounds painful, a special instrument called a biopsy gun inserts and removes the needles in a fraction of a second, minimizing discomfort. A core needle biopsy of the prostate can be obtained either through the rectum or through the perineum (the skin between the rectum and the scrotum).

TRANSRECTAL BIOPSY

A transrectal biopsy is the most common biopsy technique. This method involves inserting the biopsy needles through the rectum to withdraw sample tissue.

Transrectal ultrasound–guided biopsy. Transrectal ultrasound (TRUS) produces a fairly accurate image of the prostate for urologists to study. Biopsies almost always use TRUS to guide the biopsy needle to the tissue area they want to sample. Biopsies done without TRUS are rare.

Transrectal ultrasound–guided biopsy allows the biopsy needle to be precisely guided in real time. Ultrasound images of the prostate are taken through a lubricated probe inserted into the rectum. The small probe sends sound waves into the prostate to create echoes that are sent to a computer and translated into a picture. A small needle is placed into the guide and tissue specimens are taken from different areas of the prostate with an automated biopsy gun.

Most patients who undergo transrectal ultrasound–guided biopsy of the prostate experience some discomfort. You may feel a dull pressure as the transrectal probe is inserted in the rectum. While the biopsy cores are being taken, you may feel a quick, sharp pain. An anaesthetic jelly may be inserted into the rectum to numb the area and reduce discomfort during the procedure. For more sensitive patients, an anaesthetic agent can be injected through the rectal wall. In rare cases when patients require extensive biopsy sessions, intravenous sedation can be used to reduce discomfort.

PERINEAL BIOPSY

Some doctors will perform a biopsy through the perineum, the skin between the rectum and the scrotum. The doctor will place his or her finger in the patient's rectum to feel the prostate and then insert the biopsy needle through a small incision in the skin of the perineum. The doctor will use a local anesthetic to numb the area. This method has been almost entirely replaced by TRUS-guided biopsy (see previous page).

HOW SHOULD I PREPARE FOR A CORE NEEDLE BIOPSY?

A prostate biopsy takes about 15 minutes and is usually done in the doctor's office. During the biopsy, the patient lies either on his left side on an examination table or sits, leaning backward slightly with legs apart, in an examination chair.

There are only a few precautions to take before undergoing a core biopsy of the prostate:

- **Avoid vaccinations.** Undergo any scheduled vaccinations 2 weeks before or after the biopsy since they may cause fever. If you have any flu-like symptoms, such as chills and fever, the biopsy should be postponed because of the danger of complications due to infection.

- **Stop taking blood thinners.** Anticoagulant drugs (blood thinners) such as warfarin (Coumadin), clopidogrel (Plavix), or aspirin may need to be stopped a few days before the biopsy because of an increased risk of persistent bleeding after a biopsy. (Non-steroidal anti-inflammatory drugs, also known as NSAIDs, do not increase the risk of bleeding.) Low molecular weight heparin can be used instead. Discuss this with your doctor well before your procedure.

- **Begin any preventive antibiotics.** An oral antibiotic may be given to protect against potential infection after a biopsy. The antibiotic is started either a day before or the day of the procedure, and the patient takes the prescription antibiotic for a few days.

- **Use enemas if recommended.** Cleansing enemas are not routinely administered before a biopsy, but if used they should be given both the night before and the morning of the procedure.

WHAT IS A FINE NEEDLE ASPIRATION BIOPSY?

In a fine needle aspiration (FNA) biopsy, a very thin needle is used to extract fluid and cells. Experienced urologists and pathologists may perform prostate FNA biopsies in some selected cases (although it is not often used for prostate cancer).

The needle is placed by hand into a suspicious mass that has been felt on the surface of the prostate gland. Cells are drawn out (aspirated) with a vacuum syringe. FNA biopsy samples are sometimes difficult to interpret, and existing tumors may not be detected.

Another application of fine needle aspiration that is not used very often is extracting tissue from enlarged lymph nodes. A specially trained doctor called a radiologist will sometimes do this type of FNA, relying on a CT scan image (a specialized type of x-ray) to guide the long, thin needle. A syringe attached to the needle takes a small tissue sample from the node.

HOW SHOULD I PREPARE FOR A FINE NEEDLE ASPIRATION BIOPSY?

It is not necessary to have an enema before a fine needle aspiration biopsy. Anticoagulation (blood thinning) therapy should be paused or replaced with the blood-thinning medication heparin before a FNA biopsy (again, speak with your doctor).

Complications are rare, but potentially include rectal and urethral bleeding, bloody ejaculate, and infections associated with chills and fever. Your doctor will therefore likely prescribe an antibiotic before the procedure.

WHAT TO EXPECT AFTER A BIOPSY

After a biopsy, the patient rests for 2 to 3 hours. Blood pressure and pulse are checked periodically. Patients should avoid strenuous activities for the remainder of the day.

Many men report mild discomfort in the area of the prostate during the first 48 hours following the biopsy. Some men may also notice a small amount of blood in their urine or rectum during bowel movements for up to a week. A small amount of blood in the semen is also common for up to a month after a biopsy. This is not dangerous for you or your sexual partner.

Notify your doctor immediately if:

- you have persistent bleeding or you think you are losing a lot of blood
- you develop fatigue or a fever over 100 degrees F
- you experience any other major problems, such as increased pain or an inability to urinate

Prostate biopsy will not cause infertility and/or erectile dysfunction (problems achieving or maintaining an erection).

CHAPTER 8

WHAT IS TRANSRECTAL ULTRASOUND (TRUS)?

Naveen Kella, MD
Kevin M. Slawin, MD

DOCTORS USE ULTRASOUND TECHNOLOGY, which involves the use of sound waves and their echoes, to produce pictures of internal organs or masses. Transrectal ultrasound (TRUS) is a specific type of ultrasound that can be used to create an image of the prostate to determine if cancer is present. TRUS can also be used to guide the needles during a biopsy of the prostate. In this chapter, we'll discuss how this technology works and how it is applied to detect prostate cancer.

Transrectal Ultrasound (TRUS)

During a transrectal ultrasound (TRUS), an ultrasound machine produces images called sonograms by generating high-frequency sound waves that go through the body. As the sound waves bounce off internal organs and tissues, they create echoes. Solid tumors have different echo patterns than normal tissues. Through a transducer (a wand that produces the sound waves and detects echoes), TRUS emits sound waves to make an image of the prostate on a video screen. When this small probe is placed in the rectum, sound waves enter the prostate and create echoes that are picked up by the probe. A computer turns the pattern of echoes into a picture.

TRUS provides a fairly accurate image of the prostate for urologists to study. TRUS allows urologists to examine all regions of the prostate gland. In addition, TRUS can potentially provide experts with information about other parts of the

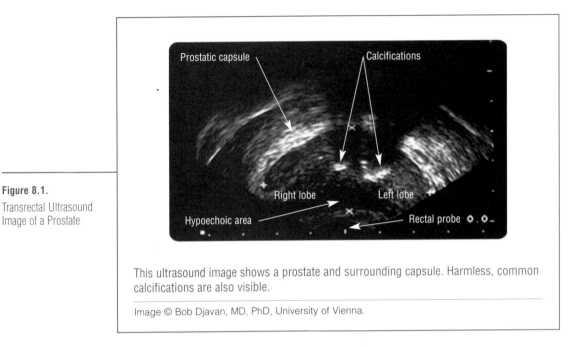

Figure 8.1.

Transrectal Ultrasound Image of a Prostate

This ultrasound image shows a prostate and surrounding capsule. Harmless, common calcifications are also visible.

Image © Bob Djavan, MD, PhD, University of Vienna.

body associated with the prostate, such as the seminal vesicles (glands at the base of the bladder that release fluid into the semen during orgasm), as well as the extent of a cancer.

Experts studying ultrasound images for suspicious areas will likely pay special attention to less reflective areas in the image, since prostate cancer is often less reflective than normal tissue.

When TRUS was developed, many urologists studied the potential use of ultrasound as an additional mode of screening for cancer. However, most doctors now feel TRUS by itself is not a better screening tool than the combination of prostate-specific antigen (PSA) test and digital rectal exam (DRE), so it is not recommended as a routine test to detect prostate cancer early.

TRUS is most commonly used during a prostate biopsy (see chapter 7). Prostate tumors and normal prostate tissue often reflect sound waves differently, so TRUS is used to guide the biopsy needles into exactly the right area of the prostate.

WHAT IS INVOLVED?

TRUS is an outpatient procedure that lasts 5 to 15 minutes. Patients usually undergo TRUS in the doctor's office. Physicians often instruct their patients to have a cleansing enema the night before the procedure in order to reduce interference with the ultrasound imaging. Oral antibiotics are usually prescribed if the procedure will be done along with a prostate biopsy.

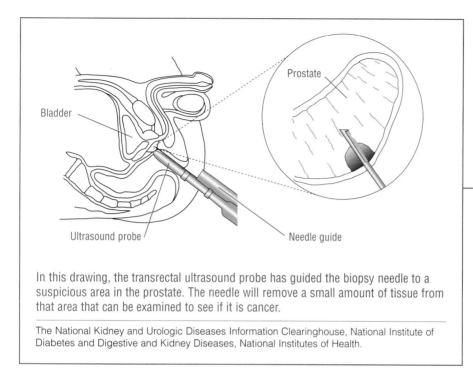

Bladder

Prostate

Ultrasound probe

Needle guide

Figure 8.2.
Transrectal Ultrasound
and Prostate Biopsy

In this drawing, the transrectal ultrasound probe has guided the biopsy needle to a suspicious area in the prostate. The needle will remove a small amount of tissue from that area that can be examined to see if it is cancer.

The National Kidney and Urologic Diseases Information Clearinghouse, National Institute of Diabetes and Digestive and Kidney Diseases, National Institutes of Health.

On the day of the procedure, the doctor will use a finger to perform a rectal exam to make sure there are no rectal disorders that need to be addressed before the TRUS. A patient typically lies on his side with his knees drawn up toward his chest. The ultrasound device is a few centimeters longer than the average finger and is slightly thicker. The device is covered with a protective condom, is lubricated with gel, and is carefully inserted through the anus into the rectum.

Most patients experience only slight discomfort. You might feel some pressure when the TRUS probe is placed in the rectum. Some physicians offer the option of pain medication that may either be orally or rectally administered to prevent temporary discomfort.

The energy involved in a transrectal ultrasound signal uses no radiation and is safe and suitable for a human body. A person having an ultrasound does not feel the sound waves.

TAKING PRECISE BIOPSIES

Before ultrasound was widely used, if urologists felt any prostate abnormalities, they performed "blind," finger-directed biopsies. TRUS images help doctors identify tumors, but also guide doctors in taking precise biopsies from anywhere in the prostate. Numerous studies have demonstrated that studying biopsies of

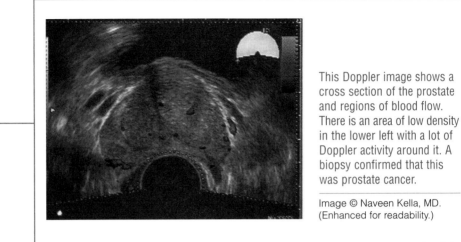

Figure 8.3.
Doppler Image
of a Prostate

This Doppler image shows a cross section of the prostate and regions of blood flow. There is an area of low density in the lower left with a lot of Doppler activity around it. A biopsy confirmed that this was prostate cancer.

Image © Naveen Kella, MD.
(Enhanced for readability.)

the entire prostate is more reliable than evaluating a biopsy of only a suspicious lesion that can be seen or felt.

With a TRUS image, a doctor can view the prostate from different perspectives and can measure the size of the gland, using this information to diagnose or treat various prostate conditions (including determining the PSA density, described in chapter 6).

DOPPLER FLOW MACHINES

Newer applications of ultrasound, Doppler flow machines, are able to show how blood flows through the blood vessels. This is important because blood flows differently through tumors than it does through normal tissue. Studies are investigating the Doppler technique's promise in pinpointing cancer, which may further help to guide prostate biopsies to the correct area of the gland.

DELIVERING TREATMENT FOR CANCER

TRUS has taken on an important role in helping doctors visualize the prostate, diagnose prostate conditions, and even treat them.

Once cancer has been diagnosed, doctors can use TRUS to help plan and deliver some cancer therapies, such as radioactive seed implants or freezing of the prostate (cryosurgery). (See chapters 21 and 24 for more information about these treatments.)

UNDERSTANDING YOUR DIAGNOSIS
OF PROSTATE CANCER

AFTER A BIOPSY, YOUR DOCTOR WILL RECEIVE AND DISCUSS your pathology report with you, outlining what was discovered about your prostate. In the following chapters we explore what is included in a pathology report and how to understand what the report means—both when the results are positive for cancer and when the results indicate that some other, non-cancerous condition is present.

If you are diagnosed with cancer, don't be afraid to ask your health care team questions about your cancer and the language they use to describe it. The terminology related to prostate cancer screening tests and results can be complicated and confusing to take in, especially when you may also be facing how cancer may affect your body and your life. Make sure you're satisfied with the explanations you get of your situation. Understanding your diagnosis and the factors that may affect your prognosis (outlook) is essential.

Your Health Care Team Is There to Help

Don't be afraid to ask your health care team questions about your cancer and the language they use to describe it.

CHAPTER 9

WHAT DOES MY PATHOLOGY REPORT MEAN?

David G. Bostwick, MD, MBA
Junqi Qian, MD

A DIAGNOSIS OF CANCER IS NEARLY ALWAYS BASED on a biopsy specimen. A pathologist is a licensed physician, usually certified by the American Board of Pathology, who diagnoses and classifies your cancer through laboratory tests such as examinations of biopsy tissue, fluid, and cells under a microscope. The testing process is sometimes referred to as pathology. The results of testing are summarized in a document called a pathology report. Pathology reports are issued after both biopsies and surgical procedures, such as a radical prostatectomy. In this chapter, we will explore the report issued after a biopsy.

The Biopsy Pathology Report

The pathologist issues a report outlining the cell type and extent of your cancer. A pathology report for a biopsy will include the information shown in Figure 9.1 on page 67, although the format may vary from laboratory to laboratory. A pathology report shows the type of cancer, the cancer grade, and whether the cancer has grown outside the prostate and into surrounding tissue, in addition to other information.

The report is issued only after the pathologist is certain of his or her diagnosis. You may want to seek a second opinion; in this case, your pathologist will send the biopsy slides themselves to the other doctor for review and interpretation, not his or her report. You can request that a particular doctor (sometimes called a consultant pathologist) or institution provide a second opinion. Consultant

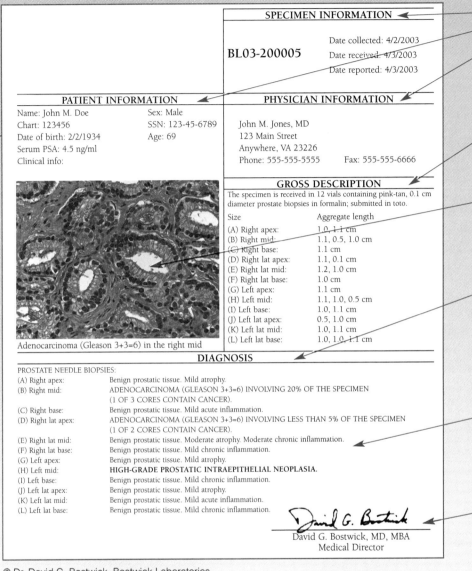

Figure 9.1.

Pathology Report for Low-Grade Prostate Cancer (with Explanatory Comments)

SPECIMEN INFORMATION

BL03-200005

Date collected: 4/2/2003
Date received: 4/3/2003
Date reported: 4/3/2003

PATIENT INFORMATION

Name: John M. Doe   Sex: Male
Chart: 123456   SSN: 123-45-6789
Date of birth: 2/2/1934   Age: 69
Serum PSA: 4.5 ng/ml
Clinical info:

PHYSICIAN INFORMATION

John M. Jones, MD
123 Main Street
Anywhere, VA 23226
Phone: 555-555-5555   Fax: 555-555-6666

GROSS DESCRIPTION

The specimen is received in 12 vials containing pink-tan, 0.1 cm diameter prostate biopsies in formalin; submitted in toto.

Size	Aggregate length
(A) Right apex:	1.0, 1.1 cm
(B) Right mid:	1.1, 0.5, 1.0 cm
(C) Right base:	1.1 cm
(D) Right lat apex:	1.1, 0.1 cm
(E) Right lat mid:	1.2, 1.0 cm
(F) Right lat base:	1.0 cm
(G) Left apex:	1.1 cm
(H) Left mid:	1.1, 1.0, 0.5 cm
(I) Left base:	1.0, 1.1 cm
(J) Left lat apex:	0.5, 1.0 cm
(K) Left lat mid:	1.0, 1.1 cm
(L) Left lat base:	1.0, 1.0, 1.1 cm

Adenocarcinoma (Gleason 3+3=6) in the right mid

DIAGNOSIS

PROSTATE NEEDLE BIOPSIES:

(A) Right apex:	Benign prostatic tissue. Mild atrophy.
(B) Right mid:	ADENOCARCINOMA (GLEASON 3+3=6) INVOLVING 20% OF THE SPECIMEN (1 OF 3 CORES CONTAIN CANCER).
(C) Right base:	Benign prostatic tissue. Mild acute inflammation.
(D) Right lat apex:	ADENOCARCINOMA (GLEASON 3+3=6) INVOLVING LESS THAN 5% OF THE SPECIMEN (1 OF 2 CORES CONTAIN CANCER).
(E) Right lat mid:	Benign prostatic tissue. Moderate atrophy. Moderate chronic inflammation.
(F) Right lat base:	Benign prostatic tissue. Mild chronic inflammation.
(G) Left apex:	Benign prostatic tissue. Mild atrophy.
(H) Left mid:	HIGH-GRADE PROSTATIC INTRAEPITHELIAL NEOPLASIA.
(I) Left base:	Benign prostatic tissue. Mild chronic inflammation.
(J) Left lat apex:	Benign prostatic tissue. Mild atrophy.
(K) Left lat mid:	Benign prostatic tissue. Mild acute inflammation.
(L) Left lat base:	Benign prostatic tissue. Mild chronic inflammation.

David G. Bostwick, MD, MBA
Medical Director

© Dr. David G. Bostwick, Bostwick Laboratories

pathologists are experts in a special field, such as prostate pathology. The consultation is usually covered by insurance.

Feel free to ask your doctor to explain your pathology report, exploring how the test results influence treatment options and how they help predict your outlook for survival. If you feel yourself becoming overloaded with information, ask your doctor to back up and explain something again or in a different way.

You may request copies of your pathology report for your own records.

- **Patient, Specimen, and Physician Information.** This information is essential in ensuring that your report doesn't get confused with that of another patient with a similar or identical name and that it gets delivered to your doctor. Every specimen is given a pathology number.

- **Gross Description.** This section describes how the sample looks without a microscope. It also identifies the area from which each biopsy was taken. (This is especially important for patients that may have biopsies from more than one area during the same operation.) The size of each biopsy is listed in centimeters (cm).

- **Photo.** This image documents the histology (the appearance under the microscope) of prostate cancer identified in one biopsy. It allows the pathologist to see which areas of the sample contained cancer and to describe the appearance of cancer cells.

- **Diagnosis.** This is the most important section of the report—it includes the "bottom line" diagnosis (see Right mid and Right Lat Apex). This is determined by what the pathologist saw under the microscope, including: the type of cancer (adenocarcinoma) and its grade (Gleason 6), as well as its size (as indicated by percentage of specimen involvement; 20 percent and less than 5 percent), and the number of biopsy cores containing cancer (1 in 3 and 1 in 2). This cancer is low grade (well differentiated).

- **Other findings.** In addition to cancer, prostate tissue may show other abnormalities. High-grade prostatic intraepithelial neoplasia was found during this patient's biopsy. This premalignant lesion of the prostate co-exists with cancer in more than 80 percent of cancer cases. Prostatitis and atrophy were also found.

- **Final report.** A final report is issued only after the pathologist is satisfied that the diagnosis is certain. However, if you want a second opinion, your pathologist will send the biopsy slides themselves for review and interpretation, not his or her report.

PATIENT, DOCTOR, AND SPECIMEN INFORMATION

The patient information on a pathology report includes the patient's name, social security number, date of birth, age, and the medical record number issued by the hospital. The PSA level and other information may also be included.

Specimen information includes the date the biopsy was performed and the unique number of the specimen issued in the laboratory. Each specimen is given a number. The number BL03-200005 in Figure 9.1 means that 200,004 other pathology specimens have been analyzed in the hospital's (this hospital is coded as "BL") pathology department during the year (in this case, 2003). At the end of the year, numbering starts again, beginning with BL04-000001.

GROSS DESCRIPTION

The pathologist first examines the biopsy specimen without a microscope. The appearance of the sample before further processing is called the gross description ("gross" refers to what can be seen without a microscope). The gross description includes the tissue sample's size, color, consistency, and other characteristics. The specimen may even be photographed for documentation (see Figure 9.1).

LOCATION AND MULTICENTRICITY OF CANCER

The urologist usually documents for the pathologist the sites within the prostate from which the biopsy cores were obtained. Often more than one needle core specimen was taken from the same site, and the pathologist reports each specimen separately to provide information about the location and multiple sites of cancer (multicentric cancer), if they exist.

DIAGNOSIS

This section of the report includes information relied upon by your doctor, specifically the final diagnosis, to help in determining appropriate treatment. The diagnosis is determined by the factors listed below.

CANCER TYPE

Based on the origin and histologic appearance (the structure as seen through a microscope), prostate cancer can be classified into the following types: adenocarcinoma, squamous cell carcinoma, transitional cell carcinoma, small cell carcinoma, and other rare types of cancer. See page 6 of chapter 1 for more information. The most common type is adenocarcinoma, which originates in the cells that line the prostate. When we talk about prostate cancer, usually we are referring to adenocarcinoma. (Figure 9.1 is a biopsy report showing adenocarcinoma.)

CANCER GRADE

The cancer grade is a measure that indicates how aggressive the cancer is likely to be based on what usually happens with cells that look like yours. The Gleason grading system used to establish prostate cancer grades is based on the microscopic appearance of cancer cells present in your prostate biopsy (see page 70).

A Gleason *grade* ranges from 1 to 5 based on how much cancer cells look like normal prostate cells. Those that look a lot like normal cells are graded as 1, and those that look the least like normal cells are graded as 5. A Gleason *score* or *sum* is helpful when a prostate cancer has areas with different grades. A grade is assigned to each of the two areas that make up most of the cancer. These two grades are added together to give a Gleason score between 2 and 10. The higher the Gleason score, the more likely the cancer is to grow quickly and the more likely it is to spread beyond the prostate. The first area is the most commonly seen grade and the second area is the second most commonly seen grade. The two grades are added to produce a Gleason score of between 2 and 10. Therefore although both a 3 + 4 and a 4 + 3 result in a Gleason score of 7, the 4 + 3 is more aggressive.

The pathologist examines the cancer cells under the microscope, studying the shape and architecture of tumor cells. The extent to which cancer cells resemble normal prostate cells and glands is called differentiation. Cancer that closely resembles normal prostate cells and glands is well differentiated. This tends to be the slowest-growing and least dangerous cancer. Poorly differentiated cancer, in contrast, is often very aggressive and fast-growing. See Figure 9.2 for photos of well differentiated cells and poorly differentiated cells.

Pathologists also report the relative amount of high-grade cancer (Gleason patterns 4 and 5—see Figure 9.2) whenever they are present.

The lower your Gleason score, the better your prognosis is likely to be. But ultimately, your prognosis depends upon several additional factors, including the cancer stage (the extent of spread of tumor within the body), and others.

TUMOR VOLUME

There are several ways of measuring the volume (size) of cancer in needle biopsies, including the number of positive cores and the percentage of biopsy cores affected by cancer. The amount of cancer in the needle biopsy helps predict the volume of tumor in the prostate only for those with a great amount of cancer in multiple needle biopsies. A large amount of cancer indicates a higher likelihood of spread outside the prostate and metastasis to lymph nodes. However, a low tumor presence on a needle biopsy does not reliably predict low-volume tumor in the prostate. Usually if more than 30 percent of biopsy cores show tumor involvement, the tumor is considered high volume, though this criterion is not official.

THE 5 GLEASON GRADES

The Gleason grading system assigns a number from 1 to 5 based on how closely the arrangement of cells in the cancerous tissue resembles normal prostate tissue.

- **Grade 1:** cancer cells look most like normal cells. These are also called well differentiated or low grade. Grade 1 cancer tends to be less aggressive than higher-grade cancers.
- **Grades 2–4:** cancer is more moderately differentiated. The cancer cells may have invaded the surrounding prostate. Prostate cancer is most commonly grade 3.
- **Grade 5:** cancer cells are also called undifferentiated or high grade and bear no resemblance to normal prostate cells.

GLEASON GRADES

Grade 1: Well-differentiated (very rare)

Grade 2: Well-differentiated

Grade 3: Moderately differentiated

Grade 4: Poorly differentiated

Grade 5: Undifferentiated

TUMOR SPREAD

Biopsies help determine how far prostate cancer has spread, if at all, beyond the prostate. The locations of biopsies containing cancer are listed within the Diagnosis section of the pathology report.

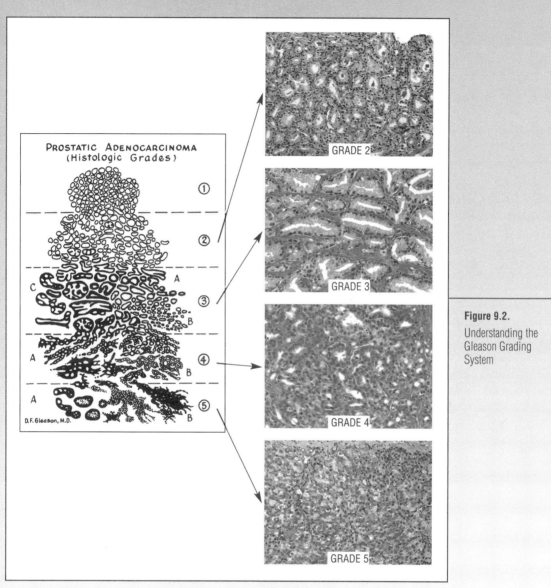

PROSTATIC ADENOCARCINOMA
(Histologic Grades)

D.F. Gleason, M.D.

GRADE 2

GRADE 3

GRADE 4

GRADE 5

Figure 9.2.
Understanding the
Gleason Grading
System

© Dr. David Bostwick, Bostwick Laboratories

Cancer near or in the nerves (perineural invasion). Perineural invasion is the presence of cancer very near or surrounding nerves. Some doctors believe perineural invasion reduces the chance of being cured of cancer after treatment, but not all experts agree with this conclusion.

Questions to Ask Your Doctor About Your Biopsy Report When It Indicates Cancer

- What type of cancer do I have?
- What is the Gleason score of my cancer?
- How many needle biopsies were taken, how many had cancer in them, and how much cancer did they contain?
- Who did the pathologic examination of my biopsies?
- Can you recommend someone who can offer a second opinion?
- Was there any evidence of cancer extending outside of the prostate?
- Where was the cancer within the prostate?
- Did the pathologist provide you with a photograph of the cancer to document its appearance? (The photograph documents the microscopic appearance of prostate cancer and allows the pathologists to show urologists and patients the type of prostate cancer.)
- Was any inflammation, prostatic intraepithelial neoplasia (PIN; possible precancerous cells), or any other condition found in the biopsies?
- Was there any evidence of perineural invasion?
- Should we obtain special studies such as DNA ploidy to further assess the aggressiveness of the cancer?
- Are there any other tests or scans I should consider having?

Cancer spread through the capsule (extraprostatic extension). Extraprostatic extension (cancer that penetrates through the prostatic capsule, or edge), also called capsular invasion, capsular penetration, or capsular perforation, is indicated by cancer invading fatty tissue (this is rare), invading the muscular wall, or growing near the epithelium of the seminal vesicles. Some biopsies target the seminal vesicles to search for evidence of extraprostatic extension. Extraprostatic extension may affect treatment decisions. For example, many physicians would recommend against having a patient with extraprostatic extension undergo surgery to remove the prostate because all the cancer is not likely to be removed during the surgery.

DNA PLOIDY

A tumor is classified as either diploid or aneuploid. The ploidy is a measure of how much DNA (deoxyribonucleic acid, the genetic "blueprint" found in the nucleus of each cell that holds genetic information on cell growth, division, and function) is contained in each cell. Patients with diploid tumors (which contain a normal amount of genetic material, or DNA) have a more favorable outcome than those with aneuploid tumors (which contain an excessive amount of DNA). However, the ploidy pattern of prostate cancer is often mixed.

DNA ploidy is a separate analysis and usually does not appear on the same pathology report unless your doctor orders it. A report of abnormal DNA ploidy analysis will include where the ploidy was performed, how many tumor cells were examined, and the DNA ploidy.

NON-CANCEROUS RESULTS

It is possible that the results of your biopsy as reported in your pathology report will reveal a diagnosis other than prostate cancer. We'll discuss that possibility in chapter 10.

CHAPTER 10

WHEN ARE SUSPICIOUS RESULTS NOT A DIAGNOSIS OF PROSTATE CANCER?

David G. Bostwick, MD, MBA

AS EXPLAINED IN CHAPTER 3, A RANGE OF urinary and other symptoms can cause a man to visit his doctor. Often, fortunately, men are examined and determined to have benign (noncancerous) conditions. The two most common prostate conditions, benign prostatic hyperplasia (BPH) and prostatitis, may cause symptoms (such as urinary problems) men fear are due to prostate cancer. But the symptoms are rarely caused by prostate cancer and by themselves do not increase the risk of developing prostate cancer. Prostatitis, BPH, and atrophy (conditions we'll discuss later in this chapter) are not associated with an increased risk of prostate cancer. High-grade prostatic intraepithelial neoplasia (PIN), the most likely precursor of prostate cancer, is a risk factor for cancer.

However, sometimes screening and other tests result in a misdiagnosis of prostate cancer. The process of accurately diagnosing prostate cancer can be tricky. (This is a reason why second opinions—having your biopsy slides reread—are so valuable for men diagnosed with prostate cancer; see chapter 12.) For example, the PSA test is valuable in indicating that a problem might exist and require additional testing. But because both benign and malignant conditions may cause a rise in PSA levels, the PSA test by itself doesn't show whether cancer is present or absent. It is also possible that rare microscopic findings may be mistaken for prostate cancer, including normal parts of the anatomy, such as the seminal vesicles (glands at the base of the bladder that release fluid into the semen during orgasm), as well as a wide variety of other prostate changes. And other prostate conditions may look like prostate cancer under a microscope and may be mistakenly identified as cancer; this is what is referred to as a "false positive" result.

Suspicious (Benign) Test Results

BENIGN PROSTATIC HYPERPLASIA (BPH)

Benign prostatic hyperplasia (BPH) is the noncancerous enlargement of the prostate (see chapter 3 for more information). Like prostate cancer, BPH may cause the prostate-specific antigen (PSA) level in the blood to rise. BPH may be diagnosed after a man reports symptoms such as weak urination, difficulty urinating, or an inability to urinate, or because of a rise in his PSA. Because a larger percentage of PSA tends to circulate in the "free" or unbound form when due to BPH than when due to prostate cancer (see chapter 6 for more information), doctors may be able to differentiate BPH from prostate cancer through more specific PSA testing. We are not sure what causes BPH to develop. Symptoms can be monitored and treated with medications or surgery if necessary.

PROSTATITIS

Like BPH, a diagnosis of prostatitis is usually made when a man has frequent urination, urgent urination, and discomfort in the prostate area. Most men have areas of mild inflammation, or swelling, in their prostate glands. However, when the inflammation is severe, is extensive, or causes a rise in PSA, it is referred to as prostatitis. (The suffix "itis" indicates an inflammatory condition; "arthritis" is inflammation of the joints, for example.) There is a wide spectrum of prostatitis, much of which is rare and poorly understood.

Further testing, such as cultures of urine and any prostatic secretions, may allow for diagnosis. Prostatitis may be caused by bacteria or other infections, tissue disruption after a biopsy, or other factors. The cause of some types of prostatitis is not known. (Antibiotics help treat some types of prostatitis. Other potential treatments include medications and sitz baths, which involve sitting in warm water.)

SEVERE PROSTATITIS

Severe prostatitis disrupts the microscopic architecture of the prostate, making interpretation difficult for a pathologist. Rarely, severe prostatitis is incorrectly diagnosed as high-grade prostate cancer. Pathologists may use special stains, such as prostate-specific antigen (PSA) and prostatic acid phosphatase (PAP), when examining severe prostatitis under the microscope to differentiate between cases of prostatitis and cancer.

PROSTATIC INTRAEPITHELIAL NEOPLASIA (PIN)

Prostatic intraepithelial neoplasia (PIN; see chapter 2 for more information) is a diagnosis made by a pathologist when a biopsy shows certain changes in the microscopic appearance (for example, size and shape) of prostate gland cells. These changes are classified as either low grade, meaning they appear almost normal, or high grade, meaning they look abnormal.

PIN does not cause symptoms or elevate PSA. The condition begins to appear in men in their twenties, and almost half of all men have PIN by the time they reach age 50.

PIN is sometimes misinterpreted as prostate cancer. It is not a cancerous condition, but a man who has had high-grade PIN diagnosed through a prostate biopsy has a 30- to 50-percent chance of also being diagnosed with prostate cancer at some point. Therefore men diagnosed with high-grade PIN are watched carefully and often have repeat prostate biopsies.

ATROPHY

Atrophy, or gradual cell damage, becomes more common and more extensive with age, particularly after the age of 40. With the help of a microscope, atrophy can be seen in portions of healthy men's prostates. (More extensive atrophy can also be seen in the prostates of men who have had hormone therapy or radiation.) A pathologist may confuse atrophy with cancer.

OTHER CANCERS

It is also possible to mistakenly identify one type of cancer as another. Cancer that has spread to the prostate from nearby areas, such as bladder cancer, may be mistakenly diagnosed as prostate cancer if first noticed in the prostate.

AFTER THE DIAGNOSIS:
WHAT NOW?

A DIAGNOSIS OF CANCER BRINGS WITH IT A VARIETY OF challenges—not only physical challenges, but practical and emotional ones too.

For example, you may be facing challenges such as choosing a doctor and a treatment center, maintaining medical records, shifting work duties and schedules, keeping up with insurance requirements, and planning for financial needs. Don't let these matters overwhelm you. The chapters in this section can help.

The following chapters also explore how to cope with the emotions you may be feeling right now, how you may be able to build the support network you need, and how to communicate with others.

This portion of the book contains a special section *written especially for family, friends, and caregivers* that provides practical advice and tips on coping with the situation and helping you get through it.

Explore Ways of Coping and Building Support

A diagnosis of cancer brings with it a variety of challenges— not only physical challenges, but practical and emotional ones too.

CHAPTER 11

COPING WITH YOUR DIAGNOSIS AND MOVING FORWARD

Christian J. Nelson, PhD
Stan Rosenfeld
Andrew J. Roth, MD

AFTER YOUR DOCTOR TOLD YOU THAT YOU HAD PROSTATE CANCER, among the first thoughts that crossed your mind may have been *Why did this happen to me?* and *This isn't fair.* You might have also wondered, *Is this a mistake? Will I die? How will my family handle this?* You may have worried about how prostate cancer could affect your life and your future.

You are not alone. In the United States, 1 man in 6 will be diagnosed with prostate cancer during his lifetime, so you're part of a group of hundreds of thousands of men coping with prostate cancer. (See *Finding Support* on page 84 for information about groups that get together to talk and learn about prostate cancer issues.)

In this chapter we'll explore ways to cope with your feelings about diagnosis and treatment, and how to equip yourself with the knowledge you need to face the future.

Coping With Feelings About Cancer

It's normal to feel angry, anxious, confused, depressed, or numb. You may also feel a sense of grief or a loss of control after a cancer diagnosis. You may waver between these feelings from one moment to the next.

Men cope in different ways. Some men face their diagnoses head on. They may plow forward and make decisions without becoming distracted by fears of what might happen. Other men may feel overwhelmed or generally negative. Many men find that their outlook and ability to cope fluctuate. The way one man

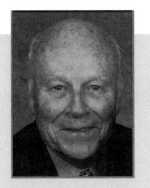

Coping With Emotions

Although it's difficult, try to retain your sense of humor. My wife and I tried to laugh even during the "not so good" days. When the doctor asked me to come in for an "autopsy" I declined and told him it sounded too final. I asked him if he would come in for an autopsy if he was in my shoes and I suggested a biopsy instead. We both had a good laugh.

— *Harry*

While from the outside I appeared to be a very upbeat person, to the point that my coworkers could hardly believe I was going through cancer treatments, inside I was angry. I was mad at the cancer, mad at the doctors for doing this to me. I didn't communicate well with my wife and was experiencing symptoms of depression while I was at home. I was also angry about my sexual situation.

— *Kent*

copes may not work for someone else. *There is no "right" way to cope with cancer.* In time, you will discover the best way for *you* to deal with your diagnosis. It may be helpful to try different coping strategies (some examples are given below and explained in more detail throughout this chapter) to find out which ones might be helpful for you:

- Express emotions and concerns.
- Maintain a balanced emotional response.
- Become informed and participate in decisions.
- Reach out for support.
- Try to find new appreciation for different elements of your life.

TALKING ABOUT EMOTIONS

Some men may want to talk to close friends or family members about their diagnoses and how they feel. Others may feel uncomfortable expressing their emotions. Some may be reluctant to share worries or concerns with people they care about because they want to protect them. This can make prostate cancer a lonely experience, even if you are surrounded by friends and family. Talking with loved ones and close friends about your cancer may help you deal with the wide variety of emotions cancer can introduce.

You can also talk with members of your health care team about how you feel. If you are interested, they may be even able to suggest a counselor who has experience in helping people with cancer sort out and come to terms with troubling feelings and concerns. Support and education groups can help as well (see page 84).

WHY DO I FEEL DEPRESSED?

It is normal to feel sad when you are faced with a cancer diagnosis. You may be feeling unsure about what the future holds and may feel hopeless. Many men find that these feelings resolve over time as they make treatment decisions and undergo the treatment they select.

It may be especially difficult to try to feel positive now, when you are experiencing natural and sometimes uncomfortable emotional reactions to the stress of your diagnosis. But throughout your decision-making and treatment processes, you will likely be able to appreciate and experience positive life experiences without ignoring the sadness or anxiety you may feel about having cancer.

Emotional distress that lasts for weeks to months and interferes with your ability to concentrate, function socially or at work, or with your ability to experience pleasure may not be temporary blues about your diagnosis; it may be clinical depression. Other signs of clinical depression include:

- persistent sad or "empty" mood almost every day for most of the day
- loss of interest or pleasure in ordinary activities
- eating disturbances (loss of appetite or overeating), or significant weight loss or gain
- sleep disturbances (inability to sleep, early waking, or oversleeping)
- noticeable restlessness or being "slowed down" almost every day
- decreased energy or fatigue almost every day
- feelings of guilt, worthlessness, and helplessness
- difficulty concentrating, remembering, making decisions
- thoughts of death or suicide or attempts at suicide

If you think you may be experiencing clinical depression, talk with your doctor or another health care professional. *If you are considering suicide, seek help immediately.* There are many effective medications and non-drug ways to treat depression. You are not alone; as many as 1 in 4 people diagnosed with cancer experience clinical depression.

WHY AM I ANXIOUS?

Worry and anxiety are common reactions to a prostate cancer diagnosis. You may worry about selecting the best treatment or feel anxious about coping with potential complications of treatment. For example, you may be worried about the sexual side effects of the treatment or what impact treatment might have on urinary functioning.

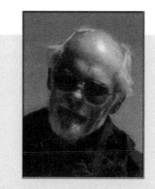

Coping With Emotions

My wife and I advise designating "cancer-free" days when the patient and his loved ones are not allowed to talk about cancer, make phone calls related to cancer, research cancer, or otherwise focus on the subject.

– *Will*

Four days after my diagnosis I wrote my first poem about my experience. Writing poems helped me record what I learned and, importantly, helped me keep my attitude positive. After a while, I showed a few of them to friends. Then I showed them to a man who had been recently diagnosed with prostate cancer. He said he found them helpful in sorting through some of the questions and feelings he himself had had about prostate cancer. He was reading articles and books by doctors who took a factual and technical approach. He also wanted to read what a fellow patient had to say.

– *Tom*

Some men may focus on their prostate-specific antigen (PSA) test results after treatment and consider them markers of life or death rather than helpful guides to help identify potential problems and deal with them promptly. They may worry so much about what will happen with their cancer that they stop enjoying life or finding meaning in their lives.

Some men become anxious about medical procedures or treatment side effects. Medications such as steroids or hormonal agents can cause anxiety or depression to become more severe. Severe anxiety can hold you back from dealing with your illness and may get in the way of properly treating the disease.

It is important to let your doctor know if you feel unusual anxiety or irritability, or if you are having difficulty sleeping. Counseling and/or medication may help you feel more comfortable.

FINDING SUPPORT

Although your loved ones may provide invaluable support, they may not be able to completely relate to your experience. Support groups for men with prostate cancer allow men to talk with others who are going through a similar range of emotions, curiosity, and learning. It may be easier for you to talk about issues like impotence, urinary function, and cancer recurrence with men who have similar concerns. Support group members may also have ideas about ways to discuss these same subjects with your loved ones or health care providers.

Groups are different. They offer varied levels of involvement and avenues for finding information and support. Groups meet in person or share thoughts and questions online. You might visit several groups before determining whether support groups are right for you and if so, which one you prefer.

Reaching Out to Others

I began facilitating a Man to Man support group when my father was diagnosed with cancer. His cancer recurred and he passed away after multiple treatments, but through the support group I learned how generous men are in sharing their experiences and reaching out to others.

— *Morris*

The American Cancer Society's Man to Man program helps men cope with prostate cancer by offering education and support for men and their family members. A core component of the program is the self-help and/or support group. Volunteers organize free weekly, bi-monthly, and monthly meetings where speakers and participants learn about and discuss information about prostate cancer, treatment, side effects, and how to cope with prostate cancer and its treatment. Many Man to Man groups invite wives and partners to attend meetings. In other locations, wives and partners may meet separately in a group setting called Side by Side. For more information about Man to Man or to locate a program in your area, see the *Resources* section in the back of this book or contact the American Cancer Society (800-ACS-2345; http//:www.cancer.org).

SPECIAL POPULATIONS: AFRICAN-AMERICAN MEN AND YOUNGER MEN

All men diagnosed with prostate cancer face challenges. However, younger men and African-American men from diverse backgrounds facing prostate cancer may find themselves coping with additional obstacles.

AFRICAN-AMERICAN MEN

African Americans are affected by prostate cancer more often than men of other races in the United States (see page 15). Researchers are looking into the causes of this disparity, and experts are reaching out to try to prevent and detect prostate cancer early in this group of men. The American Cancer Society recommends that African-American men begin testing at age 45.

Let's Talk About It (LTAI) is a free community-based program developed by the American Cancer Society and 100 Black Men of America to increase awareness and knowledge of prostate cancer among African-American men. Contact the American Cancer Society for more information (800-ACS-2345 or http://www.cancer.org).

YOUNGER MEN

While men who develop prostate cancer at young ages share some concerns with men diagnosed at older ages, such as survival, treatment decisions, and body image, they also have unique concerns. They tend to be more concerned about potency and fertility than men in their 60s and older, and they may need more information about juggling work and family responsibilities and dealing with financial burdens caused by cancer.

If you are a young man diagnosed with prostate cancer, you may want to ask your health care team about support groups that specifically address these concerns. Contact the American Cancer Society for information about Man to Man prostate cancer support groups near you.

Moving Forward

The time between diagnosis and the beginning of treatment can be confusing and quite stressful. With a new diagnosis of prostate cancer you may feel shaken; you may view your health and your expectations or dreams for your future differently from before. Acknowledging your emotions, recognizing that they are normal, and focusing on the things that add meaning to your life may help reduce the intensity and length of any sadness, anger, or despair you may feel and may help you cope with your prostate cancer.

The remainder of this chapter is designed to help you move forward and begin to manage your emotional reactions to cancer and treatment. In the next chapter we'll discuss some of the practical aspects of the learning process: interviewing doctors, asking questions, and getting second opinions.

TAKE CARE OF YOURSELF

Stress and anxiety were part of your life before you had cancer, and having a healthy, optimistic outlook may have helped you cope with stress and upsetting situations. However, no studies have shown that a more positive outlook affects the biology of a cancer in a positive or negative way. Your prostate cancer isn't affected by your personality or attitude. But your quality of life is. Cultivating a constructive and positive attitude when feasible may help you cope with the challenges you're facing.

Sometimes taking care of yourself means finding things other than thoughts of cancer to occupy your time and attention. Even if you discover you can't do things the way you always have because of treatment side effects, don't simply eliminate the enjoyable activities from your life. If you can't exercise as much or as hard as you did in the past, or if you feel you are too busy with doctor's visits to schedule the activities you used to love doing, consider fitting in fewer or shorter "dates" to do the things you enjoy.

Choosing a doctor you can trust, following his or her directions as best you can, making good lifestyle choices such as quitting smoking, drinking alcohol only in moderation, exercising, and eating healthfully can all make you feel better overall and provide you with a greater sense of control over your body and life.

TAKE YOUR TIME

It is okay to take the time you need to adjust and become educated about your situation and your options before heading into treatment. Most prostate cancers grow slowly, and experts generally agree that in most cases, taking time to get a second opinion or make decisions about treatment does not create dangerous delays.

Many treatment options exist for prostate cancer, each with potential benefits and risks. Treatment decisions are personal; only you can make them. Your personal preferences and needs and the importance you place on lifestyle choices and treatment's effects on them cannot be dictated by your doctor. Most men want to be able to look back on their treatment and know that they made the most informed decisions possible and chose what felt right for them.

You have time—time to cope with your emotions, time to educate yourself about this disease, time to talk to others who have been through it, time to explore your treatment options, time to organize your thoughts, and time to find the right medical team for you.

EDUCATE YOURSELF

Congratulate yourself for what you're doing right now, because the more you learn about prostate cancer, the better your understanding of possible treatment options will be. Gaining a better understanding of prostate cancer and its treatment is helpful for many men. Arming yourself with information may allow you to feel more in control, and exploring your options and seeking out information will help you become a constructive partner in the treatment and care process.

Every man's situation and cancer is different, and there are no absolute answers or guarantees. Doctors may be able to generalize about how men in situations similar to yours reacted to treatment, for example, but no one can predict the outcome for an individual.

Consider your typical response to new information. Would knowing more about your cancer help you understand and deal with it, or would it overwhelm you? Some men want to participate fully in treatment decisions and understand every detail of their cancer. They may feel empowered by collecting information and learning about cancer and treatment. Others are more comfortable simply following their doctors' instructions; they may become stressed and confused when faced with too much information. Try to understand what your needs and limits are. You may find it helpful to allow yourself a finite period of information gathering to see how much is enough; if you find that you become more anxious as you face more details, give yourself permission to stop searching.

Ask your health care team about resources that may have been helpful to other men with prostate cancer. If you feel overwhelmed by the amount of information available, you may want to ask a family member or a friend to help you digest it before you approach your health care team with questions and concerns. Support groups can also help you assimilate the information you have obtained.

For a comprehensive list of cancer information sources, see to the *Resources* section in the back of this book.

DECIDE WHO TO TELL

You may not be ready or may not want to tell friends, other family members, or coworkers about your cancer. Or you may want to let family or friends know that you appreciate their concern and let them know how they can help. People who care about you will want to support you. It may be helpful to think through how you'll share your diagnosis with others when you're comfortable doing so. See chapter 13 for more information on talking to friends, family members, and children about your cancer.

CHAPTER 12

MAKING THE MEDICAL SYSTEM WORK FOR YOU

Katherine C. Meade

PROSTATE CANCER AND ITS TREATMENT involve many personal issues. Your priorities are the most important factors to consider during the decision-making progress. The cancer is in *your* body, and you need to be comfortable with the treatment decisions you make. Which are most important to you: An extended life? Lowering the risk of long-term side effects? Not having your routine interrupted?

A qualified and supportive medical team can help you throughout treatment and recovery. In this chapter we'll explore how you can play an active and valuable role in forming this health care team and in making decisions about your treatment and care.

Becoming Part of Your Medical Team

The medical professionals and support personnel who will coordinate and provide your care will guide your treatment, be in charge of any procedures you receive, and help you make decisions. It is important to find doctors you trust and feel comfortable with to help you manage your cancer. Your health care team members should allow you to be active in treatment decisions if you would like to be.

THE MEMBERS OF YOUR MEDICAL TEAM
AND WHAT THEY DO

Your health care team will be made up of several people, each with different expertise to contribute to your care. One of your cancer care team members will take the lead in coordinating your care. Most prostate cancer patients initially choose a urologist to lead the team (see page 92). Later if a man chooses radiation as his primary treatment, he may transfer his care to the radiation oncologist. It should be clear to all team members who is in charge, and that person should inform the others of your progress. This alphabetical list will acquaint you with the health care professionals you may encounter, depending on which treatment option and follow-up path you choose, and their areas of expertise:

ANESTHESIOLOGIST

An anesthesiologist is a medical doctor who administers anesthesia (drugs or gases) to make you sleep and be unconscious or to prevent or relieve pain during and after a surgical procedure.

DIETITIAN

A dietitian is specially trained to help you make healthy diet choices before, during, and after treatment. A registered dietitian (RD) has at least a bachelor's degree and has passed a national competency exam.

MEDICAL ONCOLOGIST

A medical oncologist (also sometimes simply called an oncologist) is a medical doctor you may see after diagnosis. The oncologist is a cancer expert who understands specific types of cancer, their treatments, and their causes. He or she may help people with cancer make decisions about a course of treatment. Oncologists most often become involved when you need chemotherapy, but can also prescribe hormonal therapy and other anticancer drugs.

NURSES

During your treatment you will be in contact with different types of nurses.

Registered nurse. A registered nurse has an associate or bachelor's degree in nursing and has passed a state licensing exam. She or he can monitor your condition, provide treatment, educate you about side effects, and help you adjust to prostate cancer physically and emotionally.

Nurse practitioner. A nurse practitioner is a registered nurse with a master's or doctoral degree who can manage prostate cancer care and has additional training in primary care. He or she shares many tasks with your doctors, such as recording your medical history, conducting physical exams, and doing follow-up care. In most states, a nurse practitioner can prescribe medicines with a doctor's supervision.

Clinical nurse specialist. A clinical nurse specialist (CNS) is a nurse who has a master's degree in a specific area, such as oncology, psychiatry, or critical care nursing. The CNS often provides expertise to staff and may provide special services to patients, such as leading support groups.

Oncology-certified nurse. An oncology-certified nurse is a clinical nurse who has demonstrated an in-depth knowledge of oncology care. He or she has passed a certification exam. Oncology-certified nurses are found in all areas of cancer practice.

PATHOLOGIST

A pathologist is a medical doctor specially trained in diagnosing disease based on the examination of microscopic tissue and fluid samples. He or she will determine the classification (cell type) of your cancer, help determine the stage (extent) and grade (estimate of aggressiveness) of your cancer, and issue a pathology report so that you and your doctor can decide on treatment options. (See page 68 of chapter 9 for more information about cancer grades.)

PERSONAL OR PRIMARY CARE PHYSICIAN

A personal physician may be a general doctor, internist, or family practice doctor. He or she is often the medical doctor who may have performed your initial PSA tests and DREs or who may have discovered signs of prostate cancer. This general or family practice doctor may be a member of your medical team, but a specialist in prostate cancer is most often a patient's cancer care team leader.

PSYCHOLOGIST OR PSYCHIATRIST

A psychologist is a licensed mental health professional who is often part of the medical team. He or she provides counseling on emotional and psychological issues. A psychologist may have specialized training and experience treating people with cancer.

A psychiatrist is a medical doctor specializing in mental health and behavioral disorders. Psychiatrists provide counseling and can also prescribe medications.

RADIATION ONCOLOGIST

A radiation oncologist is a medical doctor who specializes in treating cancer using therapeutic radiation (high-energy x-rays or seeds). If you choose radiation, this member of your medical team evaluates you frequently during the course of treatment and at intervals afterward. The radiation oncologist will usually work closely with your urologist. He or she helps you make decisions about radiation therapy options. A radiation oncologist is assisted by a radiation therapist (see next page) during treatment and works with a radiation physicist, an expert who is trained in ensuring that the right dose of radiation treatment is delivered to you.

The physicist is also assisted by a dosimetrist, a technician who helps plan and calculate the dosage, number, and length of your radiation treatments.

RADIATION THERAPIST

A radiation therapist is a specially trained technician who works with the equipment that delivers radiation therapy. He or she positions your body during the treatment and administers the radiation therapy.

RADIOLOGIST

A radiologist is a medical doctor specializing in the use of imaging procedures (for example, diagnostic x-rays, ultrasound, magnetic resonance images, bone scans, and others; see chapter 15) that produce pictures of internal body structures. He or she has special training in diagnosing prostate cancer and other diseases and interpreting the results of imaging procedures. Your radiologist issues a radiology report describing the findings to your urologist, medical oncologist, or radiation oncologist. The radiology images and report may be used to aid in diagnosis, to help classify and determine the extent of your prostate cancer, to help locate tumors during surgery and radiation treatment, or to look for the possible spread or recurrence of the cancer after treatment.

RADIOLOGY TECHNOLOGIST

A radiology technologist is a trained health care professional who assists the radiologist by positioning your body for x-rays and other procedures and developing and checking the images for quality. The radiologist then reads these images.

SOCIAL WORKER

A social worker is a health specialist, usually with a master's degree, who is usually licensed or certified by the state in which he or she works. A social worker is an expert in coordinating and providing social services. He or she is trained to help you and your family deal with a range of emotional and practical challenges, such as finances, child care, emotional issues, family concerns and relationships, transportation, and problems with the health care system. If your social worker is trained in cancer-related problems, he or she can counsel you about your fears or concerns, help answer questions about diagnosis and treatment, and lead cancer support groups. You may communicate with your social worker during a hospital stay or on an outpatient basis.

UROLOGIST

A urologist is a physician who has specialized knowledge and skill regarding problems of the urinary tract and male reproductive organs. Seek out a urologist who specializes in urologic oncology, specifically of the prostate. Some urologists

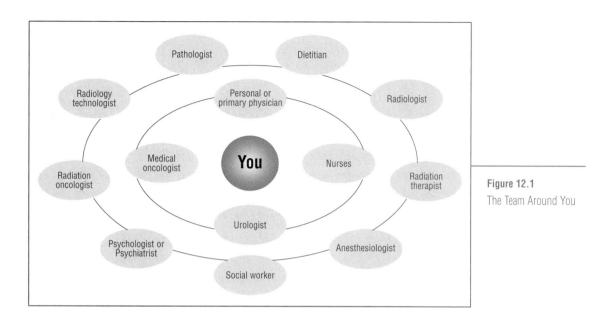

Figure 12.1
The Team Around You

focus on using diagnostic procedures to determine the location or extent of your prostate cancer. Others may specialize in surgery to remove tumors and, if necessary, surrounding tissue. Your urologist will work closely with surgical nurses, your anesthesiologist, medical oncologist (if part of your team), and radiation oncologist. He or she will issue a surgical report.

Choosing a Doctor

Choosing a doctor with excellent skills who you are comfortable with is essential. Your doctor's skill is important. But your doctor is not just a technical expert; he or she is also an ally. Keep in mind that your relationship with your doctor may extend for years after your treatment if he or she provides you with regular follow-up care.

A variety of treatments exist for prostate cancer, so it's a good idea to seek the opinion of doctors who specialize in different treatments before deciding upon one. At a minimum, you may want to speak to a urologist, a radiation oncologist, and possibly a medical oncologist who specializes in prostate cancer before deciding which type of treatment to undergo.

Medical doctors doing research have usually published their findings in medical journals, so you might ask for copies of articles to learn about a doctor's philosophy and approach.

Several organizations can help you locate prostate cancer specialists, including the American Cancer Society, the National Cancer Institute, the American College of Surgeons, and the Association of Community Cancer Centers (refer to the *Resources* section in the back of this book for contact information).

In this section we explore various factors to consider as you choose the members of your health care team.

TYPES OF PRACTICES

A solo practice means that patients see the same doctor on each visit, which provides continuity. A group practice, on the other hand, may offer more resources, expertise, and availability of care.

AFFILIATIONS

Because doctors can send patients only to those facilities where they have admitting privileges, people seeking treatment should know where doctors are affiliated—meaning the hospitals and/or institutions where patients will go for surgery or other care.

A teaching affiliation, especially with a respected medical school, may indicate that the doctor is a respected leader in the field. Academic physicians who maintain practices are often in close touch with experts around the country and are usually well versed in the latest therapies. But they may also spend more time teaching or conducting research than other doctors.

BOARD CERTIFICATION

Board certification means that a doctor has been trained and has taken certification exams in a specialty area. Fellows are doctors with years of specialty training who are eligible for board certification but are gaining additional training and experience in a subspecialty.

The American Board of Medical Specialties (ABMS) maintains a list of all board-certified doctors. If the doctor subscribes to the ABMS service, you can obtain information about his or her certification status and a list of certified specialists by geographic area. You can also look up specialists in *The Official American Board of Medical Specialties (ABMS) Directory of Board Certified Medical Specialists* (carried by some libraries; call 866-ASK-ABMS or visit the American Board of Medical Specialties web site at http://www.abms.org).

RECOMMENDATIONS

Friends, members of your place of worship, participants in support groups, and coworkers may offer recommendations about doctors. You may also want to call the better hospitals in your area for a list of prostate cancer specialists. Once you have identified the specialist you would like to see, don't be surprised if it takes several weeks to get an appointment. Remember, you have time to choose the right doctor. Finding someone with an excellent reputation is more than likely worth the research and the wait.

Several organizations, including the National Cancer Institute, American Urological Association, and American College of Surgeons (ACoS) Commission on Cancer, offer physician directories. See the *Resources* section of this book for more information.

Choosing a Treatment Center

The process of evaluating a treatment center is related to your search for a doctor and a treatment team, so only general guidelines are included again here.

COMPREHENSIVE CANCER CENTERS

You might want to seek treatment at a National Cancer Institute-approved comprehensive cancer center, especially if your cancer is considered a particularly complex case. Before attaining recognition from NCI as a comprehensive cancer center, an institution must meet high standards and pass a thorough review. Comprehensive cancer centers conduct programs in basic research, clinical research, and prevention and control research, and offer outreach and educational programs for people in the community and health care professionals. There are more than 30 comprehensive cancer centers in the United States; all of them see patients. (Contact the NCI at 800-422-6237 or look within the Cancer Centers list at http://www3.cancer.gov/cancercenters/centerslist.html for more information.)

THE COMMISSION ON CANCER OF THE AMERICAN COLLEGE OF SURGEONS' APPROVAL

To determine the quality of cancer care at a treatment setting, ask whether the Commission on Cancer of the American College of Surgeons has approved the cancer diagnosis and treatment program offered there. If it has, you'll know that it meets stringent standards and offers total cancer care, including lifetime follow up. You will also know that whether you receive your treatment in a large internationally known facility or a small local setting, the facility's ability to deliver quality cancer care is under close scrutiny. (Call 312-202-5085 or view the list at http://web.facs.org/cpm/default.htm for more information.)

Evaluating Doctors' Practices

When evaluating a doctor's practice, you may want to consider some of the issues below. You can find this information by talking with doctors, nurses, and other patients.

- Appointments should be easy to make.
- The office environment should be clean, comfortable, and convey a sense of both efficiency and concern.
- The doctor's staff should treat you courteously and respectfully.
- Waiting times should not be excessive.
- Examinations and conversations should take place in private and should not be rushed.
- Your doctor should be open to the contributions of other health professionals, such as physicians in other specialties, social workers, nurses, home care providers, or dietitians. He or she should be willing to make referrals.
- The doctor, nurses, and other assistants should take time to answer your questions and to provide instruction and education as needed.
- Phone calls should be returned quickly.
- The results of lab tests or other diagnostic procedures should be reported promptly and copies mailed, if requested.

QUESTIONS TO ASK WHEN CHOOSING A DOCTOR AND A HOSPITAL

Before committing yourself to a doctor's care, first determine that he or she is qualified and able to deliver the type of care you require. You may want to ask questions about experience, affiliations, and other issues that might impact your care.

Experience and Training

- Are you board certified?
- How long have you been in practice?
- What is your specialty? Do you have a subspecialty?
- What training have you had in treating prostate cancer?

- How many men have you treated for prostate cancer?
- How many men have you treated in the past year?
- What treatments have you used? What have the results been?
- How many times a month do you perform the procedure you are recommending?
- How many patients are you currently treating or following up with?
- What percentage of your patients have prostate cancer?

Office Visits and Care

- What can I expect from office visits?
- May I tape record our conversations so I can review the details later?
- May I bring a friend or family member to my appointments to take notes?
- What are your office hours? Can you be contacted outside those hours? How?
- Who sees your patients when you are on vacation?
- Are you or others in your practice involved in clinical trials of new treatments?

Affiliations and Referrals

- Which hospitals are you affiliated with?
- Which hospital do you prefer to admit your cancer patients to? Why?
- What other types of doctors will be on my care team? Could you tell me the names of any specialists I should see? Will you handle the referrals to these specialists?
- Can you suggest a prostate cancer expert who can offer me a second opinion?

Communication and Records

- Who on my cancer care team should I consider my main contact, and how do I get in touch with that person if I have questions or concerns?
- Is this person available to talk with my family about their concerns?
- May I receive copies of correspondence, tests, and reports?

AFFILIATED DOCTORS

The easiest way to informally assess a quality hospital is to determine which well-respected doctors work there—good doctors are seldom affiliated with substandard hospitals. After you have selected skilled doctors whom you trust and respect, the choice of a hospital usually follows automatically. Probably the simplest way to evaluate a hospital is to ask doctors in the community what they think of it.

ACCREDITATION

At the very least, a quality hospital is accredited by the Joint Commission on Accreditation of Healthcare Organizations. Accredited hospitals are listed in the *American Hospital Association Guide to the Health Care Field*, found in many public libraries. Surprisingly, about 1 hospital in 4 fails to earn accreditation. The extent and variety of services available in a facility is a key measure. The best hospitals offer:

- a postoperative recovery room
- an intensive care unit
- anesthesiologists
- a pathology lab, diagnostic lab, and blood bank
- round-the-clock staffing
- a tumor board (a group of medical professionals who meet and collaborate on patients' diagnoses and treatment)
- social work services
- respiratory therapies, physical therapists, and rehabilitation services
- advanced diagnostic and therapeutic equipment (for example, CT scans and radiation therapy)

Getting a Second Opinion

Because different prostate cancer treatments are performed by doctors with different specialties, you should consider getting second opinions from physicians who perform each of the treatment options you are potentially interested in receiving. Many people also get a second pathology reading by a pathologist who specializes in reading prostate cancer biopsies (see chapter 7 for more information about biopsies).

Asking your doctor to refer you to another doctor for a second opinion doesn't indicate that you don't respect his or her diagnosis and recommendations. Most doctors are accustomed to this request. Your body and your life are going to be affected by your choice of treatment, and it's understandable that you'd want to have confirmation about the diagnosis and care plan. Your doctor wants you to receive the most accurate diagnosis and valuable treatment possible. He or she may help arrange an appointment with another specialist. Your health insurance company will often pay for additional opinions (although you should always check with a representative beforehand to be sure).

If you seek a second opinion of your pathology report, ask your pathologist for your slides. Then take or send the slides to the pathologist who will provide the second opinion.

Designating Your Personal Advocate

It may be exhausting to handle all aspects of your medical treatment alone. You may want to consider choosing an advocate—someone who can help you through the process by asking questions or taking notes during doctor's visits or even by helping you make appointments or cope with financial or other issues. Choose someone you trust and who also listens well and will be available when you need help. Discuss your needs with this person and think of him or her as a partner accompanying you on your prostate cancer journey.

Although you may want to choose a family member as your personal advocate, keep in mind that relatives may sometimes become too emotionally involved to objectively represent your concerns. If your family member has difficulty dealing with medical issues, you may be able to find an effective advocate in your circle of friends, a member of your place of worship, or a person involved in a prostate cancer support organization.

Whomever you choose, be sure your personal advocate understands that ultimately only you can decide your treatment and recovery path.

> **Caregiver Advocates**
>
> Caregivers and loved ones should try to go to the doctor with the patient when discussing treatments and side effects. Going with a patient to a support group is also helpful. Being involved will help everyone understand the situation, how to cope, and what lies ahead.
>
> — Gordon
>
> I served as the advocate for my husband when he was dealing with his cancer. We formed an effective team and the clinicians appreciated that we were both present for all appointments and procedures.
>
> — Nancy

DETERMINE THE AMOUNT OF INFORMATION YOU WANT TO HEAR

Let your personal advocate and members of your medical team know how much information about your cancer and treatment you want to be told directly and how much detail you want. Doctors differ in how much information they give to people with cancer and their families, and people differ in the amount of information they need or want. It is up to you to tell your doctor if he or she is giving you and your advocate too much or too little information. If you would like to have your treatment team keep your advocate or another person informed about your illness and treatment, make sure to let the team know.

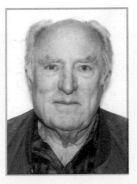

Communicating With Doctors and Asking Essential Questions

Don't simply take the treatment recommendation of the diagnosing doctor. Each man should do his own research, and plenty of it, to understand his options. When consulting doctors, ask them about their success rates, number of procedures performed, and potential side effects.

                                    – Max

Several days prior to your doctor's visit, let him or her know the topics you'd like to discuss and any questions you'd like answered. This offers you the opportunity to think through things that may be on your mind and allows the doctor time to develop responses. My oncologist appreciates the challenge presented by my questions (or at least he says he does!).

                                    – Craig

Communicating With Your Health Care Team

Tell your doctors and caregivers about any concerns you may have so they can help you find a solution. Only you know what you're feeling. Well-intentioned doctors, family members, and friends cannot meet your needs if you do not make them known.

It is okay to be assertive to get the information and care you need. If you don't understand something, ask that it be repeated, rephrased, or explained. You might say, "I'm having trouble grasping what you said—would you mind telling me again, and could you put it another way?" Another useful tactic is to repeat what was said and ask for confirmation: "Let me see if I have it right. You're saying that…" It is the health care professional's job to make you feel comfortable with the information you're getting and to be sure you understand the disease and the treatment options available to you.

Don't feel embarrassed to ask any question on your mind. Prepare a list of questions ahead of time, asking the most important ones first. Let your doctor know if you expect to play an active role in your treatment decisions and if you are researching your options; show him or her that you are an educated patient and that you want him or her to be a supportive partner.

RETAINING INFORMATION

You may want to keep track of the details your medical team provides, both for your own reference and to potentially aid other members of the team. Bringing your personal advocate with you to the doctor's office may not only help you communicate, it may also reduce the stress you would feel when taking in information and making decisions alone.

A large amount of in-depth information about your health and care is exchanged during meetings with members of your treatment team. Processing and documenting this information may be difficult if you are unfamiliar with the terms used or you feel anxious. You might want to write down the name and position of each person on your medical team you deal with and detail the information they share with you. When you can, get information in writing rather than verbally so you can refer to it later.

RECORDING INFORMATION

You or your personal advocate will probably find it helpful to take detailed notes during appointments and phone calls with your health care team. It may be even more helpful to tape-record your appointments with your doctor (with permission) as well as consultations and second-opinion sessions. Tape-recording sessions allows other loved ones to hear accurate details after the fact and prevents calls to the office to have information repeated or reworded, as much of your confusion can likely be cleared up if you review the taped material again. Tape-recording medical conversations can improve a person's ability to understand treatment, especially concerning tests and their results.

TAKING ENOUGH TIME

Of course, it's important to be aware that doctors often have busy schedules and may not be able to spend as much time with you as you'd like, especially if you give them a long list of questions from out of the blue. Arrange for office visits or phone calls that allow adequate time for discussions. Tell your doctor at the beginning of the visit that you have questions. If you still have questions at the end of the visit, say so and schedule another appointment or phone call to address them.

Your doctor should take your questions seriously. He or she should be interested in your concerns and not make you feel rushed. If your doctor does not respond this way, bring it up at your next visit. Feeling informed may help you feel confident about your treatment plan and your doctor. Make sure that your doctor has answered all your concerns and questions, no matter how small. It may take more than one visit to discuss all of your concerns since new questions may come to mind.

> **Records Are Valuable Narratives**
>
> Record basic data during or immediately after each of your contacts with medical professionals or insurance representatives. You can use your records to refresh your memory about details and to tell others what was said, what tests were done, what arrangements were agreed upon, etc. Three years into my treatment I refer to my records occasionally, not only to retrieve facts, but to read the narrative of my ongoing experience. (There are a few things I'd like to forget, but it's all memorable.)
>
> — *Craig*

Participating in Your Medical Care

As you begin treatment, remember that you are an active member of your cancer care team. You can play an active role by talking openly with your medical team, keeping organized records of your medical information, and knowing and understanding your rights as a patient.

Understanding Your Rights as a Patient

According to the American Hospital Association's (AHA) *Patient Care Partnership: Understanding Expectations, Rights and Responsibilities*, you have a right to high-quality health care and a clean and safe environment. You have the right to be involved in your care, including receiving understandable information about diagnosis, treatment, and prognosis, and the opportunity to discuss and make decisions about these things. As a patient, you have the right to: know the identity of those involved in your care, have your privacy protected, have your goals and beliefs taken into account as much as possible, and consent or decline to participate in clinical studies. You have the right to know the immediate and long-term implications of treatment choices, including financial implications, and to receive help with your bill and filing claims. Before leaving the hospital, you should receive information and resources to prepare you for post-hospital care and coping. If you feel that these rights are not being met, bring it to the attention of your health care team.

Maintaining Your Medical Information

From the time you are diagnosed with prostate cancer, you'll be communicating with your medical team and receiving and requesting medical information. Knowing the details of your cancer and treatment can help you deal effectively with your treatment experience.

Some people feel more in control and confident when they have access to details about their care and treatment. Others find tracking such details overwhelming. If you or a loved one is interested in retaining a file of your medical information, you may want to follow some or all of the suggestions here.

Doctors keep a record of key facts about your care to make future decisions about how to treat other illnesses or a recurrence of cancer. Remember that your medical records belong to you.

No one is grading you on how organized your notes are. You'll simply want to have an organizational system that allows you to find answers when you need them. One way to organize your medical information is to create the following sections and organize them in a three-ring binder with dividers or in an accordion file:

1. Ongoing treatment log. You may want to maintain a detailed diary of events and information related to your treatment, listing:

- dates of visits to doctors and the name(s) of the treatment center(s) visited

- the names of those in the office with whom you had contact

- information given to you about your cancer and your care

Note the dates and specific details of all biopsies, procedures, and treatments, for example:

- the results of your biopsies with number of cores (also known as samples or sticks), percentage of cancer in each core, staging, and Gleason score (the report from the pathologist should contain this information)
- any changes in your diet or your exercise regimen
- all diagnostic tests you receive (for example, bone scans, and MRIs) with dates and results
- a surgical pathology report if you choose to have surgery (see chapter 9), with comments from a pathologist about surgical margins, lymph nodes, location and size of cancer, and Gleason score
- if you choose to have radiation, the type of any radiation and the exact location of the radiation treatment field, as well as the total amount of radiation you received
- when treatments began and ended

You can also record your symptoms here. Be specific and quantify as much as possible. Rather than say "I was feeling sick," note details, such as "I ached in my lower back and groin at a level 5 on a pain scale of 1 to 10." Make notes about any problems or side effects you experience.

This portion of your notebook will allow you to answer your doctors' questions about your treatment history and your response to treatment.

2. Medical team member directory. Collect information from your medical team, making sure you know the names, office addresses, phone numbers, fax numbers, and e-mail addresses (if applicable) of all of your doctors, present and past. (Not all doctors use e-mail. If you are interested, you may want to ask for a doctor's e-mail address and policy about communicating with patients this way.) You might use a plastic business card holder to organize the information.

As you meet new members of your medical team, ask them for information and organize it in your file. Copy this information and submit it to your various doctors' offices and treatment centers for your permanent file.

3. Personal information directory. This section should include personal information such as: your date of birth and social security number and those of your partner or spouse, work phone numbers, names and phone numbers of people to call in an emergency, baby sitters, and anyone you may need to contact in a pinch. You should also consider filing details of your medical history here, in case you may need them. See page 104 for a sample.

GEORGE BROWN
Date of Birth: 1/31/42   SSN: 000-00-0001

Allergies: allergic to penicillin
Medical history:
- appendix removed 2/75
- history of high blood pressure
- father had prostate cancer

Prostate cancer diagnosis/treatment:
- 12/1/02 diagnosis; PSA 7, Gleason 7, bone scan negative, Dr. Roger Doyle
- Nerve-sparing radical prostatectomy, Northpoint Hospital, Dr. Jerry Jones, 2/20/03
- Kegel exercises begun 1/19/03
- Catheter removed 3/5/03. Slight dripping but stopped 3/25/03
- Used pump on penis to encourage blood flow 6/1/03
- Morning erection 7/1/03
- PSA 7/31/03 <(less than) .01

CONTACTS:
Joyce Brown (wife)
Date of Birth: 7/2/46   SSN: 000-00-0002
George and Joyce at home: 404-555-1234
George at work: 404-555-3456
Joyce at work: 404-555-6789

George's medical team:
Dr. Roger Doyle, urologist: 404-555-3870
Dr. Michael Short, oncologist: 404-555-1492

Call in an emergency:
Daughter and son-in-law Jenny and Craig Smith at home: 404-555-9068
Craig at work: 404-555-6418
Granddaughter Elizabeth's baby sitter Sarah Long: 404-555-6520

Neighbor:
Frances Clarke at home: 404-555-9962
at work: 404-555-4518

Scout (the dog):
North Avenue Kennel: 404-555-4387

4. Insurance information. File your insurance information in the binder so it will be handy when you need it. In this section, file:

- your insurance policy number and the address and phone number of your insurance company
- the names of those with whom you have had contact at the insurance company
- a copy of your health insurance policy or certificate and your benefit booklet
- copies of materials you received when you enrolled in the insurance plan and updates you've received since then

You need a copy of your actual policy so you'll know which services and treatments are covered. Review your policy carefully. Make sure the information is clear to you. Your insurance agent and benefits director are good sources of information. If you have trouble understanding the information or want confirmation of information, call your state insurance commissioner's office for help.

Keep copies of all correspondence between you and your insurance company and Medicaid or Medicare. Whenever possible, communicate in writing, by fax, or by e-mail so you have a written record. But if you speak to a representative over the phone, jot down:

- the name and title of the person with whom you spoke
- the date and time of the call
- a detailed summary of the conversation. Be aware that many insurance companies record their calls.

Also file:

- bills
- statements
- explanation of benefits (EOB)
- payment records

Include specific information about the procedures, tests, and medicines that were paid for and those that were not.

5. Consultations, letters, and phone calls. Include:

- letters from one doctor to another
- any second-opinion conference summaries you obtain
- a phone call log, including the name and title of the person with whom you spoke, the date and time of the call, and a detailed summary of the conversation

6. Reports. Place in this section:

- the name of the exact kind of cancer you have
- the date you were first diagnosed and dated reports of PSAs, biopsies, x-rays, and bone scans
- operative reports from all surgeries and the pathology reports on tissue

7. Medicines. In this section, list:

- the names of prescribed medicines and dates they were prescribed; be sure to include all medications, including those for other conditions such as high blood pressure, diabetes, or depression

- notes about when you are supposed to take them and doses (also note any doses you miss)
- what the medicines are meant to do
- any side effects or other symptoms that should be monitored
- any problems you should report immediately, and to whom
- any vitamins, herbs, or over-the-counter medicines you are taking

8. Calendar. A calendar showing a year on a single page allows you to see at a glance the overall progress of your treatment. It also shows you the larger picture—for example, when your surgery, radiation, and/or hormone treatments are—and it allows you to schedule vacations, business trips, and other obligations between treatments.

9. Follow up. In this section, include all recommendations from your medical team about checkups, tests that should be done at checkups, and the follow-up schedule. For example, you will be having PSA tests at regular intervals.

10. Maintaining your health. This is the place for information or hints about staying well or caring for yourself before, during, and after treatments. Information to file here includes, for example, catheter care. Also file general wellness plans, dietary suggestions, and exercise guidelines.

11. Potential problems. Ask members of your medical team about short-term and long-term risks or problems that may result from the disease or treatment, such as your risk of urinary blockage, impotence, or incontinence. Should you be concerned if your PSA starts to rise? What problems should you look out for? When should you call your doctor? Take notes about what you can do to be alert and prevent potential future health issues.

12. Community resources. File the addresses, phone numbers, and Web sites of local and national organizations and other resources in this section. Include news, advice, and tips you've received from these organizations and pages you've printed out from the Internet. Refer to the *Resources* section in the back of this book for valuable prostate cancer resources for cancer patients and their loved ones.

13. Questions. Keep a record of the questions you have about your care and the answers you receive. Date each entry for future reference.

By maintaining a comprehensive set of your medical records, you'll be making sure that everyone involved in your treatment—including you—is as informed as possible.

Having your own records in hand allows you to refer to the details of your cancer and its treatment. But keeping track of medical records is only one of many ways to be a valuable team member stay involved in your care.

CHAPTER 13

BUILDING YOUR
SUPPORT NETWORK

Jenevie D. Clark-Dorsey, MS HED
Michael A. Diefenbach, PhD
James A. Talcott, MD, SM

MOST PEOPLE HAVE AN INFORMAL GROUP of people they rely on in their lives. You may already recognize which of your friends or loved ones are good at offering practical advice and which others are better at simply listening to you.

It may help to consider establishing a more organized support network at this point, a group of people who can help you get through this period in your life. Potential participants may include medical professionals, as well as people who are willing to offer advice, drive you to appointments, or just listen, such as family members, friends, religious leaders or members of your house of worship, or other men who have had prostate cancer. Consider what you've learned about prostate cancer and try to think through your future emotional, logistical, educational, and physical needs.

Your family and friends are likely to play a large role in your support team. In this chapter we'll explore the potential effects of your cancer on those close to you, how to discuss your situation with people in your life, and how to include loved ones and other important people in your support group.

Cancer's Effect on the Family

A diagnosis of cancer affects everyone in the family. Your partner may be worried about how you will cope with recovery after treatment and may wonder if you are depressed about issues such as impotence and mortality. Family members are likely to experience many emotions—which may differ from yours—while trying to provide you with loving support.

Your partner may not know how to best support you physically and emotionally throughout treatment and recovery. By including your partner in the process of discovery and decision-making, you can face and address issues such as side effects and sexual intimacy as a team. Learning what to expect may also lessen any anxiety your partner may be feeling. (See also the section *Supporting the Person with Cancer: A Guide for Family, Friends, and Caregivers* on page 113.)

Although it may be awkward at first to share your diagnosis with children and grandchildren, some men find that once family members are informed, they want to help. They may attend appointments with you or call or visit when you may be feeling down.

You will likely also want to discuss with your father, brothers, and sons their own increased risk of developing prostate cancer and explain that the American Cancer Society recommendations for prostate cancer screening suggest that men at increased risk begin testing at age 45. (See chapters 2 and 4 for information about risk and early detection guidelines.)

There is no right or wrong way to involve your family and friends in your life as you face prostate cancer. However, open communication will not only allow others to provide you with support, it will help those close to you understand what you are feeling and what to expect during and after treatment.

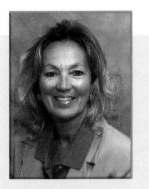

Facing Challenges Together

We handled his diagnosis much as we have handled other major incidents in our lives—together. We talked about it, listened to each other and heard each other's concerns, then made a decision that was best for us as a couple, as partners.

— *Sandy*

Talking About Cancer

The very nature of prostate cancer and the intimate region it affects makes it a difficult, often embarrassing, topic for men to talk about. Members of your medical team are experts in understanding sexual and urinary functioning after treatment, and are an excellent resource for disease- and treatment-related information. Medical team members may be experienced in talking about personal issues and should be sensitive to emotions, but when it comes to talking about thoughts or fears about cancer, some men prefer to reserve such intimate discussions for close friends or family members.

If you would like suggestions about how to talk to others and help them understand your situation, ask members of your health care team, your support group, or a religious leader for help or a referral, or contact the American Cancer Society (800-ACS-2345 or http://www.cancer.org).

TALKING WITH YOUR FAMILY ABOUT CANCER

Sharing feelings about your diagnosis with those who care about you may help you cope with your prostate cancer. You will need time to sort through your thoughts and concerns about cancer, but the sooner you discuss them with your loved ones the better. Loved ones are dealing with their own fears about your well-being and may be anxious about what they should or should not express to you, especially if they are unsure how you feel. Talking to your family may help everyone get their feelings out in the open so any fears and concerns can be addressed.

Sometimes men do not want to burden loved ones with their concerns. A protective attitude may be more harmful than beneficial. Your immediate family is concerned about your well-being, and if you do not share feelings with them, they might worry even more. Remember, your family is on your side and they want to help. When you need them, let them know.

TALKING WITH CHILDREN ABOUT CANCER

Because prostate cancer generally affects older men, many men face situations in which they must talk to their adult children about their prostate cancer (see *Talking With Your Family About Cancer*, above).

If men are diagnosed at a young age or begin families at a later age and are diagnosed with prostate cancer, they may find it necessary to talk to young children about cancer. It's impossible to shield children from all of the stressful parts of life. Even if you don't discuss your cancer with your children, they will probably have a sense that something is wrong. You may want to be the first person to tell young children you have prostate cancer, explaining about the disease and its effects, to the extent that is appropriate for their age and comprehension. All children need to know the following basic information: the name of your cancer (you may simply tell them "prostate cancer"), the part of

Finding Support

For probably the first 6 months, it was very difficult to express to Stuart some of the frustrations and overwhelming feelings I felt. I felt like expressing my emotions would be an additional burden on him. We joined a gay/lesbian/ transgender support group that was very helpful. I think the experience certainly has strengthened our relationship a great deal. I feel it really reinforced our commitment.

— *Larry*

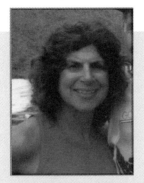

Finding Support

Partners of prostate cancer patients who want to talk about their specific needs and private issues can lean on others facing similar challenges. Through Side by Side, a complement to the American Cancer Society Man to Man support groups, partners listen to educational speakers, share stories, and explore various coping strategies. Facing struggles together helps.

— Sandi

I am co-facilitator of a Man to Man prostate cancer support group because I believe that the importance of these groups cannot be overstated. The sharing that comes from spouses and other family members who attend is so valuable. There is so much information and wisdom available from members of these groups that cannot be obtained through a purely medical perspective.

— Dave M.

the body where the cancer is, how the cancer will be treated, and how their own lives may be affected by the disease and treatment.

TALKING WITH FRIENDS OR COWORKERS ABOUT CANCER

When deciding when and with whom to share information about your diagnosis, think about if others might be affected by your prostate cancer and your needs. For example, you might need to adjust your work schedule to accommodate certain treatment regimens, and your coworkers might need to take on more responsibility while you are away from work. You will find it much easier to ask for and receive assistance if you have already told them about your situation. It may be helpful to tell one person you are close to and ask for their advice about or help in telling others.

Be prepared for some friends and coworkers to react with embarrassment or not know the right things to say to you. They may avoid the subject altogether. Those around you may be unsure about how to appropriately offer you support. You can help overcome awkwardness by talking with others about how your situation will affect your activities with friends or your work life and discussing how you hope to cope with any challenges. Educating others about prostate cancer may also help them cope. You may want to tell them the basics your treatment, your schedule, and your hopes to get through this successfully. You might also tell them they can't get cancer just from being around you.

Assembling a Support Team

A cancer diagnosis often raises emotional and practical challenges, and support and reassurance from others can help you stay grounded and calm as you face these challenges. (See chapter 11 for more information about coping with feelings and concerns about cancer.)

The support you need may come from your family, friends, religious leaders or members of your house of worship, social workers, therapists, colleagues, or support organizations. Your ideal support group may be made up of any combination of people, but its primary function is to help where and when you need it.

You will probably naturally look to your family members and friends for support. They may help you in many intangible ways, such as listening and helping you inform others about your condition and your needs. They may also provide tangible support by hugging you, driving you to and from treatment, or cooking meals.

You might also consider looking to a support group for emotional strength and practical help. (See chapter 11 for more information.) Support groups may offer you the answers and understanding you need—now and throughout your treatment and recovery. Although each man's situation, life, and cancer are different, talking to other men about prostate cancer may help. You may want to contact the American Cancer Society (800-ACS-2345 or http://www.cancer.org) or talk to your doctor for a list of support groups in your area. Additional resources are listed in the *Resources* section of this book.

Supporting the Person With Cancer

Your family and friends, and caregivers will likely be important members of your support team. Each of these people will be going through challenges of their own as they help you to deal with prostate cancer. The following section is written especially for them. You may want to share the information in it with them or have them read it themselves.

Finding Support

Healing starts by reaching out to whatever support group structure you have, and you identify that support in a day-by-day process, I think. You look to your family members, you look to support groups, you look to communities and virtual communities. And I believe the Internet has played a huge role in providing men with the kind of support that is most necessary, which is the willingness to discuss issues on an intimate level, no holds barred.

— Taras

When you are told you have prostate cancer, you will probably be shocked. Don't panic. You may need to go through the necessary internal steps of denial, depression, bargaining, etc. before you accept your diagnosis. I found it helpful to form my own support group of prostate cancer survivors I knew to cope with the significant emotions involved.

— Alfred

SUPPORTING THE PERSON WITH CANCER:
A GUIDE FOR FAMILY, FRIENDS, AND CAREGIVERS

YOU PROBABLY AREN'T SURE EXACTLY HOW to deal with your friend or loved one's diagnosis of prostate cancer, how to talk about the subject, or how to cope with the emotional and practical challenges his illness has raised. Whether you are a family member, friend, caregiver, neighbor, or coworker, this section is for you.

You don't have to be the person with cancer's partner, best friend, or primary caregiver to play an active part in his care and recovery. Knowing that other people care is extremely important. The most important thing you can do is to let him know you care.

You may feel strongly about how you want to help the man with prostate cancer, and you almost certainly want to protect him from pain and suffering. You face the challenge of being available and supportive without being intrusive. Make sure to follow the lead of the man with prostate cancer about how you could be most helpful to him.

Talking About Cancer

It may help to allow the man with prostate cancer to guide your initial conversations after diagnosis. He may want to talk in great detail about his situation and options, or he may need time to adjust without discussing it. You may want to keep in mind the following goals when talking to him:

- Start slowly. It may be difficult to discuss important personal topics.

- Resist the urge to assure him with statements like "You'll be fine," "Everything's going to be okay," or "Don't worry." Saying such things may indicate that you don't want to think about the unpleasantness of cancer, and that he can't truly confide in you.

- Understand that men and women often communicate in different ways, and make allowances for those differences. In our society, women sometimes express their feelings more than men. It may be helpful to openly discuss differences in how men and women express feelings and how they like to be supported.

- Remember that you don't have to agree with your friend or loved one. Two people aren't always in the same emotional state or at the same level of acceptance at the same time. There's no simple answer to many problems, especially if they are long standing.

Supporting Treatment Decisions

As you probably realize, there is an incredible amount of information available about prostate cancer. Not all of it is helpful, accurate, or relevant, and the volume of information itself may be overwhelming. The man with cancer may ask for your help in gathering and interpreting information to discuss with his health care team. But he may be confused or frustrated if he receives unsolicited or conflicting information. The person with cancer is ultimately responsible for understanding his situation and choices.

Remember that deciding upon a cancer treatment can be complicated. It involves assessing likely outcomes, evaluating risks, and considering personal goals. Should the growth of the cancer be slowed or stopped? Would potential treatment side effects be acceptable in order to treat the cancer? Is watchful waiting without active treatment preferable for now?

Prostate cancer is often slow growing, and aggressive treatment may cause serious and enduring side effects that profoundly affect a man's quality of life. Therefore doing everything possible to eradicate cancer may not always be the best option. Listen to your friend or loved one, talk through your mutual concerns, and try to support his personal treatment decisions.

Taking Care of the Person With Cancer: What Caregivers Need to Know

Learning as much as possible about what is happening and what might happen can reduce any fear you have of the unknown and help you to realistically prepare for the future. Talk with health care professionals and with other people who have cared for someone with cancer and ask them questions. You may also want to read other parts of this book to learn more about prostate cancer.

Caregiving and Offering Support During Treatment

As a caregiver or member of your loved one's support team, you should be aware of the person with cancer's course of treatment, the possible physical and emotional side effects that may result, and what your responsibilities as a caregiver will be. Write down any instructions you receive from doctors. Before you leave the office or hospital with your loved one, make sure you understand exactly how to follow the instructions and what your role should be.

You can make caregiving and supporting the person with cancer easier by accepting others' offers to help and providing *specific* suggestions for things they can do. Ask them to help you run a particular errand, provide a home-cooked meal, or help with a certain responsibility around the house. Friends can't help if they don't know what to do.

Caring for someone you love who is physically or emotionally affected by treatment may be difficult. Taking over responsibilities, changing habits and routines, and worrying about what will happen may result in fatigue or caregiver burnout. The more you care for your own needs of rest, nutrition, enjoyment, and relaxation, the better you will be able to help the person you are caring for and the more likely it is that you'll have a positive outlook and a healthy body.

Transitioning to Recovery

Recovering from treatment may be a challenge for some men. You can help the man with prostate cancer by continuing your support and allowing him to slowly regain his life and daily routines. Celebrate holidays and family occasions and milestones—religious rituals, birthdays, graduations, athletic or academic accomplishments—and pursue shared activities with your family. Start new traditions and create new memories of family gatherings, outings, or celebrations.

RESUMING PHYSICAL INTIMACY
WITH YOUR PARTNER

Partners of men with cancer face unique opportunities and challenges as they look toward their loved one's recovery. Prostate cancer treatment often carries side effects such as impotence or incontinence, which may affect your emotional and physical relationship. (See chapter 30 for more information about adjusting to life after cancer and coping with intimacy and sexuality challenges.)

Although maintaining physical intimacy is important to your sense of closeness, you may be concerned that sex will injure your partner. You may also feel awkward about physical contact because you think pursuing it would be insensitive if your partner is not ready. Although you feel bad about it, you may also respond negatively to the physical changes in your partner. The following are some suggestions for re-establishing intimacy with your partner:

- Don't be upset if your partner does not seem interested in physical intimacy right away. Sometimes people with cancer initially shy away from physical closeness.

- Touching, holding, hugging, and caressing are ways to express the acceptance and caring that is so crucial to your partner. This shows love and expresses your belief in his continued desirability.

- Your willingness to look at the changes in your partner's body and willingness to touch him will make the path to regaining sexual intimacy easier.

- If you need more help, a professional counselor can help you work out your feelings toward your partner, about the disease, or about how your life has been affected.

If your partner has withdrawn from you, try to prevent a cycle of misunderstanding by reaching out gently and repeatedly. Provide the reassurance that cancer will not destroy your love or your intimate relationship.

Life After Cancer

As your loved one begins to look to the future and the rest of his life, you will probably begin to focus on yours as well. You and your loved one can make new plans for yourselves and your family and look forward to creating new memories and dreams for the future. (See chapter 30 for more information about quality of life and relationships after treatment.)

If you find it difficult to move beyond your loved one's experience with cancer, seek out a support group where you can feel free to share your experience with others who have gone through it as well.

CHAPTER 14

TAKING CARE OF PRACTICAL MATTERS: WORK, INSURANCE, AND MONEY

Charles L. Bennett, MD, PhD,
Nicolle S. Gorby, E. Allison Lyons

COPING WITH A CANCER DIAGNOSIS IS A CHALLENGE IN ITSELF, and worrying about paying your medical bills and balancing work and treatment schedules may cause you additional stress. This chapter will explore some of the practical issues that may arise and ways to handle them.

Employment and Workplace Issues

You are not required to inform your coworkers about your medical condition. You may choose to tell only those with whom you are comfortable. Because you see your coworkers regularly, they may be able to provide you with important, constant support. But it is your right to choose whether you wish to divulge information about your diagnosis.

Although your coworkers will most likely be concerned about your cancer and want to help, some prejudice may exist, especially in a competitive work environment. In order to protect against discrimination, it may be important to keep a log of when you have shared information about your illness and with whom. Keep another record of your job performance evaluations. You may want to consider talking to a union representative, if available, about illness and the workplace.

Keep in mind that you may need to talk to your employer about your illness at some point in order to discuss options such as flexible work time, job sharing, or telecommuting.

THE AMERICANS WITH DISABILITIES ACT (ADA)

The Americans With Disabilities Act (ADA) is designed to protect the workplace rights of those who are disabled and receiving medical treatment for serious illnesses. The ADA prohibits discrimination based on your cancer diagnosis. Additionally, many states have their own laws prohibiting discrimination. It's important to know what is, and what is not, covered under the ADA when considering your particular situation.

- For information regarding your rights under the ADA, go to the U.S. Department of Justice's ADA home page at http://www.ada.gov or call 800-514-0301.

- For information about job accommodations, call the U.S. Department of Labor's Office of Disability Employment Policy's Job Accommodation Network at 800-526-7234 or visit http://www.jan.wvu.edu.

- If you want to file a complaint against an employer for discrimination based on a disability or for more information, call the U.S. Equal Employment Opportunity Commission (EEOC) within 180 days of the alleged discrimination (or up to 300 days depending on state and local laws) at 800-669-4000; 800-669-6820 (TTY); or http://www.eeoc.gov.

- You may also consult an employment discrimination attorney.

Before bringing a claim under the ADA, it is important to note that often you may have to forgo rights and benefits under other laws such as Social Security Disability, which requires that an employee be totally disabled. You cannot be totally disabled to qualify as a disabled person under the ADA.

TAKING TIME OFF FOR TREATMENT

When planning your treatment schedule, ask your doctor if you will need to take time off from work. Prostatectomy will require time off for surgery and recovery, while external radiation therapy will require you to visit the doctor's office every day for multiple weeks. Other appointments for follow-up doctor visits, lab and imaging tests, or other treatments such as chemotherapy may also require time off. Side effects from treatment may also affect your energy level and ability to work.

After addressing these issues with your doctor, meet with your employer to plan a schedule that will work the best for you both. By planning ahead you will be able to ensure that your responsibilities are covered during any absences. Make a list of all your projects and duties and assess the amount of time needed

Questions to Ask About Work

You may want to ask your doctor about the work schedule you can expect to maintain during treatment.

- Will I be able to work throughout my treatment?
- If I have to stay home to recover from surgery or other treatment, how long will I be away from my job? Can I expect to feel up to doing some "telecommuting" by doing some work by phone, mail, or e-mail?
- Will any of my abilities to perform my job be impaired as a result of treatment?
- How will I know if I am overdoing it at my job?
- Do I need to give my place of employment any special forms or other documentation from my doctor before taking time off from work?

for completion. Review this list with your manager and plan a method for completion, including delegation of responsibilities if needed. Also make sure that all appropriate paperwork is completed prior to your absence.

While you may need to be away from the office for an extended period during your treatment and recovery, you may find you are able to keep in touch with your work by phone, mail, and e-mail, and you may even be able to work a few hours a day. However, it is probably wise to assume that while you are out, you will need to make arrangements for other people to perform the majority of your work.

THE FAMILY MEDICAL LEAVE ACT (FMLA)

The Family Medical Leave Act (FMLA) allows you to take up to 12 weeks of unpaid leave to take care of yourself or a family member and protects your job and health benefits during leave. Upon your return, you must be restored to your original job or to an equivalent job with the same pay, benefits, and other terms of employment. However, you must meet certain criteria to qualify. For more information about FMLA or to file a complaint, contact the U.S. Department of Labor's Employment Standards Administration, Wage and Hour Division (866-4-USWAGE or http://www.dol.gov/esa/whd/fmla/).

QUESTIONS TO ASK ABOUT INSURANCE PLANS

Consider the issues below when evaluating an insurance plan, posing them to an insurance agent if necessary:

- What specialties are offered under this plan?
- Do I need to be referred before seeing a specialist?
- What is the monthly premium and the co-pay and/or deductible?
- How are care providers outside of the insurance network covered?
- Are there restrictions for pre-existing illnesses?
- Which types of prostate cancer treatments are covered?
- What out-of-pocket costs will I have to cover?
- Can I appeal for additional coverage if I need it?

Insurance and Your Rights

PRIVATE INSURANCE OPTIONS

Many employers offer insurance programs. They vary in co-payments, coverage, deductibles, freedom in choosing providers, and referral policies. Private insurance programs may also be available to individuals, but individual coverage is usually more costly.

Learn what your plan covers, and to what extent. Be sure you know whether you can qualify for reimbursement of out-of-pocket costs through a plan such as a flexible spending plan. If you have any questions about your policy, contact the toll-free help number to receive more information. Also make sure you understand how bills are submitted and paid, and make sure to submit your bills and payments as you receive them. If you become overwhelmed, contact a caseworker or a financial counselor for help.

If you don't have insurance, you can ask for help through your doctor's office or a social worker at the clinic or hospital where treatment will be administered.

SHORT-TERM AND LONG-TERM DISABILITY INSURANCE

Some employers offer short-term and/or long-term disability insurance benefits that provide employees with at least a partial paycheck while they are out of the office—for example, during prostate cancer treatment. Ask your human resources department about eligibility, any enrollment cost, and how much of your salary the benefits pay.

STATE RISK POOLS

State legislatures create health insurance risk pools as a safety net for those who have been denied health insurance coverage due to pre-existing illnesses or whose only insurance options are above their financial means. Benefits are comparable to those of standard private insurance companies, including a choice of deductibles or co-payments. These plans often have waiting limits for those with pre-existing conditions, though generally not longer than 12 months. Risk pools usually cost more than insurance provided through an employer.

CANCER INSURANCE

If you purchased this type of insurance through your workplace prior to your cancer diagnosis, it may cover some of the gaps of your private insurance. Cancer insurance has several limitations: some plans only pay for inpatient hospital care, while others have fixed dollar limits and many even impose time limits before you can be covered. It is important to thoroughly research a particular policy before enrolling. Make sure to find out if the policy you are investigating is one that covers out-of-pocket costs in addition to deductibles and patient co-pays, and if it includes coverage for situations such as hospital confinement, external beam radiation, and National Cancer Institute (NCI) evaluation and treatment.

MEDICAL SAVINGS ACCOUNTS (MSAS)

Medical savings accounts (MSAs) are another way in which some individuals may obtain health care coverage. MSAs are tax-free savings accounts that may be used to pay out-of-pocket expenses that arise during medical treatment. MSAs are available to individuals who are self-employed or work for a small firm with 50 or fewer employers. An employer or public payer makes contributions to an individual's MSA, allowing the individual to purchase low-cost insurance with high deductibles or co-payments. The balance in an MSA can be used to then pay out-of-pocket costs.

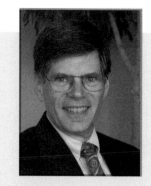

Short-Term Disability Helps

In my company, once I used up all my sick leave, the rest was covered under short-term disability. I received a paycheck for the 7 weeks I was away from the office. I did substantial telecommuting, however.

— Tom

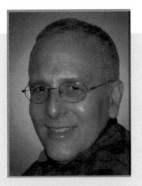

Frustrated with Health Insurance Issues

It was ironic that I was covered by insurance until I needed coverage. I was laid off less than a year after my surgery and stayed on COBRA for 18 months. Then I moved to a HIPAA plan. The options have been very expensive.

— Bob

Providing Insurance Companies with Background

I was diagnosed in my 40s. I was self-employed, and I did have insurance issues. But I found that, if necessary, it is possible to provide your provider with an overwhelming amount of substantiation—physicians' reports and scientific abstracts—that reinforce the treatment decision you want to make. The insurance companies look at this information.

— Taras

FLEXIBLE SAVINGS ACCOUNTS

If this type plan is offered through your employer, you can have money from your paycheck deducted before taxes and put into an account. The money can be used to reimburse yourself for your co-payments and other out-of-pocket costs for doctor visits, prescriptions, and certain types of over-the-counter products.

EXTENDED EMPLOYEE HEALTH CARE PLANS

CONSOLIDATION OMNIBUS RECONCILIATION ACT (COBRA)

If you have been out of work for less than 60 days, you should be able to keep medical insurance through the Consolidation Omnibus Reconciliation Act (COBRA). COBRA temporarily continues group rate health coverage for former employees, retirees, and their spouses. Though this coverage is more expensive than employee group rates (because the employer is no longer paying for part or all of it), it is less expensive than individually purchased insurance. Services included under the plan may include inpatient and outpatient hospital care, physician care, surgery, and other major medical benefits and prescription drugs. Check with your previous employer or health plan to find out if you qualify.

HEALTH INSURANCE PORTABILITY AND ACCOUNTABILITY ACT (HIPAA)

The Health Insurance Portability and Accountability Act (HIPAA, or the Kennedy-Kassenbaum Act) protects an individual's employer-provided insurance when the person changes jobs, regardless of preexisting medical condition. Under HIPAA, an employer must include a new employee in the company's group insurance plan within 12 months, regardless of an employee's preexisting medical condition, even if the condition will be expensive to treat and may increase the firm's insurance premiums. Furthermore, insurance companies must make coverage available to individuals who leave group plans.

FEDERAL INSURANCE PROGRAMS

VETERANS AFFAIRS (VA) HEALTH CARE SYSTEM

If you served active duty in the military before 1980 or have performed 24 continuous months of active service since 1980, you may be eligible for the Department of Veterans Affairs (VA) health care benefits. To enroll, a veteran must complete a 10-10EZ form (call 800-222-VETS or visit http://www.va.gov/1010ez.htm to obtain the form). Medical benefits include hospital care and outpatient services, treatment, procedures, supplies, prescription medication, and other services as needed. Veterans who have injuries or conditions that are not service-connected will have to complete an annual means test to determine a co-pay based on family income and net worth.

MEDICARE

Individuals over the age of 65 who paid (or whose spouse paid) Medicare taxes automatically receive Medicare Part A. Part A covers access to inpatient hospital care, critical access hospitals, skilled nursing facilities, hospice care, and some home health care for free. If you do not automatically qualify, you can also buy Part A by calling the Social Security Administration at 800-772-1213.

You can purchase additional insurance, Medicare Part B, to cover doctors' services, some drug coverage (such as most chemotherapy drugs; other medicines may also be covered), and outpatient hospital care. The premium increases up to 10 percent for every year after 65 that you do not enroll. To sign up during the general enrollment period, which lasts from January 1 to March 31, call 800-772-1213.

MEDIGAP

Medigap is private health insurance that covers the gaps in Medicare services. You can enroll up to six months after you qualify for Medicare Part B. At this time, private companies are not allowed to deny you coverage. Though you can enroll at a later date, you may be required to take a physical exam, and the insurance company may elect not to sell you the policy. Before purchasing Medigap it is important to balance financial terms with services provided. (A list of services not covered by Medicare is available at http://www.lawsguide.com/mylawyer/guideview.asp?layer=3&article=285.)

MEDICAID

In conjunction with the federal government, each state provides health care for persons with low incomes. Since this program is administered on a state-by-state basis, the eligibility rules and services provided vary. Contact your state

Medicaid office to determine whether you qualify for this program. It is possible to "spend down," or incur large medical expenses that reduce your income, to qualify as a "medically needy" person to receive Medicaid. Some patients may be required to pay a minimal deductible or co-pay for these services, except for those persons in a hospital or nursing home. Services the state is required to provide include inpatient and outpatient hospital services, physician services, nursing facility services, home health care, laboratory and x-ray services, and ambulatory services.

If you are 55 years old or above and need care provided in day health centers (which provide health, therapeutic, and social services), hospitals, and nursing homes, contact the Program of All-Inclusive Care for the Elderly (http://www.cms.hhs.gov/pace/default.asp). If you qualify, you may ask about this program by calling your local Medicaid office.

MEDICARE-MEDICAID RELATIONSHIP

If you are eligible for Medicare but are unable to afford additional coverage, supplemental coverage may be available through Medicaid. Additional services may include nursing facilities beyond Medicare's 100-day limit as well as prescription drugs. Call your state Medicaid program to determine if you are eligible.

SUPPLEMENTAL SECURITY INCOME (SSI)

Supplemental Security Income (SSI) is a federal program that provides a monthly benefit for the disabled, those over 65 years of age, or the blind. There are limits on eligible individuals' income and assets; SSI recipients' assets may not exceed $2,000 for an individual or $3,000 for a couple, excluding small allowances for the value of a home, automobile, and life insurance policies. SSI recipients are allowed to earn $65 per month before their payments are reduced by 50 cents for each dollar earned. There are no work mandates for SSI recipients. For more information, contact Social Security at 800-772-1213 or http://www.ssa.gov/notices/supplemental-security-income/.

SOCIAL SECURITY DISABILITY INCOME (SSDI)

If you are not able to work due to a disability, you may want to find out if you have long-term disability insurance through your former place of work. This type of policy may cover up to 60 to 70 percent of your income. If you have been working for a long time, call the Social Security Administration at 800-772-1213 to find out if you qualify for SSDI. The qualification list is quite narrow, so if you are rejected the first time, you may want to reapply or appeal your rejection. Benefits begin 6 months after a disability.

PATIENTS WITHOUT HEALTH CARE

HILL-BURTON FREE OR LOW-COST MEDICAL CARE

Facilities designated as Hill-Burton centers are required to provide a specified amount of services to people who are unable to pay. If your income is less than twice the United States Department of Health and Human Services Poverty Guidelines, you may qualify for free or reduced medical care (call 202-690-7507 with questions or visit http://aspe.hhs.gov/poverty/poverty.shtml). Hill-Burton facilities include hospitals, nursing homes, and outpatient clinics. To find a Hill-Burton facility in your area, call 800-638-0742. At your first visit, request the facility's individual notice, which will describe whether you will qualify for this type of care and will outline the care provided.

THE MEDICINE PROGRAM

The Medicine Program is a volunteer organization that provides prescription medication to individuals if they meet sponsor criteria. Basic requirements include that the applicant does not have insurance for outpatient prescription drugs, does not qualify for a government program that would provide these drugs, and has an income that makes it difficult to purchase these drugs. To enroll, fill out a program application form (available at 573-996-7300 or http://www.themedicineprogram.com/info.html).

CLAIM DISPUTES

Keep all copies of your health care bills, the amount you paid, and the amount that your health insurance company was supposed to pay. Submit all bills in a timely manner. If you are having trouble with these tasks, hospitals, clinics, and your doctor's office may help complete forms and work with your insurance company. Ask about this service.

If your insurance company decides not to cover some of your claims, or if your claims are denied, work with your hospital or doctor's office to determine the cause of the denial. If it is based on the interpretation of the policy language, obtain the specific wording and work with your doctor's office or hospital to appeal this decision. If you have any questions, call your insurance company.

Complaints may also be filed against your private insurance company at the state and federal level. Contact your state insurance commission if you feel you have been treated unfairly; you may be paid restitution if the commission agrees. In addition, many of these departments will work with your insurance company and health care provider to obtain coverage for procedures that have been denied. You can file a complaint at the federal level about private insurance at the Employee Benefits Security Administration at 866-267-2323 or http://www.dol.gov/ebsa.

If hormonal therapy is used for treatment, you may be able to obtain these drugs for little or no cost if you are found to be in financial need (see chapter 22 for more information about these medications):

- **Zoladex or Casodex.** If your income is less than $18,000 ($24,000 as a couple) you may qualify for a free supply of Zoladex shots or a 3-month supply of Casodex (800-698-0085 or www.astrazeneca-us/drugassist/).

- **Eulexin.** A phone interview is required (Schering Plough Oncology, 800-521-7157) to receive the proper paperwork and determine if you qualify to receive Eulexin once a month for 3 months through your doctor.

- **Lupron.** If you do not have insurance and have been denied Medicaid you may qualify for free Lupron shots. You must call for an application (TAP Pharmaceuticals, 800-830-1015, option 2) to be completed by your doctor.

- **Trelstar.** You may qualify for a 30-day supply (Pharmacia Treat First Oncology Program, call 877-744-5675 to have an application faxed to your doctor). Your doctor must renew your supply each month and you must send in a new application each year.

- **Eligard.** If your income is below 125 percent of the federal poverty guidelines and you do not receive other financial help for medication you can apply for a 3-month supply (Sanofi-Synthelabo Needy Patient Program, 800-446-6267, option 2). Each doctor may only have 6 patients enrolled in this program each year and patients can be enrolled for only 6 months a year.

- **Viadur.** To find out more information about Bayer's programs and their guidelines call Bayer Pharmaceuticals, 800-998-9180. If you qualify, you will receive a card to bring to the pharmacy when picking up your medication. A new application must be sent in every 6 months.

- **Plenaxis.** In order to receive Plenaxis, your physician must first enroll in PLUS (Plenaxis User Safety) Program by calling 866-PLENAXIS (866-753-6294). After enrolling, your physician can request information about assistance programs.

- **Nilandron.** If your income is below the Aventis Poverty Level (family of one below $17,960 per year or family of two below $24,240 per year), you will qualify for free treatment. Your physician must complete an application located at http://www.aventisoncology.com and submit reorders after every 3 cycles of treatment.

Financial Planning

ESTIMATING EXPENSES

In order to be financially secure while receiving treatment for prostate cancer, you may want to prepare for the highest costs you may face. This involves creating a financial plan that includes your estimated income and benefits, expected costs, management of your investments, and a plan for your estate. The Federal Citizen Information Centers offer information about handling debt, including medically acquired debt, and can be contacted at 800-FED-INFO (800-333-4636).

To estimate your income and benefits, include your total household income, including both your income and your spouse's. Also include a list of all assets you could liquidate if you had to stop working, including life insurance policies, home equity, stocks, bonds, and other financial accounts.

Treatment costs can vary widely throughout the country. To accurately estimate expected costs for your treatment, talk to your doctor or contact another patient who has dealt with prostate cancer who may be able to provide you with information. Include insurance deductibles, coinsurance co-payments, and other out-of-pocket costs such as travel expenses for treatment, home health care, and any other additional services.

INVESTMENTS

When considering your investments, you may want to move your money into more secure investments that would be relatively easy to liquidate should you need cash. Short-term and limited-term investments, such as money market accounts at a bank or a money market mutual fund can provide income, for example. Consult a financial advisor about how best to invest your finances and maintain your savings.

PLANNING YOUR ESTATE

You may also want to plan your estate. This is an important process for everyone, not just those undergoing cancer treatment. Your estate plan should include the following:

- a will: a document that directs how and to whom your assets will be distributed

- durable power of attorney: someone who will handle your finances if you are no longer able to do so

- health care proxy: a person who will make decisions about your health care if you are not able to do so

INCOME AND EXPENSES WORKSHEET

Estimate Your Income and Benefits. Include:

- your salary   _____
- your partner's salary or contributions to household   _____
- other regular income   _____

Now determine what sources of income you would have if you had to stop working because of your treatment:

- _____   _____
- _____   _____

List the worth of each asset that you would consider selling or liquidating:

- life insurance policies   _____
- home equity   _____
- stocks and bonds   _____
- other   _____

Estimate Your Expenses

Refer to your insurance worksheet for specific dollar amounts. Estimate your:

- insurance deductible   _____
- coinsurance   _____
- co-payment   _____

Keeping in mind your doctor's highest estimates of hospital stays, number of treatment sessions, duration of treatment, and your likely health status, estimate the following costs:

- highest possible out-of-pocket medical expenses   _____
  - travel costs   _____
  - flights   _____
  - lodging   _____
  - cabs or rental cars   _____
  - food   _____
  - parking   _____
- greatest possible number of hospital stays   _____
- prescription drug costs   _____
- experimental treatments not covered by your medical coverage   _____
- home health care costs   _____
- lost wages   _____
- services such as babysitting, cooking, or cleaning   _____

Financial resources are available to help while you are in treatment; this chapter lists several resources for financial assistance.

- living will: a document that specifies the types of medical treatment you would or would not want if you are not able to communicate these choices

Make sure to discuss all of these decisions with your spouse and meet with an attorney who specializes in estate planning if possible. These documents may also be drafted at a legal clinic or nonprofit group. Call the American Cancer Society for names and organizations that can help you. Make sure to review this information periodically and make any necessary changes to ensure they continue to reflect your wishes.

SOURCES OF INCOME OR ASSISTANCE

If you have financial trouble, there are many places you can turn for help. The Consumer Credit Counseling Service (800-251-2227) can help you make a payment plan to your creditors. The following also lists options for liquidating your current assets.

LIFE INSURANCE

Life insurance can provide one way of increasing your assets to pay for health care. The primary way to use your life insurance to gain immediate access to resources is called living benefits, in which you gain the value of a policy through accelerating the policy's death benefit. You may sell the insurance policy to a viatical provider or obtain loans from the insurance company or from a third party against the value of the policy held.

A viatical provider buys insurance from people who have a short life expectancy, by giving cash for their policy. After purchasing the policy, the company continues to pay the premiums until the individual passes away, at which point the viatical provider obtains the remaining money from the policy. A doctor normally has to certify the life expectancy of the individual, and the lump sum is usually 60 to 80 percent of the face value of the policy and is received tax-free. Before making this type of decision, talk to your partner or other relatives as well as a lawyer or a financial planner in order to decide if this is the best financial option for you.

HOME EQUITY LOANS AND CONVERSIONS

If you are at least 62 years old and either own or nearly own your house, you may be able to liquidate your home equity. Equity is the difference between how much your house is worth and how much you owe on your mortgage. You may take out a home equity loan, or second mortgage, which must be repaid. Or you may take out a reverse mortgage, in which you are paid a percentage of the amount of equity in the home. This money does not have to be repaid as long as you live there. Interest and service charges apply. This may disqualify you from some federal aid programs. You can receive more information from a financial advisor or the AARP (800-456-2277 or http://www.aarp.org).

RETIREMENT

You can use some money from your retirement plan before retiring by qualifying for the hardship provision in your plan. Contact the human resources department at your workplace to find out how to use this option.

FAMILY LOANS

If your relatives would like, they can help you financially. If you are loaned money, make sure to outline a repayment period and an interest rate, which must be at least the minimum federal rate or else there may be tax consequences. Family members can also give a tax-free gift up to $11,000 a year or pay medical bills without a cap if payments are made directly to the medical facility. (Limits and terms of tax-free gifts may change; ask a financial advisor for up-to-date information.) Be aware of the possibility that such gifts or loans may affect your relationship. You may want to discuss expectations and feelings with the family member considering making a potential gift or loan.

HELP FROM OTHER ORGANIZATIONS

Various non-profit, religious, and civic organizations provide help for people with cancer. The Salvation Army, United Way, and other organizations listed under "social services" in the phone book may be able to help you with your out-of-pocket expenses by providing free meals, transportation, and other home care services.

WELFARE OFFICE

County boards of assistance, Aid to Families with Dependent Children, and Food Stamps programs can all be contacted to obtain information concerning state and federal funds available to cover necessary expenses.

BANKRUPTCY

Bankruptcy is a final option if you are unable to keep up with your medically acquired debt. If you decide to take this step, make sure to contact an attorney, legal aid clinic, or non-profit agency. Bankruptcy is a complicated process.

STAGING
AND PROGNOSIS

IF YOUR PROSTATE BIOPSY CONFIRMS YOU HAVE CANCER, your doctor will order more tests to learn more about the cancer within the prostate and whether it has spread to nearby tissues or other parts of the body. This process of staging will provide essential information about your cancer and will help you to know which treatment options are most appropriate. It will also give you a better idea about your prognosis, or likely outcome.

Every man's situation is unique, and every man has a different experience with prostate cancer. This is the time to gather information about your cancer and consider what it may mean for your body and your future. You won't find a one-size-fits-all approach to your decisions in the following pages, but you will find the foundation for understanding your cancer so you'll be prepared to make the best possible decisions for your cancer and your life.

Every Man's Situation Is Different

This is the time to gather information about your cancer and consider what it may mean for your body and your future.

CHAPTER 15

STAGING

Peter R. Carroll, MD
Hedvig Hricak, MD, PhD
Maxwell V. Meng, MD
Sangtae Park, MD
Darko Pucar, MD, PhD

I F YOUR PROSTATE BIOPSY CONFIRMS A CANCER, more tests may be done to find out the cancer stage—that is, how widespread the cancer is. The stage of a cancer is one of the most important factors involved in determining treatment options and predicting a patient's outlook for survival.

What Is Staging?

Staging is the process of gathering information from digital rectal examinations (DREs), biopsies, and diagnostic imaging tests (studies that produce pictures of what is going on inside your body) to determine more about the cancer within the prostate and whether it has spread to nearby tissues or other parts of the body.

Your doctor will use your DRE results, prostate-specific antigen (PSA) level, and Gleason score to decide which other tests (if any) to order as part of the staging process. Men with a normal DRE result, a low PSA, and a low Gleason score may not need other tests because the chance that the cancer has spread is so low.

THE TNM STAGING SYSTEM

A staging system is a standardized way for cancer care professionals to describe the extent to which cancer has spread, if at all, when it is first diagnosed. While there are several different staging systems for prostate cancer, the most widely used system in the United States is the TNM system. It is also known as the Staging System of the American Joint Committee on Cancer (AJCC). If your doctors use another staging system, such as the Whitmore-Jewett system, which stages prostate cancer as A, B, C, or D, ask them to translate it into the TNM system or to explain how their staging will help determine your treatment options.

In TNM staging, information about the primary tumor (T), nearby lymph nodes (N), and distant organ metastases (M) is combined and a stage is assigned according to the specific TNM grouping.

The stages described below are based on the *AJCC Cancer Staging Manual*, Sixth Edition, published in 2002. However, some doctors may be using the slightly different 1997 version. This can be confusing, so be sure to ask which version your doctor is using.

The results of diagnostic tests are integrated to determine prostate cancer TNM stage as follows:

T CATEGORIES

There are two types of T classifications for prostate cancer: the clinical stage and the pathological stage. While clinical stage is determined for all prostate cancer patients, pathologic stage is usually determined only for patients treated with surgery.

The clinical stage of a person's cancer is determined based on information from a doctor's examination and diagnostic tests. The pathologic stage is determined by information from the surgical removal of the cancer and lymph nodes. Occasionally a biopsy can demonstrate if prostate cancer has spread outside the capsule (the outer edge of the prostate) or into the seminal vesicles (the glands at the base of the bladder that release fluid into the semen during orgasm).

An important factor in prostate cancer clinical tumor staging is whether or not your tumor is palpable (that is, the doctor can feel the tumor) during a digital rectal examination. The letter T followed by a number from 0 to 4 describes the spread of the tumor within the prostate and to nearby pelvic organs:

T1: Your doctor cannot feel the tumor or cannot see it with imaging such as transrectal ultrasound.

T1a: The cancer is found incidentally during a transurethral resection (TURP) for benign prostatic enlargement. Cancer is present in less than 5 percent of the tissue removed.

T1b: The cancer is found during a TURP but is present in more than 5 percent of the tissue removed.

T1c: The cancer is found by a needle biopsy done because of an elevated PSA.

T2: Your doctor can feel the cancer during a digital rectal exam (DRE), but it still appears to be confined to the prostate gland.

T2a: The cancer is in one half or less of only one side (left or right) of your prostate.

T2b: The cancer is in more than half of only one side (left or right) of your prostate.

T2c: The cancer is in both sides of your prostate.

T3: The cancer has begun to spread outside your prostate and may involve the seminal vesicles.

T3a: The cancer can be felt during a DRE; it extends outside your prostate on one side, but not to the seminal vesicles.

T3b: The cancer can be felt during a DRE; it extends to the seminal vesicles.

T4: The cancer has spread to tissues next to your prostate (other than the seminal vesicles), such as the bladder sphincter muscles that help control urination, the rectum, and/or the wall of the pelvis. To detect this advanced tumor stage, it is usually necessary to use imaging tests in addition to a DRE.

N CATEGORIES

The letter N followed by 0 or 1 indicates whether the cancer has spread to lymph nodes near the prostate.

N0 means that your cancer has not spread to any lymph nodes.

N1 means the cancer has spread to one or more regional (nearby) lymph nodes in the pelvis.

Imaging tests such as magnetic resonance imaging (MRI; see page 139) or computed tomography (CT; see page 138) are necessary to detect the spread of prostate cancer to nearby lymph nodes, since these nodes cannot be felt during the DRE.

M CATEGORIES

The letter M followed by 0 or 1 indicates whether the cancer has spread to bones or distant organs, or to lymph nodes that are not next to the prostate.

M0 means that the cancer has not spread beyond the regional lymph nodes.

M1 means the cancer has spread beyond the regional lymph nodes.

M1a means the cancer has spread to distant (outside of the pelvis) lymph nodes.

M1b indicates spread to the bones.

M1c indicates spread to other organs such as the lungs, liver, or brain (with or without bone disease).

Imaging tests are necessary for the detection of metastatic disease. Prostate cancer most commonly metastasizes to the bones, where it can be detected with a bone scan. Metastases to the liver, lungs, or brain (other common locations) can be detected by either CT or MRI. CT is more widely available and is therefore used more often.

STAGE GROUPING

Once the T, N, and M categories have been determined, this information is combined with the Gleason score in a process called stage grouping. The overall stage is expressed in Roman numerals from I (the least advanced) to IV (the most advanced). This is done to determine your outlook for survival.

Stage I: T1a, N0, M0 and minimally aggressive tumor with a low Gleason score of 2 to 4.

Stage I cancer is contained within the prostate and has not spread to lymph nodes or other places in the body. Stage I cancer is found during a transurethral resection; it has a low Gleason score (2 to 4), and less than 5 percent of the tissue is cancerous.

Stage II: T1a, N0, M0 with a higher Gleason score of 5 to 10, or T1b to T2c, N0, M0, regardless of Gleason score.

In stage II, the cancer is contained within the prostate and has not spread to the lymph nodes or elsewhere, and one of the following is true:

- It was found during a transurethral resection. It had an intermediate or high Gleason score of 5 or higher, or more than 5 percent of the tissue contained cancer.
- It was discovered because of a high PSA level, cannot be felt on a DRE or seen on transrectal ultrasound, and was diagnosed by needle biopsy.
- It can be felt on a DRE or seen on transrectal ultrasound.

Stage III: T3, N0, M0, any Gleason score.

Stage III cancer has begun to spread outside the prostate and may have spread to the seminal vesicles, but it has not spread to the lymph nodes or elsewhere in the body.

Stage IV: T4, N1, or M1, regardless of other categories.

One or more of the following apply to Stage IV cancer:

- The cancer has spread to tissues next to the prostate (other than the seminal vesicles), such as the bladder's external sphincter, the rectum, and/or the wall of the pelvis.
- It has spread to the lymph nodes.
- It has spread to other, more distant sites in the body.

TNM information used with the permission of the American Joint Committee on Cancer (AJCC®), Chicago, Illinois. The original source for this material is the *AJCC® Cancer Staging Manual*, 6th edition (2002). Springer-Verlag New York, Inc., New York, New York.

Tests to Determine the Spread of Prostate Cancer

If a prostate biopsy confirms that cancer is present, additional tests, such as physical exams and imaging studies, may be done to find out how far the cancer has spread within the prostate, to nearby tissues, or to other parts of the body.

PHYSICAL EXAM

The physical exam, especially the digital rectal exam (DRE), is an important part of prostate cancer staging. By doing a DRE your doctor can sometimes tell if the cancer is only on one side of the prostate, if it is present on both sides, or if it has probably spread beyond the prostate gland. See chapter 5 for more information about DRE.

Your doctor may also examine other areas of your body to see if the cancer has spread outside your pelvis. In addition, your doctor will also ask you about symptoms such as bone pain, which may indicate that the cancer has spread to your bones.

IMAGING STUDIES

Imaging studies (also called radiographic studies) produce pictures of internal body structures and can provide valuable information about the extent and location of cancer. Information gained from radiographic studies is used in combination with other information such as the PSA level and Gleason grade.

Imaging studies that may be used to help determine the stage of your prostate cancer include: a ProstaScint scan, radionuclide bone scan, computed tomography (CT, or "CAT scan"), magnetic resonance imaging/spectroscopy (MRI/MRS), ultrasound, intravenous pyelogram (IVP), and chest x-ray.

PROSTASCINT

Advances in immunology (the study of how the body resists infection and certain other diseases) have led to the development of the ProstaScint scan, which has the potential to detect the location of microscopic prostate cancer cells in the body.

An antibody is a protein produced by immune system cells and released into the blood to defend against foreign agents. ProstaScint uses a purified monoclonal antibody (a special kind of antibody manufactured in the laboratory) that recognizes human prostate cancer cells. After this antibody—which is connected to a radioactive tracer—is injected into the body, the entire body is scanned in a process similar to a routine bone scan (see next page).

The imaging test was designed to detect cancer that has spread outside the prostate gland to the lymph nodes or other soft tissues. However, ProstaScint scanning may be valuable in a limited number of patients who are thought to be at high risk for metastases despite normal results in conventional tests, such as CT. It may be performed either before or after initial treatment to help decide the next course of therapy in those whose PSA levels indicate cancer may remain or has recurred. Use of the ProstaScint scan in combination with conventional tests such as CT may improve its accuracy.

At this time, the ProstaScint scan requires further refinement before doctors and patients make decisions based on test results. Newer monoclonal antibodies have been developed that can identify cancer cells better, and it is likely that such imaging will be applied more widely in the future.

RADIONUCLIDE BONE SCAN

Because prostate cancer can spread to the bones, a whole body bone scan may be ordered by your doctor to see if metastasis to the bone is evident. The technical name for this procedure is radionuclide bone scan. It involves the injection of a radioactive tracer material, followed by scanning under a detector. The scan is based on the principle that bony abnormalities, including cancer metastases, absorb the tracer and "light up" on the scan. Often, a previously broken bone or a non-cancerous area of the bone can mimic cancer within the bone. Therefore, your doctor may order x-rays, a CT, or a biopsy of these areas to determine if cancer is truly present.

Because of PSA testing, prostate cancer is often diagnosed at an early stage. Therefore bone scans are not necessary for most patients. Current recommendations are that bone scans be considered in men who are thought to be at high risk for bone metastases, including those with a PSA greater than 10 ng/ml, those with cancer stage T3 or T4 or a Gleason score above 7, those with bone pain, and those with an abnormal blood test for alkaline phosphatase (a non-specific blood test for an enzyme that is released from diseased bone).

COMPUTED TOMOGRAPHY (CT)

Computed tomography (also called CT or CAT scan) uses a combination of x-rays and powerful computers to produce two-dimensional cross sections (often called slices) of the body. A patient having a CT scan lies down on a table that moves the entire body horizontally in and out of a circular, doughnut-shaped x-ray machine. In the evaluation of men with prostate cancer, CT scans can detect abnormalities in the kidneys, ureters, bones, and lymph nodes.

A CT urogram is a special type of imaging test that allows doctors to examine the kidneys or ureters. It involves the injection of intravenous contrast material before pictures are taken.

In prostate cancer staging, CT of the pelvis and abdomen (as opposed to a CT urogram) has been used to look for spread of the cancer beyond the prostate through the capsule (extracapsular extension), seminal vesicle invasion, lymph node involvement, or metastasis to the bones.

Fortunately, more men are undergoing PSA screening and are detecting cancer early. As a result, most men currently diagnosed with prostate cancer have low- or intermediate-risk disease (defined by PSA, Gleason score, and clinical stage), and CT is generally not useful in detecting extracapsular extension or lymph node involvement.

Although CT is not recommended routinely for all patients, men with high-risk disease features—such as a DRE suggesting extensive cancer, high PSA (over 20 ng/ml), or a high Gleason score (over 8)—may benefit the most.

MRI AND MRS

Magnetic resonance imaging (MRI) uses a combination of powerful magnets, radiofrequencies, and computers to produce detailed images of the prostate and surrounding areas. MRI works at the atomic level, because atoms behave in a predictable manner under the influence of the powerful magnets inside the MRI machine.

After a prostate biopsy confirming cancer, your doctor may order an MRI to better understand the extent of the cancer in the prostate and to determine whether extracapsular extension or seminal vesicle invasion is present. MRIs can be performed in two ways in prostate cancer patients, with the patient simply lying down on a table (as in CT scans) or with a separate probe placed in the rectum during the MRI, called endorectal MRI.

The power of MRI lies in its ability to provide a higher resolution picture of the prostate than CT and TRUS. In prostate cancer studies, conventional MRI of the abdomen and pelvis has been used to detect lymph node involvement or abnormalities in abdominal organs, as well as in the prostate.

Endorectal MRI focuses specifically on the prostate and is used to determine the extent of cancer in the gland and whether any extracapsular extension is present. Endorectal magnetic resonance spectroscopy (MRS) is a closely related test that was developed to further refine the endorectal MRI test. MRS works by detecting the levels of different metabolic compounds within the prostate tissue (such as choline, citrate, and creatine), which exist at different levels in cancerous tissues and noncancerous tissues.

Although endorectal MRI and MRS are promising, neither is widely available nor widely used in the United States for the evaluation of men with prostate cancer. One reason is that interpretation of the MRI/MRS scans requires a highly specialized radiologist with extensive experience. In addition, more studies are needed to define which prostate cancer patients would benefit most from MRI/MRS.

ULTRASOUND

Ultrasound creates an image of the structures inside the body using sound waves; there is no radiation exposure during the test. By sending sound waves through the front of the abdomen, the ultrasound can provide views of the prostate as well as the volume of urine within the bladder. Through the back and side of the body, the ultrasound can provide views of the kidneys. In prostate cancer patients, ultrasound can be separated into two categories, abdominal and transrectal.

Abdominal. In a case of advanced prostate cancer, the kidneys and bladder may become obstructed by local growth within the prostate or by enlarged lymph nodes in the pelvis. In these cases, abdominal ultrasound is a safe, fast way to detect this potential problem and help determine if additional treatment is needed. CT is an alternative to ultrasound that is more commonly used for this purpose.

Transrectal. As described in chapter 8, transrectal ultrasound (TRUS) is performed by placing a probe into the rectum. The doctor most commonly uses the ultrasound picture to guide a biopsy needle into specific areas of the prostate. The number of biopsy tissue cores that contain cancer and the extent of cancer in those cores is related to the likelihood of cancer beyond the prostate (as well as the risk of recurrence after conventional treatment, such as surgery or radiation).

Many studies have shown that the ability of conventional TRUS to identify areas of prostate cancer depends on the experience of the doctor performing the procedure. Even in the most experienced hands, the accuracy of cancer detection and staging using TRUS is poor, and visualization of cancer on TRUS is typically accurate 50 percent of the time. TRUS findings can suggest spread of the cancer outside the prostate or to the seminal vesicles; however, the only way to confirm this is by directed biopsy or removal of the prostate gland.

Color Doppler, power Doppler, and contrast-enhanced ultrasound were developed as refinements to the standard TRUS, which is sometimes described as "gray-scale" TRUS. These new ultrasound machines detect blood flow patterns, which may be increased in cancerous areas. These tests require expensive machines, can take longer to perform, and may require intravenous injection of contrast materials. Moreover, although they were initially thought to improve the diagnosis and staging of prostate cancer, they have not yet been shown to offer any

Table 15.1. IMAGING RECOMMENDATIONS

Imaging Test	When It Is Recommended
Chest x-ray	• Patient has advanced disease or a high PSA level • Patient has chest or rib pain, shortness of breath • As a pre-operative preparation
Intravenous Pyelogram (often replaced by Ultrasound or CT Urography)	• Patient has current or recent kidney stones • Suspect blockage of the urinary tract • Patient has blood in the urine
Transrectal Ultrasound	• Patient is eligible for biopsy • To direct biopsies • In assessment of prostate volume • (Consider color Doppler for directed biopsies if available)
Computed Tomography	• As part of staging for very high-risk patients (i.e., clinical T3 stage, Gleason score greater than 7, PSA greater than 20 ng/ml) • For specific indications to look at the kidneys or ureters (CT urography) • To check dose of radiation after prostate brachytherapy • Patient has blood in the urine
MRI/MRS	• As part of staging for select intermediate and high-risk patients
Bone Scan	• As part of staging when PSA is greater than 10 ng/ml, or for high-risk patients (T3 or T4, Gleason score greater than 7) • Patient has elevated alkaline phosphatase • Patient has bone pain
ProstaScint	• For high-risk patients (T3, Gleason score greater than 7, PSA greater than 40 ng/ml) • With PSA recurrence after treatment, especially when other tests are inconclusive

major advantages over traditional TRUS, and there is no strong evidence to support the routine use of these alternative ultrasound tests. Further studies are needed before color, power, and contrast TRUS may be recommended for all patients.

In some cases TRUS may be recommended after surgery or radiation to determine if the cancer has returned in the treated area of the prostate. In these cases, TRUS primarily helps guide the biopsy needle to areas which are of concern for cancer recurrence.

INTRAVENOUS PYELOGRAM (IVP)

The intravenous pyelogram (IVP) is a test in which a contrast material (a substance such as a dye used to make a radiology image clearer) is injected into a vein. Because various body tissues absorb contrast material differently, an image produced using contrast material shows differences between types of tissues, allowing abnormalities such as tumors to be seen more clearly. IVP is useful in detecting blockage in the kidneys or ureters. IVP currently plays a limited role in evaluating patients with prostate cancer.

Some people are severely allergic to the contrast agent (iodine contrast) required for IVP, and those with underlying kidney problems or diabetes may suffer kidney damage from the contrast material. If an evaluation of the kidneys is requested, IVP is usually replaced by ultrasound or computed tomographic (CT) urography.

CHEST X-RAY

X-rays are a type of radiation that can be used at low levels to produce an image of the body on film. A chest x-ray can detect abnormalities in the heart, lungs, and major blood vessels of the chest and ribs. If advanced disease or a high PSA level is found, a chest x-ray may be ordered, especially if a man has symptoms such as rib pain or a chronic cough that could indicate spread to the lungs or ribs. A chest x-ray is also done before most operations that require general anesthesia to ensure no abnormalities within the lungs (such as pneumonia) are present.

Modern-day imaging often plays an important role in the clinical staging of prostate cancer. You and your doctor should discuss the reasons for tests that are ordered and the limitations of those tests. Your doctor will evaluate imaging tests that are likely to be valuable in your situation; decisions about imaging tests will be made based upon your specific situation, including Gleason score, PSA level, and clinical stage.

CHAPTER 16

LYMPH NODE BIOPSY

Peter R. Carroll, MD
Viraj A. Master, MD, PhD
Maxwell V. Meng, MD
Nadeem U. Rahman, MD

THE LYMPHATIC SYSTEM DEFENDS THE BODY against disease and infection. It is made up of lymph vessels and lymph nodes. Lymph vessels carry fluid from different areas of the body to the heart. They also serve as channels for immune cells to move around the body. The lymph nodes are small bean-shaped collections of immune system tissue along the lymph vessels that house immune system cells and help fight infections.

Lymph Nodes and the Spread of Cancer

Occasionally, cancer cells can move beyond the tissue where they first developed and metastasize (travel though the body). When prostate cancer spreads outside the prostate gland, it typically moves to the pelvic lymph nodes first. Therefore, some patients who have been diagnosed with prostate cancer may have their pelvic lymph nodes and/or other tissue sites in the body removed and tested.

Generally, early stage prostate cancers and low Gleason grade cancers do not spread to lymph nodes. If prostate cancer has spread to the lymph nodes, you and your health care team will explore the most effective treatments for your situation.

This chapter explores different methods of lymph node analysis.

Lymph Node Biopsy (Lymphadenectomy)

Lymph node biopsy is primarily a diagnostic procedure, important for staging the cancer and determining appropriate treatment.

Lymph node biopsy of the pelvis may also be called pelvic lymphadenectomy, node dissection, or pelvic lymph node dissection. This procedure is used less frequently than it was two decades ago because the widespread use of prostate-specific antigen (PSA) screening has allowed for earlier detection and a lower incidence of spread to the lymph nodes.

Doctors use results from PSA testing, the prostate biopsy, physical exam, and imaging studies to determine which patients are at higher risk for spread to the pelvic lymph nodes and therefore may benefit from lymph node biopsy. A careful discussion between you and your doctor about potential lymph node biopsy should take into account whether you are at risk of metastases to the lymph nodes, how the information gained will influence subsequent treatment, and the risk of complications (see page 146 for information about potential complications).

WHEN ARE LYMPH NODES REMOVED FROM THE BODY?

Fewer than 10 percent of patients who undergo radical prostatectomy will have lymph node metastasis. Most of those who undergo pelvic lymph node removal have the procedure during a radical prostatectomy to determine if cancer has spread. However, if another method of local treatment is chosen, such as radiation or cryotherapy, node removal may be done beforehand as a separate operation in an effort to determine the true extent of the cancer. If cancer has spread outside the prostate, lymph node removal is typically not used to treat cancer itself because cancer has already spread through the bloodstream and may be developing in other parts of the body.

Several methods of lymph node removal are available, all of which can be performed safely. The best technique for lymph node removal is the one that you and your surgeon are most comfortable with. See Table 16.1 for a summary of various methods and their advantages and disadvantages.

OPEN LYMPHADENECTOMY

In the traditional open lymphadenectomy procedure, an incision is made in the abdomen below the belly button and extended down 3 to 5 inches toward the pubic bone. The pelvic lymph nodes are removed and may be examined under a microscope.

For men choosing radical prostatectomy (see chapter 20), open lymphade-nectomy is often done immediately before the prostate is removed, because the results of the examination of the nodes removed during the open lympha-denectomy may affect the radical prostatectomy. If no cancer is found in the lymph nodes, the doctor will proceed with prostate removal. If cancer is found in the nodes, the doctor may leave the prostate in place because prostatectomy is unlikely to cure the cancer (but could cause significant side effects). You and your urologist should discuss these possibilities and what factors affect them before you undergo an open lymphadenectomy.

When lymph node removal is not accompanied by removal of the prostate, in-hospital recovery generally averages 1 to 2 days. A drain that comes through the abdomen may be left in place after surgery for a day. You should expect to return to your usual level of physical activity within a month, but may resume being relatively active within a week of surgery.

LAPAROSCOPIC LYMPHADENECTOMY

In laparoscopic lymphadenectomy, a minimally invasive surgery, surgeons may remove the lymph nodes using telescopic instruments. Several small abdominal incisions allow slim telescopes and operating instruments to be inserted into the body. With a laparoscopic procedure, a man's return to regular activities is generally quicker, and there may be less pain and scarring than with other, more invasive procedures. One potential disadvantage of laparoscopic lymphadenectomy in comparison to open lymphadenectomy is the longer amount of time required to perform this procedure.

MINILAPAROTOMY LYMPHADENECTOMY

Minilaparotomy lymphadenectomy, first performed in 1992, is very similar to traditional open lymphadenectomy, but the incision is smaller (between 2 to 3 inches). Minilaparotomy lymphadenectomy is a faster procedure than laparoscopic lymphadenectomy and avoids much of the pain and potential scarring associated with an open lymphadenectomy.

FINE NEEDLE ASPIRATION (FNA) OF LYMPH NODES

A fine needle aspiration (FNA) is the least invasive method of searching for metastatic prostate cancer. In this procedure, a cytologist (a specially trained pathologist) inserts a very thin needle into the enlarged lymph node and uses a syringe to withdraw some cells from the tissue, which is then examined under a microscope.

Table 16.1. ADVANTAGES AND DISADVANTAGES OF DIFFERENT METHODS OF LYMPH NODE ANALYSIS

Method of Lymph Node Analysis	Information Obtained	Time to Full Recovery	Incision	Pain	Anesthesia
Open Lymphadenectomy	complete	4 weeks	5 inches	moderate	yes
Laparoscopic Lymphadenectomy	complete	1 week	several, ½- to 1-inch	mild	yes
Mini-laparotomy Lymphadenectomy	complete	4 weeks	3 inches	mild	yes
Fine Needle Aspiration	limited	immediate	none	minimal	no

FNA relies on the presence of large lymph nodes in locations that can be reached safely with a needle. FNA is performed if a lymph node is visible and enlarged on imaging studies (such as CT or MRI) and the doctor has a suspicion that prostate cancer has spread.

The advantages of FNA are that is causes very little pain and allows for rapid recovery. The biggest disadvantages are the possibilities that not enough cellular material may be removed to make a diagnosis or that the needle may not sample the area with cancer, providing a "false negative" result.

FNA is rarely used for men with early stage prostate cancer or for those who are considering prostate removal or radiation therapy, but it may be useful for men who have more advanced disease and multiple enlarged lymph nodes that are likely to harbor prostate cancer.

WHAT ARE THE POTENTIAL COMPLICATIONS OF LYMPH NODE BIOPSY?

Only about 5 percent of people with prostate cancer undergoing lymphadenectomy experience side effects or complications, all of which are generally temporary. The body tolerates the removal of these pelvic lymph nodes very well and quickly adjusts. However, potential side effects may include:

146

- lymphocele: This is a collection of lymph fluid in the area where the nodes were removed. Symptoms usually develop within 3 weeks and may include constipation, urinating more often, or having difficulty urinating.

- lymphedema: This is the buildup of lymph fluid in tissues. In rare cases, removing the lymph nodes may prevent fluid from returning to the bloodstream. This results in chronic swelling, tightness, and limited range of motion in the leg on the side of the body where the affected lymph nodes are located. Lymphedema cannot be cured, but your doctor or nurse can let you know about precautions that may help prevent it.

- nerve damage: It is possible to injure a nerve during lymph node biopsy and affect the movement of the legs. The injury usually heals in several months.

- cardiovascular complications: With any surgery there is an extremely low likelihood of serious potential complications, including heart attack, stroke, clots in the legs, clots in the lungs, and others. Death is also a remote possibility.

CHAPTER 17

WHAT COMBINATION OF FACTORS PREDICT MY OUTCOME?

Harry B. Burke, MD, PhD

A S A PERSON DIAGNOSED WITH PROSTATE CANCER, you'll need to make decisions about your disease that will affect your life in many ways. To make these decisions, you need to know what to expect in terms of his disease and its treatment so that you can discuss your options with your doctor and loved ones.

In the last 10 years a great deal of research has gone into predicting outcomes and providing men with prostate cancer with the kind of information they need to make informed decisions. In order for men to use these predictions wisely, they need to understand what is behind the predictions they are receiving.

What Is a Prognosis?

Doctors cannot foretell a person's future health with perfect accuracy, so they provide a man with prostate cancer with a prognosis, a prediction of the probable course of his disease and an indication of the likelihood of recovery from that disease. A favorable prognosis means the cancer is likely to respond well to treatment. An unfavorable prognosis indicates that the cancer is expected to be difficult to treat and control.

A prognosis is not absolute. Cancers don't always grow or respond to treatment as expected. A person's situation may also change (for example, if treatment is effective or a person's cancer progresses) and ongoing cancer research may provide new developments in cancer treatment and result in an improved prognosis.

Requesting prognostic information is a personal decision. Consider how you will cope with the information you may be given. It is up to you to decide how much information you want and what decision you will make next. You may want to discuss this issue with your doctor. Remember that all prognoses are only predictions. You are not a number, your situation is complex, and no one can be sure what your outcome will be.

FACTORS THAT HELP DETERMINE EXPECTED OUTCOMES

A variety of factors affect a man with prostate cancer's likely outcome, such as his age and general health. However, doctors rely heavily on certain information about the cancer to determine the likely progression of the disease and the best treatment for it. The key factors considered at diagnosis include:

- tumor volume (how large the tumor is at diagnosis)
- the location and extent of the primary tumor (TNM stage)
- pre-treatment PSA
- the Gleason score (how aggressive the cancer would likely be if it were allowed to progress without treatment)

HOW PROGNOSES ARE DETERMINED

To determine a patient's prognosis, doctors consider everything that could affect that person's disease and outcomes (these are called prognostic factors). Then they consult published studies and clinical trials to learn more about the past outcomes of other men with prostate cancer in similar situations and try to predict what might happen in an individual's case.

However, no study exactly reflects an individual's situation, and even if the group's prognostic factors are similar to an individual's, multiple studies of similar factors may provide different results (and therefore different outcome estimates for a patient).

Alternatively, doctors may rely on data from individual patients to create individualized predictions. We'll explore both of these approaches here.

Keep in mind that simplified methods of gauging the likelihood of certain outcomes may not be useful in determining your course of treatment and how it could affect your prognosis.

Facing a Prognosis

When I was diagnosed, my Gleason was 7 plus. I started out from the standpoint of, you know, "You're really in bad shape. Where are we going from here?"

– John D.

My cancer was detected early. When the doctor told me, "If you choose not to do anything about your prostate cancer, you may live 10 or 15 years without any threat or danger to your life," I felt quite positive.

– Tieh Huei

INDEXES AND NOMOGRAMS

Indexes and nomograms are tables and charts that help translate information into prognoses. They translate what may be a complicated set of data into a simplified prognosis, but because they are only able to reflect a small number of prognostic factors, they may produce a potentially inaccurate prognosis. Nomograms are frequently used for men with prostate cancer. Indexes and nomograms do not focus on survival, and they cannot advise doctors or patients on how to alter or improve outcome.

Indexes. An index is a system of developing probabilities of outcomes that provides a weight for each prognostic factor. The weight indicates how important that factor is in determining the outcome. Then the weights of each factor are added for a total score, which appears in a table. An individual's outcome is the one in the table associated with his total score. Using indexes provides only limited information. For example, indexes don't take into account the effects of factors on each other.

Nomograms. A nomogram is a chart representing the relationship between one or more prognostic factors and an outcome. This chart shows a numbered scale for prognostic factors and outcomes. A doctor draws a line at a number corresponding to each of a patient's prognostic factors, such as PSA or Gleason score. The point where this new line intersects the outcome line represents the patient's outcome. It is difficult to represent complex prognostic factors in a nomogram.

STATISTICAL MODELS

Another, more precise approach is to use a computer program based on a statistical model to determine prognosis. Inputting the patient's exact prognostic factors allows the program to calculate that individual's probability of having a particular outcome. This is more accurate than other approaches because it indicates an *individual's* probability rather than the *average* probability of a group of people with similar prognostic factors.

Statistical models are generally limited to physicians' use. In the future, these programs will likely become more widely available to patients through the Internet. (Some elementary versions are already available online.) Patients will be able to enter their information and receive their outcome predictions, for example, entering prognostic factors and receiving a probability of recurrence and survival over the next 15 years.

Keep in mind the several limitations of statistical models. Statistical models are built around past results. Therefore, men's outcomes from 10 or 15 years ago—when biopsy rates were unavailable, radiation doses were different, and hormonal therapy was not as widely used—may not accurately reflect the future of men today. Most numbers used in statistical models are from major academic centers; it cannot be assumed that results at other treatment centers will be the same. It is also important to keep in mind that the future of an individual with prostate cancer is not dictated by numbers; many complex factors determine prognoses and a man's prognosis may change over time as his prognostic factors change.

HOW PROGNOSES ARE EXPRESSED

Doctors use statistics to help predict prognoses, and numbers to express those results. These numbers are usually expressed as a probability over time—for example, that a patient has a 90 percent chance of surviving 10 years.

Survival statistics indicate how many people with a certain type and stage of cancer survive the disease. The most common measure used is the 5-year relative survival rate.

SURVIVAL RATES

Five-year and 10-year survival rates refer to the percentage of men who live at least 5 or 10 years after their prostate cancer is first diagnosed. Relative (also known as disease-specific) survival rates exclude patients dying of other diseases. This means that anyone who died of another cause, such as heart disease or a car accident, is not counted. Because prostate cancer usually occurs in older men who often have other health problems, relative survival rates are generally used to produce a standard way of discussing prognosis.

Unfortunately, it is impossible to have completely up-to-date survival figures. To measure 10-year survival rates, records must be available for patients diagnosed at least 13 years ago (10 years of follow up plus the time it takes to assemble the data). The death rate (also called the mortality rate) from prostate cancer has been decreasing, in large part because more men are being diagnosed at earlier stages, where they have a broader range of treatment options available to them. This means that men diagnosed recently probably have more positive prognoses than what is reflected by the numbers available now.

It is easier for some people to cope if they know the survival rates for their cancer type, stage, and grade; others become confused and afraid when informed of statistics for their cancer. If you would like such information, your doctor is familiar with your individual situation and is most capable of explaining information about your likely outcomes.

TREATMENT OUTCOME PREDICTIONS

Before choosing a course of action, you probably want to know which treatment will offer you the lowest chance of recurrence and spread, and the highest chance of survival. Doctors know a great deal about the long-term success and side effects of treatments like prostatectomy and external beam radiation, but they know less about the long-term success and side effects of newer treatments. If results are only available for 5 or 10 years following a particular therapy, doctors are not able to accurately predict beyond that 5-year or 10-year period.

The expected outcomes for prostate cancer treatment options are found in the treatment chapters of this book.

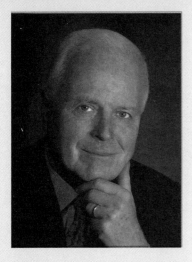

RICHARD RIORDAN,
CALIFORNIA SECRETARY FOR EDUCATION, FORMER MAYOR OF LOS ANGELES

I found my "quarterback," a doctor who helped me evaluate and make treatment decisions.

DIAGNOSIS

WHEN I WAS MAYOR of Los Angeles, I was diagnosed with prostate cancer. I wasn't depressed or afraid. On the way home from my diagnosis, I bought a bottle of champagne to share with my wife. It just felt like the thing to do—to celebrate life.

My cancer was caught relatively early, and my prognosis was excellent. I was familiar with others' experiences, and I read a lot about it. When I told others about my diagnosis, I was matter-of-fact and optimistic. We all die someday, and worrying too much about it puts a burden on you and on those around you.

I asked around for a doctor without bias toward or against certain treatments. That's how I found my "quarterback," a doctor who helped me evaluate and make treatment decisions and referred me to other experts. I decided on radiation treatment.

TREATMENT

I forced myself to exercise every morning when I was in treatment. I jogged in a park near my treatment center before my 7:30 appointments, and then headed to work by 8 o'clock. I avoided fatigue and didn't let myself miss a beat.

Hormone injections can cause hot flashes, but they only last a minute or two. When I was in the middle of a major speech once as mayor and had a hot flash come on, I was able to continue as though nothing had happened. I woke up hot at night sometimes, too.

ADVICE FOR LOVED ONES

My advice to those with a loved one who has prostate cancer: Let them know that you are there for them. Don't pretend the cancer doesn't exist, but relate to the man with prostate cancer as you would have before. While I coped with diagnosis and treatment, I was focused on getting through it on my own with my loved ones, and I didn't want others to feel sorry for me. That's why I didn't make it public until after my tenure as mayor was over.

AFTER TREATMENT

I probably scored a 5 out of 10 on a healthy living scale before cancer; now I probably rank a 7 out of 10. I eat more soy protein, drink soy milk, and make soy milk "cocktails," green tea, soy milk, and fruit. I also drink pomegranate concentrate.

TREATMENT OPTIONS

ONCE YOUR PROSTATE CANCER HAS BEEN DIAGNOSED, graded, and staged, you may feel pressure to make a quick decision about how to treat it. Give yourself time to absorb information about prostate cancer and treatment. Ask your health care team questions, research your treatment options, and formulate your own goals before focusing on one treatment. Choosing a prostate cancer treatment requires balancing treatment effectiveness with potential side effects such as impotence or incontinence.

Treatment options for men with prostate cancer may include surgery, radiation, hormonal therapy, cryotherapy, chemotherapy, hyperthermia, and not actively treating cancer but monitoring it through watchful waiting. In the following chapters we explore what is involved with each of these treatments, as well as their advantages, potential side effects, and typical treatment outcomes. We also explore investigational treatments and the role of clinical trials in advancing research into treating diseases, including prostate cancer.

A treatment decision is complicated, and may be difficult to make by yourself. Talk with your loved ones and friends and consider getting more than one opinion. You may want to talk with other prostate cancer patients you know or meet through support groups. Ask them about the treatment option they selected, how they reached their decision, and why it was right for them. Ask doctors about their experience and outcomes, and learn about what you can realistically expect after treatment so you will be satisfied with your decision.

Ask Questions, Research, and Set Your Goals

Choosing a prostate cancer treatment requires balancing treatment effectiveness with potential side effects such as impotence or incontinence.

CHAPTER 18

RECOMMENDED TREATMENT GUIDELINES AND INFORMATION

David K. Ornstein, MD

I N THE NEXT CHAPTER, WE'LL EXPLORE HOW TO MAKE an informed decision about treatment. But before we explore the decision-making process and treatment options, we'll provide an overview of the current prostate cancer treatment guidelines and important information. The guidelines answer frequently asked questions men have after their initial diagnosis—including how a man's age and general health affect treatment choices—and explain different treatment side effects.

Clinical guidelines outline prespecified treatment paths. One treatment path is suggested for every patient, based on each particular set of prognostic factors. The treatment path that is outlined as appropriate for an individual patient is the one most likely to offer the greatest chance of survival to the person with this set of prognostic factors. Therefore outcome predictions are the foundation of these clinical treatment guidelines.

Common Guidelines

Prostate cancer can be a confusing disease for patients and their families. It does not affect every man in the same way, and multiple effective treatments are available. Some prostate cancers are slow growing and may not cause serious health problems in a man's lifetime, while others are life-threatening.

Several credible national organizations publish prostate cancer treatment guidelines you may want to consult before making a decision about which therapy to choose. Because these are general guidelines, treatment strategies for individual patients may deviate from these recommendations. It is therefore critical that you consult your doctors about which options are best for your particular situation.

AMERICAN UROLOGICAL ASSOCIATION

The American Urological Association (AUA) and American Foundation for Urologic Disease (AFUD) provide helpful information about prostate cancer treatments and cases in which they may be appropriate (http://www.urologyhealth.org; search for "prostate cancer treatment" or treatment-related terms).

NATIONAL CANCER INSTITUTE

The National Cancer Institute (NCI) provides a treatment option overview for patients and addresses treatment options for cancer by stages. Call 800-4-CANCER or visit http://www.cancer.gov/cancerinfo/pdq/treatment/prostate/patient for more information.

NATIONAL COMPREHENSIVE CANCER NETWORK

The National Comprehensive Cancer Network (NCCN) is an alliance of 19 of the world's leading cancer centers that provides information to help patients and health care professionals make informed decisions about cancer care. Since 1995 the NCCN has assembled panels of experts to lay out guidelines for oncology professionals for all major tumor types. Recently the American Cancer Society has joined with the NCCN to help translate the NCCN Clinical Practice Guidelines into easy-to-understand versions for patients. These expert guidelines incorporate the latest available information in cancer care.

SUMMARY OF THE "NCCN PROSTATE CANCER TREATMENT GUIDELINES FOR PATIENTS"

The most current NCCN guidelines for prostate cancer patients were published in August 2004. These guidelines were generated by a panel of experts including urologic surgeons, medical oncologists, radiation oncologists, prostate cancer survivors, and American Cancer Society and NCCN professionals. Among the topics covered are: the different types of treatments available, information about clinical trials, specific information explaining the different stages of prostate cancer, various treatment paths and options for prostate cancer patients, and a glossary.

The *NCCN Prostate Cancer Treatment Guidelines for Patients* help educate men and their families so they can be informed and active participants in their prostate cancer care. These guidelines are based on the opinions of experts and the best available data, and they could change based on future research studies, so be sure

Table 18.1: FACTORS THAT HELP DETERMINE THE MOST
APPROPRIATE TREATMENT, BASED ON RISK OF RECURRENCE

A man's staging information, Gleason score, and PSA level help determine his expected risk of recurrence, which in turn can be used to help choose the most appropriate treatment.

There may be some variation in these groups. For example, men with multiple "intermediate" factors, such as T2c, Gleason 7, and PSA 15, may be shifted into the next higher risk group.

Clinical Stage		Gleason Score		Blood PSA Level	Risk of Recurrence
T1, T2a		2–6		< 10	Low
T2b, T2c	*or*	7	*or*	10–20	Intermediate
T3a	*or*	8–10	*or*	> 20	High
T3b, T4		Any		Any	Very high

Based on *Prostate Cancer Treatment Guidelines for Patients, Version IV/August 2004*, the American Cancer Society and National Comprehensive Cancer Network.

to seek out the latest version. The *NCCN Prostate Cancer Treatment Guidelines for Patients* are available through the American Cancer Society (800-ACS-2345 or http://www.cancer.org) and the NCCN (http://www.nccn.org/patient_gls/_english/ _prostate/index.htm).

TREATMENT OPTIONS FOR PROSTATE CANCER BASED ON NCCN RECOMMENDATIONS

A man diagnosed with prostate cancer and his health care team must first decide whether treatment is appropriate at all. Sometimes watchful waiting—simply keeping an eye on the cancer without actively pursuing treatment—makes the most sense. If treating the prostate cancer makes the most sense, choosing the most appropriate approach involves understanding the extent and aggressiveness of the cancer and balancing the risk of death from or suffering from complications related to prostate cancer with the risk of treatment-related side effects.

In chapter 17 we discussed the factors that affect prognoses (predictions of a man's health and lifespan). The options for initial prostate cancer treatments are determined by 2 of the factors that guide doctors in a prognosis—a patient's estimated risk of recurrence (see Table 18.1 and Table 18.2) and his life expectancy (see Table 18.2).

The treatment options for men with prostate cancer that has not spread to the lymph nodes and/or bones include watchful waiting (observation; see chapter 23), radiation therapy (external beam or seed implantation; see chapter 21), and radical prostatectomy (surgical removal of the prostate; see chapter 20).

Options for men with more advanced cancer and at higher risk of recurrence may include hormonal therapy (see chapter 22), hormonal therapy plus radiation, or radical prostatectomy with lymph node biopsy.

TREATMENT OPTIONS FOR METASTATIC PROSTATE CANCER

Patients with prostate cancer that has spread beyond the prostate to the lymph nodes and/or bones should be treated with some form of hormonal therapy:

- orchiectomy: surgical removal of the testicles
- luteinizing hormone-releasing hormone (LHRH) agents: injections that are given regularly (whether monthly, every 3 to 4 months, or at other intervals) that block the secretion of testosterone
- an LHRH agent plus oral anti-androgen: an injection to block the secretion of testosterone in combination with pills that block the action of testosterone

If a man's PSA begins to rise, indicating that the hormonal therapy is not working, or if the patient develops symptoms while receiving a combination of LHRH agents and oral anti-androgen, the oral anti-androgen should be discontinued. The most common symptoms would be pain, usually in the bones, or urinary symptoms if the man has not had his prostate removed.

TREATMENT OPTIONS FOR CANCER THAT RETURNS OR GROWS AFTER TREATMENT

The treatment that is most appropriate for a man's recurrent prostate cancer depends upon where in the body the recurrence occurs and if it has responded to hormone therapy. Various treatment options for men with recurrent prostate cancer are discussed in chapter 29.

Table 18.2. TREATMENT OPTIONS BASED ON RISK
AND LIFE EXPECTANCY

A man's treatment options are affected by his risk of recurrence and life
expectancy.

Recurrence Risk	Life Expectancy (Years)	Recommended Initial Treatment Options
Low	Less than 10	Watchful waiting
		Radiation (3-D conformal radiation therapy or brachytherapy)
Low	10 or more	Watchful waiting
		Radiation (3-D CRT or brachytherapy)
		Radical prostatectomy +/- lymph node biopsy
Intermediate	Less than 10	Watchful waiting
		Radiation (3-D CRT +/- brachytherapy)
		Radical prostatectomy +/- lymph node biopsy
Intermediate	10 or more	Radical prostatectomy +/- lymph node biopsy
		Radiation (3-D CRT +/-brachytherapy)
High	Any	Hormonal therapy (Androgen deprivation therapy) + radiation (3-D CRT)
		Radiation (3-D CRT +/- concurrent short-term ADT)
		Radical prostatectomy + lymph node biopsy
Very High	Any	Hormonal therapy (ADT)
		Radiation (3-D CRT) + hormonal therapy (ADT)

Based on *Prostate Cancer Treatment Guidelines for Patients, Version IV/August 2004*, the
American Cancer Society and National Comprehensive Cancer Network.

CHAPTER 19

MAKING AN INFORMED DECISION ABOUT TREATMENT OPTIONS

John H. Lynch, MD

FORTUNATELY, COMPARED TO MANY OTHER CANCERS, prostate cancer grows relatively slowly. This gives most men diagnosed with prostate cancer time to think about, talk about, and research their options before deciding on a course of therapy. A variety of treatment options are available, each of which may have potentially powerful effects on your cancer—and each has the potential to cause side effects that will affect your quality of life. You may want to consider the issues in this chapter as you read about treatment options and contemplate your potential treatment path.

Remember that there is no one treatment answer that is right for everyone. Not only do men have different stages and grades of cancer; they also have different goals for their treatment and their lives. Consulting people you trust and researching what may be appropriate for you will help you make an informed treatment decision you'll feel confident about. Take the time to write down your thoughts and make sure you have the answers to your important questions.

Some questions you can ask yourself as a starting point are:

- What are the pros and cons of each treatment or procedure? Do I need more information about particular treatment options? Where can I turn for that information?

A Personal Decision Only You Can Make

After diagnosis, having heard many myths about prostate cancer and treatment side effects, I decided to take my time making a decision and spent months researching. I don't necessarily recommend delaying a decision, but I do advocate educating yourself to all the facts before you decide. It's a very personal decision. No one should be making it for you.

— *Don*

- Considering all the advantages and disadvantages, which option seems to make most sense to me for my particular prostate cancer? Does my health care team agree?
- What will I need to do in my life to get through the treatment I have chosen (for example, get extra help at home or take time off from work)?
- Who makes up my support team and how will they help me?
- What steps should I take before treatment begins?
- I still can't seem to make up my mind or take action. What's bothering me? What issues are still unresolved in my mind? Who can I talk to who can help me arrive at a decision?

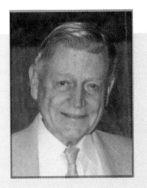

Decisions Affect Later Treatment Options

Although doctors recommended one type of treatment for my prostate cancer, I opted for another, naively thinking that I could simply have different treatment later if necessary. I didn't know that my initial treatment decision affected options down the road. If I had it to do over again, I would have understood the consequences of my treatment decisions early on, when the cancer was confined to the prostate.

— *Charles*

Consulting Your Health Care Team

Members of your health care team can help you understand likely treatment outcomes. But no one can predict exactly what you will experience. The treatment recommendation a doctor makes is based on that doctor's experience with and knowledge about comparable situations. His or her recommendation is likely to be influenced by your age and your general medical condition, the Gleason score (grade) of your prostate cancer, and the extent of the cancer. It is also influenced by whether the purpose of therapy is to cure the disease or, in situations where cure is not necessary or possible, if the goal is to alleviate symptoms and control the disease to provide for the highest possible quality of life.

Your health care team should be able to provide you with the information you need to reach a decision about the best treatment for you. Your family physician can explain any other medical conditions you have that may influence your life expectancy or that may complicate any treatments such as surgery, for example. Your urologist can provide information about the stage of your cancer, whether the cancer is confined to the prostate or has spread beyond it, and the aggressiveness of the cancer, determined by the Gleason score (see chapter 15).

Do not be afraid to consult other doctors (such as a radiation oncologist, a medical oncologist, or both) before making your decision. Do not worry about offending anyone. Your care and your comfort are the priorities, and doctors understand this.

ADJUVANT THERAPY TO REDUCE THE RISK OF RECURRENCE

Adjuvant therapy is treatment used in addition to the primary treatment to increase its effectiveness (for example, the use of chemotherapy or radiation following surgery). Adjuvant therapy is aimed at decreasing the chance that cancer will return. It is usually given within a few weeks after the primary therapy and uses combined treatments to try to destroy cancer through multiple approaches. Also called multi-modality therapy, it is pursued when there is a significant risk of recurrence, even though there is no evidence of residual cancer in the body.

Adjuvant therapy usually involves different types of cancer specialists who work together. The team usually includes a urologist, a radiation oncologist, and a medical oncologist. Adjuvant therapy could be in the form of radiation, hormonal therapy, or chemotherapy, alone or in combination.

Your health care team understands the full context of your situation, including your treatment goals, lifestyle priorities, and health status. Talk to them about adjuvant therapy and whether it may help control your prostate cancer or increase your odds of survival.

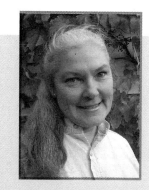

Support and Encouragement to Take Responsibility

When my partner was diagnosed with prostate cancer, I was a relative computer novice. But I joined an online prostate cancer discussion group, and I'm proud to say that many of my dearest friends are people I met through the lists. Part of what we do is encourage patients to slow down, calm down, and look carefully at all of their options before leaping into a decision they may live long enough to regret. Empowered patients are well-informed, willing to participate in their own disease management decisions, and prepared to take responsibility for their own outcomes. This empowerment provides the uplifting energy that enables patients to cope.

– Donna

Researching Treatment Options

Endless amounts of print and Web information are available about prostate cancer, and some of your friends and acquaintances may have advice of their own. Learning about your options may help ease your anxiety while also allowing you to better understand the treatment and recovery process. So where can you turn for trustworthy information?

You may want to begin your own research into treatment options and prostate cancer in general by exploring reliable printed and Internet sources, as well as other sources of cancer information and services. Be aware that information on the Internet or in print may be outdated or inaccurate. You may want to review the *Resources* section in the back of this book and consult these sources both for information and to confirm the accuracy of information from other web sites, books, and magazines.

Questions to Ask Your Health Care Team About Your Treatment Options

You may want to write down questions and bring them with you to your next doctor's appointment. The list below may be a useful starting point. If you think of issues not raised below, jot them down and ask about them too.

As you research and consult your health care team, try to continually clarify and stay focused on learning enough to reach your treatment goals. You may also want to see *Questions to Ask Your Health Care Team About Side Effects of Treatment* on page 170.

As you meet with your health care team to ask about treatment possibilities, consider taking notes about your doctors' answers. This may make it easier for you to review and process information later when you are at home, weighing your options.

Treatment Options

- What may happen if I don't get active treatment at this point (if I pursue "watchful waiting")?
- What are the chances that my cancer can be treated successfully?
- Do you feel that my medical condition or age may influence my treatment options?
- What do you feel my strongest treatment options are?
- Is there one treatment you recommend over the others? If so, why?
- If I want to consult with other doctors, who would you recommend?
- How much time do I have before I need to decide on a particular treatment?

During Treatment

- When do I need to begin treatment?
- How long will the treatment period last?

Surgery

- If I choose surgery, how long will the surgery itself take?
- What type of anesthesia do you recommend? What side effects might I experience from the anesthesia?
- How many operations like mine have you performed? What have the results been?
- How long will I be in the hospital?
- How long will I need to wear a catheter?

- What are the risks with surgery?
- What are the chances I will need a blood transfusion? Should I bank my own blood in case I need a transfusion, and if so, how many units should I bank?
- What side effects might I experience?

Brachytherapy

- How long does the procedure take?
- Will I need a catheter and for how long?
- Will I likely have additional urinary symptoms?
- How long before the radiation from the seeds wears off? Do I need to take special precautions around others?
- What side effects might I experience?

External Radiation

- How long is each treatment? How many will there be?
- What urinary and/or bowel symptoms might I have?
- What side effects might I experience?

Hormone Treatment

- What are my hormone treatment choices?
- Do you recommend using an anti-androgen?
- Will I need to have hormone treatment forever?
- What side effects might I experience?

After Treatment

- What are the chances of recurrence of my cancer with the treatment programs we have discussed?
- If the recommended treatment doesn't get rid of all of the cancer, what options will I have?
- When will you know if the treatment was effective?
- How will you determine whether the treatment was effective?
- How often do I need to have follow-up exams?
- What type of tests will you do for follow up?

Contact the American Cancer Society (http://www.cancer.org or 800-ACS-2345) or ask members of your health care team for resources on prostate cancer and treatment. You can also speak with men who have had prostate cancer and who serve as trained volunteers in the American Cancer Society's Man to Man program, or consult men in other support groups such as US TOO.

Considering the Side Effects of Treatment

Most treatments for cancer come with some risk of side effects. Any treatment or drug powerful enough to kill cancer cells may be strong enough to affect your body in other ways. It won't necessarily be simple for you to determine which treatment will be best for you and your cancer. Generally, however, you will feel more in control by being aware of the potential side effects of the treatments you plan to undergo, by understanding how common or uncommon they are, and by knowing what can be done to control or prevent the side effects.

Ask your doctor about side effects he or she would expect in your particular case. Be sure to also find out how long side effects will likely last; some are temporary while others are permanent.

POTENTIAL SIDE EFFECTS

The majority of men diagnosed with prostate cancer have localized disease. Treatments for prostate cancer that has not spread beyond the prostate can be successful both in terms of curing the cancer and in providing excellent quality of life. Regardless of which treatment they undergo, men treated for localized disease should be able to return to a productive life. No treatment should prevent a man from working or playing. Sexual dysfunction and incontinence may be treatable if they occur. Treatments such as hormone therapy can cause some mild side effects, but symptoms can be treated, allowing for a better quality of life.

Talk to the Experts About Potential Treatments

I was initially leaning toward one treatment for my prostate cancer. I met with a doctor about my options. The more research I did, the clearer it became that a different treatment was the best option for me personally. My oncologist explained my condition, procedures, possible side effects, success rates, and expected outcome. I also met with my support group and listened carefully to the experiences and side effects men had with different therapies before making my decision.

— *Eugene*

Take Control by Becoming Informed

Waiting 7 weeks until treatment, I had time to think. I realized that I was in charge of the situation. I was not being swept along, I was in control. I couldn't determine the outcome, but I could and did decide what the best course of action was for me. The side effects and recovery were as I expected. The time I took to learn about prostate cancer was well spent. I knew what I was getting into and was prepared for the results.

— *Bob*

The various treatments for prostate cancer continue to improve, resulting in fewer side effects and a better quality of life for men after treatment. But no option is perfect—every treatment carries risk. No one can predict who will and who will not have what side effects, so it is imperative that you understand the potential complications of every treatment option. As we explore each treatment in later chapters, we'll discuss side effects in more detail.

- **Radical prostatectomy** has possible complications of impotence, incontinence, bladder neck contracture or scarring, and rectal injury. Like any other major surgical procedure, prostatectomy may also potentially cause allergic reactions, bleeding, infection, pneumonia, a blood clot in a vein, a blocked artery in the lungs, heart complications, and complications from anesthesia.

- **External beam radiation** may cause impotence, urinary symptoms, rectal symptoms, fatigue, bleeding, and rectal or bladder dysfunction.

- **Brachytherapy** may cause many of the same symptoms as external radiation, including impotence, urinary and bowel problems, and the formation of a fistula, an abnormal opening between the urethra and the rectum.

- **Hormone treatment** can cause loss of libido (sex drive), impotence, hot flashes, a potential for breast enlargement and/or tenderness, a tendency to gain weight, an increase in body fat, and with long-term use, a loss of muscle mass and osteoporosis.

- **Cryosurgery** may result in impotence, urinary and rectal symptoms, scarring in the urethra, incontinence, and the formation of a fistula.

Establishing Your Treatment Goals

An important step in deciding on a treatment is determining your treatment goals and your priorities for life after treatment. You may need to consider how much risk you are willing to take in order to meet your goals. If your primary goal is to live as long as you possibly

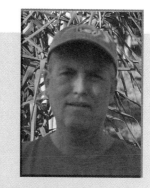

Determine Your Treatment and Look Forward

Prostate cancer makes you feel out of control. So get back as much control as possible. Talk to others and learn all you can. Too many men stick their heads in the sand and turn the responsibility over to their doctors, wife, or children and do what they are told. It's your body, your disease, and you have your own particular goals in life. Make a decision you're satisfied with, don't look back, and don't ever give up.

– Michael

Go to Source Articles

I research at the medical libraries of 2 of our local hospitals. I go back to source documents to find original information on a topic instead of relying on versions or opinions that individuals have put out on the Internet.

– Peter

QUESTIONS TO ASK YOUR HEALTH CARE TEAM ABOUT SIDE EFFECTS OF TREATMENT

- What risks or side effects should I expect from my treatment options?
- What are the chances that I will have problems with incontinence?
- Will incontinence likely be temporary or permanent? If it is permanent, can it be treated and how?
- What are the chances that I will have sexual dysfunction?
- Will I have trouble achieving erections after treatment? If so, will these changes be permanent?
- How will you treat erectile dysfunction?
- How will I know if I develop urethral scarring from surgery? How will you treat it?
- Will there be any change in bowel function? If so, how long will it last?
- What is the risk of bleeding in either the urinary tract or rectum?
- If I undergo brachytherapy, will I need to take any special precautions at home? Will I need to stay away from my young children or grandchildren?
- If I undergo external radiation, will I be likely to develop urinary symptoms or have trouble urinating?
- Is there anything that can be done to prevent or alleviate the side effects associated with hormone treatment?

WHAT "QUALITY OF LIFE" MEANS

We say that treatment side effects such as impotence or incontinence affect quality of life in important ways. But exactly what is meant by the term "quality of life"? Researchers have identified 4 key components that constitute quality of life:

- physical well-being, which includes things like strength, mobility, and fatigue
- psychological well-being, which includes feelings like happiness, sadness, anxiety, and fear
- interpersonal well-being, which includes relationships with family, friends, and caregivers
- spiritual well-being, which includes the meaning of suffering and the purpose of life

can, for example, you may decide upon a treatment with a higher risk of side effects such as impotency in exchange for the increased likelihood of living longer. If you are elderly or have significant medical problems, you may choose a treatment with a lower risk of side effects.

Think about the quality-of-life factors that will influence your decision and consider writing down your specific goals in order of priority, for example:

1. "I want to be cured."
2. "I want to live as long as I possibly can."
3. "I want to have as few side effects as I possibly can."

As you learn about your treatment options and the potential side effects that accompany them, you will want to strike a balance between your goals and likely treatment outcomes. You may find that your goals change slightly if there isn't a single treatment that is likely to help you reach every goal but if several treatment options are likely to help you reach most of your goals.

In the next chapters, we'll explore each treatment option for men with prostate cancer, including what it involves and its advantages, potential complications, and expected outcomes.

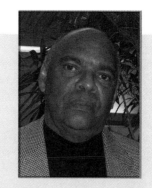

Setting Treatment Goals

I researched treatment and decided to set 3 objectives and priorities for myself: (1) Stay alive, (2) Maintain my overall quality of life, and (3) Maintain sexual function and sexual fulfillment.
— *Alfred*

Loved Ones' Role of Support for Men's Decisions

Since being diagnosed with breast cancer in 1982, I have been an advocate and educator for patients with cancer. When my husband was diagnosed with prostate cancer, he turned to me to make the treatment decision for him. After all, I was the expert. I was able to provide him with reliable research and information about what side effects to expect. But he had to make the treatment decision himself.
— *Sandy*

Table 19.1. TREATMENT WORKSHEET

Write down all potential issues that come to mind about each treatment you are considering: how long it will take, the side effects, the pros and cons, and anything else that comes to mind. As you consult your doctors and research

Radical Prostatectomy	External Beam Radiation	Brachytherapy
Length of treatment		
Hospitalization		
Survival rate		
Chance for cure		
Time off from Work		
Impotence		
Incontinence		
Other side effects		
Out-of-pocket costs		
Benefits		
Subsequent treatment options if it doesn't work		
Follow-up tests		
Notes		

treatment options, add any new issues or information that may help you make a decision about treatment. The treatment information in the chapters that follow will help you fill out this worksheet.

Combination External Beam Radiation plus Brachytherapy	Hormonal Therapy

QUESTIONS TO ASK YOUR HEALTH CARE TEAM ABOUT LIFE DURING TREATMENT

Physical Activity and Diet During Treatment

- When will I be allowed to get out of bed and walk?
- Will I be able to go up and down steps?
- When can I shower?
- Can I eat normal food?
- Are there foods I should not eat?
- Can I have alcohol?
- Is there a particular diet that is best for me?
- How should I take care of the catheter?
- Will there be much pain?
- Are there exercises that might help me regain urinary control?
- When can I travel?
- What kind of vitamins and supplements might be helpful?

Work and Play During Treatment

- How long will I be out of work?
- If I am having external radiation can I continue to work during the treatment?
- How much walking should I do?
- When can I drive my car?
- When can I travel?
- When can I resume exercise like running on a treadmill or lifting weights?
- When can I resume playing golf?
- When can I ride a bike?

Intimacy During Treatment

- Should I expect to have a decreased sex drive?
- Should I expect to experience erectile dysfunction? Does potency return? If so, will I regain erectile functioning gradually or all at once? What, if anything, can I do to try to speed up my return to potency, and how soon after treatment should I start?
- Should I avoid sexual activity for any period of time before, during, or after treatment?
- If and when sexual function returns what type of changes should I expect?

CHAPTER 20

SURGERY

E. David Crawford, MD
Jeffrey M. Holzbeierlein, MD
Arnon Krongrad, MD
Paul D. Maroni, MD
J. Brantley Thrasher, MD

S URGERY IS CONSIDERED THE GOLD STANDARD for treating patients with cancer limited to the prostate, also known as "localized" prostate cancer. When a patient decides to have a radical prostatectomy (which may also simply be called prostatectomy; surgical removal of the prostate gland) to treat prostate cancer, several different approaches can be used. We'll explore radical retropubic prostatectomy, radical perineal prostatectomy, and laparoscopic radical prostatectomy in this chapter. Cryosurgery (a specialized type of surgery that uses very cold temperatures to destroy prostate tissue) is addressed in chapter 24.

Talk to doctors about their experience with prostatectomy before proceeding. Select a surgeon who is experienced in the prostatectomy technique you choose and who is committed to helping you understand the factors involved and navigate the decisions necessary for your particular situation.

> **Feeling Comfortable with Treatment Decisions**
>
> When my biopsy showed early stage prostate cancer, I carefully selected a surgeon and had a prostatectomy. I have no incontinence, erectile function is about 50 percent unassisted, 80 percent medication-assisted. My wife and I are comfortable with our loving relationship and our sex life. I am pleased with my decision and grateful for the beautiful open vistas ahead.
>
> – *Marty*

What Is Radical Retropubic Prostatectomy?

Radical retropubic prostatectomy is the most common method of surgery for prostate cancer. Retropubic means "behind the pubic bone." The pubic bone is the

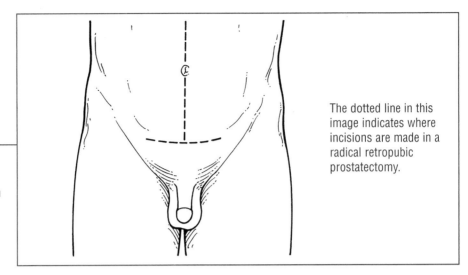

Figure 20.1.
Radical Retropubic
Prostatectomy Approach

The dotted line in this image indicates where incisions are made in a radical retropubic prostatectomy.

bone that can be felt on the lowest part of the abdomen. In a radical retropubic prostatectomy, surgeons reach the prostate through the front of the abdomen.

WHAT IS INVOLVED?

In a radical retropubic prostatectomy, the surgeon removes the prostate, the seminal vesicles, and, if necessary, the nearby lymph nodes.

The surgeon makes an incision on the lower part of the abdomen, extending from just below the belly button to the pubic bone (Figure 20.1). The surgeon can remove lymph nodes if necessary for examination under the microscope.

Removal of the lymph nodes is not routine when prostate cancer is detected early. However, the lymph nodes are usually removed if there is any abnormality. Urologists use a number of statistical tables (as described in chapter 17) to determine the risks of lymph node involvement with cancer. As a rule, when the Gleason score is below 7 and the prostate-specific antigen (PSA) value is less than 10, there is very little risk of lymph node involvement.

The surgeon carefully detaches the prostate from the urethra, bladder, and rectum and saves the gland for analysis by a pathologist. Sutures are used to reconnect the urethra directly to the bladder. The entire procedure lasts from 90 minutes to 3 hours.

Working Toward Treatment Goals

A year after surgery I have met 2 of my treatment goals and am working on the third: (1) becoming cancer-free, (2) gaining urinary continence, and (3) preventing impotence and restoring sexual function. I am still fighting erectile dysfunction despite nerve-sparing surgery and sildenafil (Viagra), but I have complete urinary control.

– Eugene

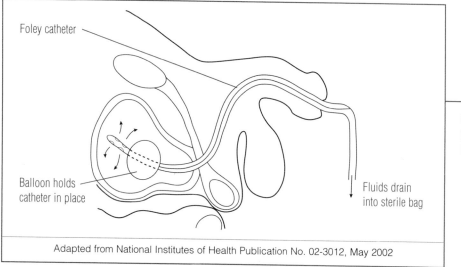

Figure 20.2.
Foley Catheter Inserted
Into the Penis

Foley catheter

Balloon holds
catheter in place

Fluids drain
into sterile bag

Adapted from National Institutes of Health Publication No. 02-3012, May 2002

CATHETERS AND DRAINS

Patients remain in the hospital for 1 to 3 days following radical retropubic prostatectomy surgery. A rubber tube called a Foley catheter (see Figure 20.3) is threaded through the tip of the penis and into the bladder during surgery. A small balloon on the end of this catheter is then inflated to keep it in place. The Foley catheter drains urine directly from the bladder out of the body, allowing the reconnected urethra and bladder to heal.

All types of prostate removal require this catheter to allow for proper healing of the bladder to the urethra. The catheter is left in place for 1 to 2 weeks. Because patients return home with this catheter in place, doctors and nurses explain the proper care of the catheter and urine collection bag before a patient leaves the hospital.

Most urologists also leave another small tube—a drain— in place. The drain is inserted into the space behind the pubic bone and comes out through the skin near the incision. The drain carries any fluid collecting in this space out of the body, thereby helping to prevent infections and giving the area a better chance to heal. This drain typically remains in place for 1 to 3 days. Removal takes a few seconds and may sting temporarily but does not usually require pain medication.

If staples were used to close the incision, they normally are removed 5 to 10 days after the operation. The Foley catheter is removed by deflating the balloon

A Friend Named Foley

They took my prostate gland but left me with a new friend, who I called "Foley" (the catheter). When you are tethered to someone in such an intimate way for 13 days, you get to be pretty tight. I was 100 percent continent immediately after saying goodbye to Foley.

— *John B.*

Nerve-Sparing Prostatectomy

Recent improvements in our knowledge about the position of the nerves that control erections (called cavernous nerves) have allowed the development of a surgical technique that attempts to save these nerves. This approach is called a nerve-sparing prostatectomy and is most easily performed with the retropubic and laparoscopic techniques. The cavernous nerves lie between the prostate and the rectum, with one group on each side of the prostate (Figure 20.2). Preserving more nerves increases the chances of unassisted post-operative erections. However, having nerves in place does not ensure unassisted erections.

In order to qualify for this type of operation, the patient must be at low risk of his cancer invading and extending past the capsule of the prostate. This risk is determined based on PSA, Gleason grade, and rectal examination. Most urologists will not attempt the nerve-sparing technique if there is a good chance that cancer tissue will be left behind. But even if a person has a low risk of nerve involvement, it cannot be determined with certainty whether the nerves can be saved until the prostatectomy procedure, when the surgeon can observe the area. Sometimes the surgeon may try to spare the nerves on only one side of the prostate if that side appears to have little cancer involvement. This may still allow a man to retain erectile functioning.

on the end of the catheter from outside the body, allowing the tube to easily come out. This procedure only takes a few seconds and usually causes only mild discomfort or none at all.

RECOVERY

Before leaving the hospital, patients must be able to eat small meals and walk around. A prostatectomy is major surgery and can disrupt a man's appetite. Good nutrition is an important factor in healing, and patients are encouraged to eat as healthfully as possible. Bowel and sleep habits can take several weeks to return to normal.

After returning home, patients typically need to take pain-control medications for a few days to a few weeks. Pain medications that contain opioids (the strongest pain relievers available, available by prescription only; morphine is one example) can cause constipation. For this reason, if you are taking opioids it is best to begin taking stool softeners sooner rather than later.

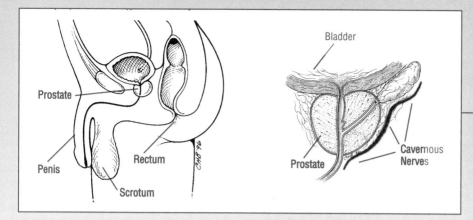

Figure 20.3.

The Position of the
Nerves That Provide
Erections

Nerve Grafts

If the nerves that control erections must be removed during prostatectomy, a man will become impotent. Some doctors are now exploring the use of nerve grafts to try to restore potency if the original nerves must be removed. A nerve graft done at the time of prostatectomy may help some men regain most or all of their ability to achieve erections (with or without the help of oral medications). This approach, done at the same time as a prostatectomy, involves replacing the original nerves with small nerves taken from the side of the foot. Men undergoing the procedure experience numbness in an area about the size of a half dollar on the outside of the ankle. This is still considered an experimental technique, and not all doctors agree about its usefulness. Further study is underway.

Avoiding daytime naps and increasing exercise will usually help you return to a normal sleep schedule. Patients generally feel well enough to return to desk work within 2 to 4 weeks following surgery (others remain out of work for a few months), but it can take 4 to 6 weeks for a man to return to normal physical activity, exercise, or heavy labor.

A small amount of discharge or urine leakage usually occurs around a Foley catheter. This is the body's response to the catheter and is not usually a sign of infection. If the discharge is more than would fill a thimble, or if urine is continuously leaking around the catheter, this may signal a problem and should be reported to your doctor. Sometimes applying a small amount of antibiotic ointment at the tip of the penis can relieve the discomfort from the catheter sticking to the skin.

The Foley catheter can contribute to bladder infections (symptoms include severe burning with urination or frequent urination), although this happens infrequently. These infections are usually not detected and treated until after the catheter is removed.

The incision used in radical retropubic prostatectomy usually heals well without any major problems, but an abdominal scar is an unavoidable consequence of this operation.

ADVANTAGES OF RADICAL RETROPUBIC PROSTATECTOMY

Radical retropubic prostatectomy is a widely accepted type of therapy aimed at curing prostate cancer. In experienced hands, this operation is safe and involves little chance of complications.

In a retropubic approach, the surgeon is able to evaluate the lymph nodes at the time of surgery (a separate incision is necessary in the perineal approach; see page 181). The retropubic incision also provides the opportunity to perform a nerve-sparing procedure. Although there are ways to save the nerves with the perineal approach (described on page 178), the required technique is much less familiar to most surgeons.

Retropubic prostatectomy is more common than laparoscopic prostatectomy, which is fairly new and is only available at a few specialized centers around the United States. The surgeon's experience is extremely important in the laparoscopic operation, and it may be difficult for many surgeons to obtain this level of practical skill.

POTENTIAL CONSEQUENCES OF RADICAL RETROPUBIC PROSTATECTOMY

All prostatectomy methods share some risks; see *Potential Complications of Any Type of Prostatectomy* on page 192 for those shared by retropubic, perineal, and laparoscopic techniques.

An additional risk specific to the retropubic approach is a rare chance of developing a hernia, either in the groin or lower abdomen area, or below the wound. A hernia is a defect in the muscles of the abdominal wall. If a hernia develops, the patient will usually see a bulge in the area, and may feel pain and pressure. The bulge can usually be pushed in while the patient relaxes the abdominal muscles. Patients with hernias are often cautioned to go to an emergency room if they are not able to push the bulge in *and* they have associated vomiting and pain. Surgical repair is usually recommended to relieve symptoms and/or to prevent intestines from becoming trapped in the hernia.

EXPECTED OUTCOMES

A man's chance of being cured by prostatectomy is largely dependent on the extent of cancer found during the pathologist's examination of the prostate after it is removed. A "cured" man is usually defined as a man with an "undetectable" PSA—that is, a PSA level so low that it can't be detected by the PSA lab test (usually after 5 or 10 years). Patients with (1) a pre-treatment PSA below 10, (2) a Gleason score of 6 or less, and (3) no cancer found outside the prostate during surgery may have cure rates in excess of 90 percent. The cure rate drops to about 40 percent if a patient has a high pre-treatment PSA, a high Gleason score, or cancer that is very extensive and involves nearby lymph nodes or organs. Currently no data supports a benefit of one surgical approach over another in terms of curing cancer.

If the PSA does not become undetectable following prostatectomy, your doctor will carefully review available information and determine if more treatment is needed. As discussed elsewhere in this book, a detectable PSA or a rising PSA after surgery does not necessarily mean that a person is going to die from prostate cancer. The most common cause of death in men with prostate cancer is not prostate cancer: it's heart disease.

What Is Radical Perineal Prostatectomy?

Radical perineal prostatectomy is the oldest surgical approach for treating prostate cancer. It is now less common than radical retropubic prostatectomy.

WHAT IS INVOLVED?

Radical perineal prostatectomy involves the removal of the prostate through an incision in the perineum (the area between the scrotum and anus, see Figure 20.4). The prostate is removed through this incision. During the procedure, which usually lasts from 1½ to 4 hours, the patient is on his back with his knees pulled toward his chest so the surgeon can access the perineum. After surgery the patient stays in the hospital for a day and will probably be away from work for approximately 3 weeks.

As with other prostatectomy techniques, after surgery, while still under anesthesia, a Foley catheter is put in the penis to help drain the patient's bladder. The catheter usually stays in place for 1 to 3 weeks to allow for easy urination while healing. Patients should be able to urinate on their own after the catheter is removed.

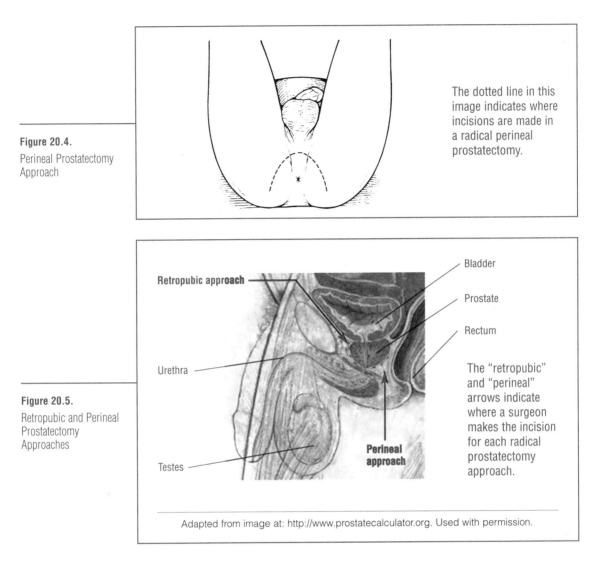

Figure 20.4.

Perineal Prostatectomy
Approach

The dotted line in this
image indicates where
incisions are made in
a radical perineal
prostatectomy.

Figure 20.5.

Retropubic and Perineal
Prostatectomy
Approaches

Retropubic approach

Bladder

Prostate

Rectum

Urethra

The "retropubic"
and "perineal"
arrows indicate
where a surgeon
makes the incision
for each radical
prostatectomy
approach.

Perineal
approach

Testes

Adapted from image at: http://www.prostatecalculator.org. Used with permission.

WHEN MAY RADICAL PERINEAL PROSTATECTOMY BE APPROPRIATE?

There are several reasons why a doctor may advise a patient to undergo a radical perineal prostatectomy rather than a radical retropubic prostatectomy or laparoscopic radical prostatectomy:

- The radical perineal prostatectomy approach is typically easier to do than the radical retropubic approach when a patient is obese, as it avoids abdominal fat (however, see the *Difficulty Maintaining Necessary Body*

Position section below; some obese men may not be able to lie in the position necessary for the procedure). There is much less fat in the perineum than the abdominal area, which can make a radical perineal prostatectomy a much simpler procedure.

- Patients who have had previous radiation to the pelvis for any reason may want to undergo radical perineal prostatectomy rather than another approach. Radiation damages both healthy and abnormal tissues, which results in dense scar tissue in the pelvis. The perineal approach avoids this scar tissue, simplifying the surgical process.

- Patients who have had previous pelvic operations such as bladder surgery, aortic or femoral vascular bypass surgery, meshed hernia repairs, or colon surgery may consider undergoing radical perineal prostatectomy so the surgeon can avoid the complexity of working around scar tissue.

WHAT FACTORS MAY NOT ALLOW FOR RADICAL PERINEAL PROSTATECTOMY?

A few patients are not candidates for radical perineal prostatectomy. A few of the other conditions that may prevent men from qualifying for this procedure are discussed below.

DESIRE FOR NERVE-SPARING SURGERY OR LYMPHADENECTOMY

Radical perineal prostatectomy is used less often than radical retropubic prostatectomy because the nerves cannot be spared as easily, and lymph nodes cannot be removed for examination using this approach. But radical perineal prostatectomy might be appropriate if a man does not want the nerve-sparing procedure or does not require simultaneous lymph node removal with surgery.

DIFFICULTY MAINTAINING NECESSARY BODY POSITION

Men who are obese may not be able to lie in the necessary position for the procedure. The doctor may check a man's ability to be in this position in his or her office by having the patient pull his knees to his chest while lying on his back. If the patient has difficulty breathing in this position, he may not be a good candidate for a perineal prostatectomy. Patients with lung problems may also have difficulty breathing in this body position.

Patients may not be able to undergo radical perineal prostatectomy if they have serious joint problems of the hip that limit its mobility, or in some cases, if they have artificial hips.

LARGE PROSTATE

Patients with extremely large prostates (greater than 100g) are also not very good candidates for radical perineal prostatectomy because it is difficult to remove such large prostates through such a small incision. (Typical prostate weight is approximately 20g for men in their 20s to 30g for men in their 50s or older due to the high prevalence of benign prostatic hyperplasia, BPH.)

HIGH-RISK PROSTATE CANCER

If cancer spreads from the prostate, it typically spreads to the pelvic lymph nodes first. Therefore it is important to sample the lymph nodes in high-risk patients to properly stage patients and determine further therapy.

Unfortunately, the radical perineal prostatectomy approach requires an additional procedure to sample the pelvic lymph nodes, and thus patients at high risk for metastasis to the lymph nodes (patients with a PSA greater than 20, Gleason score of 8, 9, or 10, or clinical stage of T3) may not be good candidates for radical perineal prostatectomy.

Fortunately, because of PSA testing, most patients today are at low risk for pelvic lymph node involvement.

ADVANTAGES OF RADICAL PERINEAL PROSTATECTOMY

PAIN LEVEL

Due to the location of the incision in radical perineal prostatectomy, patients typically have low pain levels after the procedure. Patients undergoing radical perineal prostatectomy have been shown to require less pain medication than those who undergo radical retropubic prostatectomy. (Pain level and recovery time for radical perineal prostatectomy are similar to those currently being reported by doctors using the laparoscopic technique for prostatectomy; see page 189).

RECOVERY TIME

Hospital stays are usually short, and patients are able to return to work quickly with few restrictions in their activity.

SCARRING

The radical perineal prostatectomy incision is not visible under normal circumstances (although laparoscopy typically involves smaller incisions, laparoscopic incisions are visible on the abdomen when patients are not wearing a shirt).

POTENTIAL CONSEQUENCES OF RADICAL PERINEAL PROSTATECTOMY

As noted earlier, all prostatectomy methods carry risks; see *Potential Complications of Any Type of Prostatectomy* on page 192 for those shared by retropubic, perineal, and laparoscopic techniques. The consequences listed below are more specific to the perineal approach.

RECTAL INJURIES

Injuries to the rectum are more common with radical perineal prostatectomy compared to radical retropubic prostatectomy, but when these injuries do occur, they typically do not cause long-term complications. Radical perineal prostatectomies done by surgeons who are experienced in the procedure rarely result in rectal injuries.

Any rectal injuries typically occur during the initial portion of the radical perineal prostatectomy and are often identified and repaired during the operation. Bowel preparation (using enemas and strong oral laxatives before the procedure) limits complications if a rectal injury occurs.

FECAL INCONTINENCE

A long-term complication that has been reported after prostatectomy, particularly after radical perineal prostatectomy, is fecal incontinence (the inadvertent loss of stool). In most people who experience bowel problems immediately after surgery, this condition improves within the first year after surgery.

NERVE INJURY

A potential complication unique to radical perineal prostatectomy is injury to a nerve that provides sensation to the outer portion of the foot. This injury is due to pressure on the nerve due to positioning of the leg during surgery. This complication typically resolves itself within 2 to 3 days. Recently, with the use of new stirrups for positioning, this complication has been virtually eliminated.

EXPECTED OUTCOMES

Radical perineal prostatectomy and radical retropubic prostatectomy outcomes are statistically the same in terms of recurrence, positive margins (cancer left behind after surgery), the incidence of prostate cancer outside of the prostate, postoperative complication rates, urinary function, and erectile function. While less blood is generally lost in radical perineal prostatectomy, there is a higher rectal injury rate.

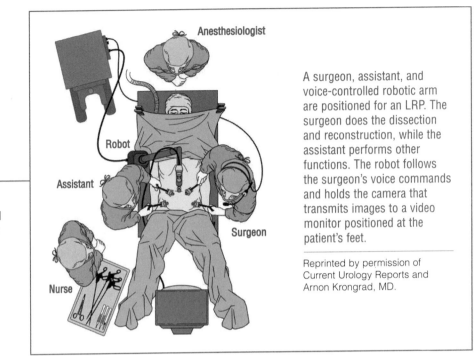

Anesthesiologist

A surgeon, assistant, and voice-controlled robotic arm are positioned for an LRP. The surgeon does the dissection and reconstruction, while the assistant performs other functions. The robot follows the surgeon's voice commands and holds the camera that transmits images to a video monitor positioned at the patient's feet.

Reprinted by permission of Current Urology Reports and Arnon Krongrad, MD.

Robot

Assistant

Surgeon

Nurse

Figure 20.6.
Laparoscopic Radical Prostatectomy (LRP)

What Is Laparoscopic Radical Prostatectomy (LRP)?

As you have read, various techniques of prostatectomy are available. These techniques are designed to, at a minimum, completely remove the prostate, seminal vesicles, and ends of the vas deferens (one of two muscular tubes that carry sperm from the testicles to the urethra).

Since computerization, fiber optics, robotics, and smaller, specialized instruments have been introduced into the operating room, a new option in prostatectomy has emerged: laparoscopic radical prostatectomy (LRP). This minimally invasive operation is the latest technical innovation in prostate cancer care.

LRP is a combination of well-established prostatectomy techniques. Early results of the technique appear promising, but it is not yet clear if it will offer any long-term advantages over other prostatectomy techniques. It is relatively new and is not widely performed in the United States at this time, although some sites with considerable experience do exist. Because the operation is technically difficult and takes some time to learn, surgeon experience is critical in determining patient outcome. Therefore, patients choosing this technique should carefully select an experienced doctor.

WHAT IS INVOLVED?

LRP integrates a variety of new technologies, including robots. Already in use in other disciplines, surgical robots today perform a range of functions in LRP. Using a robot rather than a human assistant allows for a less crowded operating table and allows the operative team a steady view of the prostate area (Figure 20.6 shows a robot used to hold the laparoscope during LRP).

In this technique, several small incisions (usually 5) are made in the abdomen, through which specially designed instruments are inserted to view and remove the prostate. One of the incisions is extended slightly to allow the surgeon to remove the prostate.

The duration of an LRP procedure depends on the expertise of the doctor, but with an experienced surgeon, the procedure takes about the same amount of time or slightly longer than other prostatectomy techniques. As with radical retropubic and radical perineal prostatectomy, operative times vary and may be longer if a patient is obese or has had previous surgery.

ADVANTAGES OF LAPAROSCOPIC RADICAL PROSTATECTOMY

The most direct primary advantages of LRP are reductions in blood loss, pain, time spent in the hospital, and recovery time. Secondary benefits include a reduced need for blood transfusions, decreased risk of anemia, and use of fewer narcotic pain medications.

> **One Man's Experience with LRP**
>
> I was concerned about after-effects of surgery and intensified my own research into treatment options. In my case, when discussing treatment options with doctors, LRP was never mentioned. But I decided laparoscopic radical prostatectomy was for me. I spoke to many men who had undergone the procedure with my doctor. Before, LRP, I used to dribble urine a little. Now, nothing. I'm tighter than a tick. My wife and I could not be happier with the whole experience and particularly the outcome.
>
> – John B.

REDUCED PAIN

LRP involves several small abdominal incisions. (While a large dressing is necessary after retropubic surgery, only small sterile gauze dots are necessary after LRP.)

This explains the most obvious benefit of LRP: less pain. Within hours of the operation a patient is usually fully awake, alert, eating solid food, and can be physically active. Strong pain relievers such as opioids are usually not necessary. Patients often have normal bowel function following laparoscopic radical prostatectomy.

BLOOD LOSS AND COMPLICATIONS

Typically much less blood is lost during LRP than in other types of prostatectomy. Men undergoing LRP are rarely asked to donate blood before the procedure, as transfusions are extremely rare. Laparoscopic prostatectomy carries a relatively low risk of cardiovascular complications (see *Potential Risks or Consequences of Any Surgical Procedure* on page 189).

PRESERVATION OF TISSUE

LRP allows for finer movements and enables a surgeon to better view the area being operated upon. This helps reduce blood loss and better preserve the tissues affected by surgery.

RECOVERY

Laparoscopic radical prostatectomy usually decreases time spent in the hospital recovering. Patients often have an appetite and want to eat following surgery, allowing intravenous lines to be removed soon after the procedure and increasing their ability to move around.

Most patients leave the hospital less than 24 hours after laparoscopic radical prostatectomy. Because of the little pain experienced and relatively normal blood counts, most patients can walk within a few hours of surgery and may leave the hospital the next morning.

POTENTIAL CONSEQUENCES OF LAPAROSCOPIC RADICAL PROSTATECTOMY

Potential Consequences of Any Type of Prostatectomy on page 192 explains the risks of a retropubic, perineal, or laparoscopic technique. Laparoscopic prostatectomy carries some specific risks and also warrants special mention regarding possible decreased risks of certain complications.

A nerve-sparing technique may be appropriate for a man undergoing laparoscopic prostatectomy. Erectile functioning after laparoscopic prostatectomy depends upon the patient's age, erectile functioning before surgery, success of the nerve-sparing technique, and other factors.

CONVERSION

Conversion is defined as abandoning the laparoscopic approach in favor of the open surgical approach in the middle of surgery. This might occur if the surgeon has difficulty after beginning the laparoscopic approach; for example, if he or she encounters excessive bleeding or scarring. Conversion rates reflect patient characteristics and surgeon experience. Speak to the surgical team about their experience and conversion rates prior to surgery.

INFECTION

Patients having LRP may in rare cases develop urinary tract infections. Because catheters are left in for varying periods, bacteria can get into the bladder. These infections are usually easy to eradicate.

INCONTINENCE

LRP in experienced hands is associated with continence rates that seem to be about as good as with other prostatectomy techniques. With LRP, many patients have temporary incontinence, but permanent incontinence is rare. Patients usually regain nighttime continence first, then morning continence, then complete continence. Some patients have no incontinence at all.

PAIN

Relative to what is experienced with other prostatectomy techniques, the pain of LRP is minor. Patients' pain may often be relieved with over-the-counter pain relievers such as acetaminophen (Tylenol). After the catheter is removed and patients become more active, they may develop pain in the perineum, the region between the scrotum and anus. Pain in the perineum is relieved by lying down, using over-the-counter anti-inflammatory medications such as ibuprofen, and taking hot baths.

EXPECTED OUTCOMES

More information is needed about LRP outcomes. At this time there is much more information available about the outcomes of other prostatectomy procedures.

LRP is essentially a prostatectomy done with modern tools. There is no evidence that the laparoscopic technique causes better or worse post-treatment survival and function than open prostatectomy, but this is mainly because there is very little long-term data on this approach. Randomized trials are needed to clearly establish comparable outcomes.

Potential Risks or Consequences of Any Surgical Procedure

Choosing any prostate cancer treatment involves taking potential risks. Surgery has successfully treated men for prostate cancer while saving lives and lifestyle in the process. However, a man with prostate cancer must carefully consider the possible impact of the surgery on his quality of life and be certain he can "live with the decision" should some rare, devastating, or merely bothersome complication occur.

Men with prostate cancer who are considering surgery should also learn about the surgeon who will be performing the procedure. Surgeons who frequently perform these operations typically have better results while minimizing complications.

The surgical process puts the body through a certain amount of trauma and potential complications. Talk to your health care team about any concerns about surgery and when to alert them to surgical side effects. For example, keep in mind that pain medications may normally cause some nausea, but make sure to alert your medical team if you experience excessive vomiting. Some common surgical complications are listed here.

ANESTHESIA COMPLICATIONS

The use of anesthesia for any surgical procedure can be associated with rare but very serious risks, including heart attack, stroke, blood clots, and death. Modern advances in anesthesia make these occurrences uncommon, but certain patients are at higher risk than others. Patients may need to be on the operating table (and therefore under anesthesia) for slightly longer times with laparoscopic radical prostatectomy than with other prostatectomy approaches, although this time will continue to shrink as doctors gain experience with the procedure.

A patient should have a careful and thoughtful discussion with his anesthesiologist about his past medical history and any previous problems with anesthesia in order to help avoid serious complications.

CARDIOVASCULAR COMPLICATIONS

This category of risk includes some of the most serious potential complications, including heart attack, stroke, clots in the legs, clots in the lungs, death, and others. Overall, the likelihood of these sorts of complications is extremely low. A patient who has risk factors for heart disease (high blood pressure, obesity, high cholesterol, tobacco use) should have a thorough cardiac evaluation before surgery, which may include an exercise stress test.

SCARRING AND PAIN

Two things are guaranteed any time an incision is made in the skin—scarring at the incision site and some amount of pain. A tremendous number of pain medications have been developed, and the goal of any care team should be to keep a patient's pain within a tolerable range. If they do not automatically do so, ask your nurses and doctors to actively address any pain that is not well controlled.

Mini-Laparotomy Prostatectomy

A new modification of the prostatectomy that is not yet widely used but deserves special mention is the mini-laparotomy prostatectomy. (Mini-laparotomy should not be confused with *laparoscopic* procedures, described on page 186.) Advances in surgical anatomy, technique, and new instruments have allowed surgeons to remove the prostate gland through smaller or "mini" incisions. The opening through which the prostate is removed can be as small as 4 inches, half the size of the traditional incision.

Smaller incisions decrease pain and recovery time after an operation. Many patients need only a few pain pills to control pain after the first night, and patients are able to leave either the first or second day after the operation. Men are typically able to return to full activity within 4 to 6 weeks.

The mini-laparotomy prostatectomy also allows for less scarring; the scar typically stops below the waistline. After the smaller incision is made, the operation is identical to that described previously. Nerve-sparing techniques can be used with mini incisions, so any person who desires surgery is a candidate for this modification. Occasionally the incision needs to be extended to manage difficult anatomy or troublesome bleeding.

Reported outcomes from about 250 patients indicate that, when this procedure is performed by experienced surgeons, blood transfusions are almost never necessary and incontinence is extremely rare. As with other prostatectomy techniques, potency varies, depending on a man's age and cancer stage.

Infections

There are many possible sources of infection after surgery. Fortunately, nearly all infections are treatable without another surgical procedure or a return stay in the hospital. Redness, pus or cloudy fluid draining from the incision site, or increased pain at the site of the incision can be a sign of a wound infection. Any wound drainage that occurs beyond the first few days and any increase in redness near the incision should be reported to the surgeon's office. Although the low-grade fevers that occasionally occur a day or two after returning home can be normal, any fever that does not respond to acetaminophen (Tylenol) may be a sign of an infection.

Pneumonia (an infection in the lungs) is a potential problem after surgery for many conditions, including prostate cancer. The risk is especially high for patients who remain in bed for several days. This risk can be lowered by doing deep breathing exercises and by getting up and walking as soon as possible after the operation (sometimes the same day).

Potential Consequences of Any Type of Prostatectomy

All surgeries put a patient at risk for the abovementioned complications. Radical retropubic prostatectomy, radical perineal prostatectomy, and laparoscopic radical prostatectomy share several additional risks. Managing these potential consequences is essential to preserving quality of life for men undergoing prostatectomies.

The major long-term complications of all types of prostatectomy are often referred to as the "2 I's" —incontinence and impotence. (For more detail about coping with side effects such as incontinence and impotence and regaining intimacy after treatment, see chapter 30.) Studies have shown that one of the reasons surgery is considered more frequently in men younger than 60 years of age is that these men fare better with regard to urinary control and erectile function as they age.

INCONTINENCE

Incontinence is an unintentional loss of urine. One of the functions of the prostate is to help control the flow of urine. After the prostate is removed, the control of urine depends largely on the strength of the urinary sphincter (the muscle that squeezes the urethra shut and provides urinary control), which can be harmed by the surgery. Historically, major incontinence following prostatectomy was a tremendous problem, due in part to the large blood loss during surgery that made it very difficult to see the urethra and where it attaches to the bladder. The reduction in blood loss with current techniques allows surgeons to preserve greater urinary function.

Regaining control of urination after the operation can take some time. Some men will leak enough urine to cause concern immediately after the catheter is removed. Patients returning to the surgeon's office for catheter removal after surgery should be prepared for this possibility by bringing a few absorbent pads. This degree of leakage lasts a few days or weeks for most men, but in some cases it can persist for several months to a year. Roughly 5 to 10 percent of men will have very bothersome incontinence that persists long after a prostatectomy.

The degree of long-term incontinence and the extent to which it impacts a man's quality of life can vary greatly. Some men are very bothered by the occasional loss of even a very small amount of urine, while other men find complete incontinence to be only a minor problem. Most men who have had a prostatectomy occasionally lose a few drops of urine during certain strenuous activities, but they do not consider themselves incontinent.

TREATMENTS FOR INCONTINENCE

There are options available to men with worrisome urinary leakage, ranging from exercises to more invasive treatments (see chapter 30 for more information):

- Men may exercise the urinary sphincter to help maintain urinary function using what are called Kegel exercises (see chapter 30).

- Biofeedback involves monitoring devices that help people consciously regulate processes that are usually controlled automatically.

- Men with moderate amounts of urine loss may be candidates for the male sling. The sling is surgically inserted and works by compressing the urethra, effectively creating a barrier to the flow of urine.

- A more common operation for men with larger amounts of leakage is the implantation of a plastic device called an artificial urinary sphincter that compresses the urethra, blocking the flow of urine. Success rates for the artificial sphincter can be as high as 90 percent.

- Bulking agents such as collagen can sometimes be injected into the neck of the bladder to thicken it and improve continence. Because injections usually do not last for long, repeat treatments may be necessary and can grow to be expensive.

A consultation with a urologist will help men understand their situations and levels of incontinence and which approaches to management may be most helpful.

ERECTILE DYSFUNCTION

Erectile dysfunction, or impotence, is another long-term complication that deserves special mention. While physicians do not agree on the precise definition of erectile dysfunction, it can generally be described as the inability to have an unassisted erection that is satisfactory for sexual intercourse.

Two bundles of nerves run along the side of the prostate and are important to the chances of regaining erections after surgery. Nearly all men will have difficulty achieving unassisted erections if both sets of these nerves are damaged or removed during treatment.

In the past, impotence was something that men had to "accept" as part of the operation. The chance of potency after prostatectomy is greatly affected by the level of erectile function before surgery and the skill of the surgeon performing the surgery. Some cancer centers that perform many nerve-sparing prostatectomies report that an impotence rate as low as 25 and 30 percent for men under 60. However, other doctors have reported higher rates of impotence in similar patients. Nerve-sparing procedures allow erections to be preserved in many men. Unfortunately, not all men are candidates for a nerve-sparing procedure because of the presumed extent of their cancer. And at least 1 out of 3 men who has a nerve-sparing procedure will nevertheless have substantially worse sexual function after the operation. Impotence occurs in 70 to 80 percent of men over 70, even if nerves on both sides are not removed.

However, there are some options for men who have erectile dysfunction following prostatectomy, either with or without the nerve-sparing procedure.

TREATMENTS FOR IMPOTENCE

Impotence is an area of tremendous research interest because it affects a large number of men. The quality of erections is something that decreases in most men as they age, whether or not they have prostate cancer. More options are available every year to effectively treat this problem; speak to your health care team if you are curious about options that may be appropriate for your situation (see chapter 30 for more information).

Most men first try an oral prescription medication to help erectile functioning. There are a variety of other over-the-counter or alternative medications available in drugstores that claim to address erectile dysfunction. While there have been scattered reports about the effectiveness of these drugs and use is rarely discouraged, there is very little scientific proof that these medications work well in men after prostate removal.

The following options can be very effective, but they may be inconvenient or otherwise bothersome:

- A penile suppository is a small pellet of medication that is placed into the tip of the penis to produce an erection.
- A penile injection involves placing a needle into a specific part of the penis and injecting medication that produces an erection.
- A vacuum device consists of a plastic sleeve that is placed over the penis and a "pump" that draws blood into the penis, creating an erection.
- A penile prosthesis is a device that is surgically placed in the penis. Prostheses may involve bendable rods or inflatable cylinders to help men achieve erections.

EFFECTS ON EJACULATION

All patients considering a prostatectomy should understand how prostate removal affects ejaculation. The prostate is designed to control the volume and direction of semen. Glands in the prostate produce fluid that nourishes sperm and provides an appropriate environment for sperm movement. Muscles in and around the prostate act like a switch, changing the flow between urine and semen.

Removing the prostate means there is no longer a means of transporting sperm to the urethra. Because the gland that provided the major bulk of semen is no longer present, a man without a prostate gland will produce little or no ejaculate. Men who have had their prostates removed still experience sexual excitement and orgasm, but there is no accompanying semen production. Any patient having a prostatectomy who wants to keep open the option of fathering children should consider banking sperm before treatment.

ORGAN INJURY

The prostate is surrounded by the rectum, ureters, and bladder, as well as various nerves, veins, and arteries. The unintentional injury of a nearby organ, most often the rectum, is possible during surgery.

A man's medical history affects the risk of injury to adjacent organs. For example, patients with a history of colon surgery or radiation already have scarring and distortion in the area, so the likelihood of injury rises.

This type of injury can usually be easily repaired, with no noticeable difference after the operation; however, on rare occasions, serious complications have occurred. These minor injuries occur in less than one percent of prostatectomies performed by most urologists.

BLADDER NECK CONTRACTURE

All surgery causes scarring. In a few cases, the scar formed at the site of reconstruction of the urethra and bladder impedes the flow of urine. Such a scar, called a bladder neck contracture, can usually be treated in a very quick, outpatient procedure, which is typically very effective.

Transurethral Resection of the Prostate (TURP)

Transurethral resection of the prostate (TURP) is an operation that involves removing a part of the prostate gland that surrounds the urethra (the tube through which urine exits the bladder). It is most commonly used to relieve symptoms of benign prostatic hyperplasia (BPH).

The procedure may also be used for some men with prostate cancer who cannot have a prostatectomy because of advanced age or other serious illnesses. TURP may be used to relieve symptoms caused by a tumor before other treatments begin. But it is not expected to cure this disease or remove all of the cancer.

THE DAY BEFORE SURGERY... THE DAY AFTER

An excerpt from a poem by Tom Morris

A typical question
All the nurses asked
Was whether I'd been able
To pass any gas.

They're checking on whether
The digestive system was accidentally cut.
If so, that could truly become
A pain in the butt.

So here's a new perspective
That sounds silly to say.
Passing gas would become
A highlight of the day.

Finally it happened.
It sounded so good.
The system was intact,
Knock on wood.

But distension and swelling
Just wouldn't pass.
An occasional Maalox
Jostled passing more gas.

I don't know if I'm typical,
But the bottom line for me.
The cancer now is gone,
I'll deal with recovery.

CHAPTER 21

RADIATION THERAPY

Michelle H. Gurel
Brian D. Kavanagh, MD, MPH
Brian J. Moran, MD
Adam Raben, MD
David Raben, MD

RADIATION THERAPY USES HIGH-ENERGY RAYS or particles to kill cancer cells. Radiation is sometimes used to treat low-grade cancer that is still confined within the prostate gland or that has only spread to nearby tissue. If prostate cancer is more advanced, radiation may be used to reduce the size of the tumor and to provide relief from present symptoms and prevent future symptoms. (See chapter 29 for more information about treatments for recurrent or advanced cancer.)

Two main types of radiation therapy are available: external beam radiation and brachytherapy (internal radiation). Both can be effective methods of treating prostate cancer, although there is more information about long-term results of treatment with external beam radiation. Both types of radiation therapy are explored in this chapter.

What Is External Beam Radiation Therapy (EBRT)?

All forms of external beam radiation involve radiation beams focused on the prostate gland from a source outside your body. External beam radiation therapy (EBRT) remains a mainstay of treatment for men with localized prostate cancer.

Recent advances in the planning and delivery of radiation allow for more precisely aimed radiation beams and fewer effects on normal tissue. In the past 10 years, radiation treatment has evolved from using conventional x-rays to more advanced methods:

- **Three-dimensional conformal radiation therapy (3DCRT)** uses special computers to precisely map the location of your prostate and administer radiation. This method increases the precision of treatment and allows for increased radiation doses without increasing complications, resulting in improved outcomes.

- **Intensity-modulated radiotherapy (IMRT)** is an advanced form of three-dimensional therapy. Radiation beams are aimed from several directions, and the strength of the beams can be adjusted to minimize the dose of radiation reaching the most sensitive normal tissues. This reduces complications while still delivering a high dose of radiation to the cancer.

- **Conformal proton beam radiation therapy**, a technique related to 3DCRT, uses a similar approach. But instead of using x-rays (also called photons), this technique focuses proton beams on the cancer. Protons are positively charged subatomic particles that can destroy cancer cells in a manner similar to x-rays, but may cause less damage to the normal tissues they pass through, which might lead to fewer side effects. So far, treatment outcomes after proton therapy appear to be similar to outcomes reported after radiation therapy using x-ray therapy.

The following discussion will focus on the advantages, possible consequences, and expected outcomes of using external beam radiation therapy to treat early stage prostate cancer.

WHAT IS INVOLVED?

Before treatments start, imaging studies such as MRIs, CT scans, or x-rays help doctors find the exact location of your prostate gland. These images are of the prostate and critical structures within the pelvis, including the bladder and rectum, so you may be asked to empty your bowels with an enema the evening before the procedure and maintain a partially filled bladder just prior to the planning procedure.

The radiation team then marks the skin with ink marks they will use later as a guide to focus the radiation in the right area. The entire planning process may take 1 to 2 hours. Patients are generally asked to return 5 to 10 days later for additional checks before the actual radiation treatments.

When it is administered in standard daily doses, external beam treatment usually takes place 5 days a week in an outpatient center over a period of 7 to 9 weeks. The radiation technician or therapist controls the machine that delivers the beams from outside of the treatment room. Each treatment generally lasts only 10 to 15 minutes and is painless.

SHORTER RADIATION COURSES

Newer radiation approaches are examining the feasibility and potential side effects of *higher* individual daily doses of radiation given over a *shorter* period, typically fewer than 6 weeks. This approach has been studied extensively for early-stage prostate cancer and the treatment outcomes reported so far seem to be equivalent to those of standard external beam radiation and radical prostatectomy.

An even newer external beam treatment technique, stereotactic body radiation therapy, is under investigation in a few centers. The large, precise radiation dose is directed at a small tumor area and allows the course of treatment to be reduced to 6 to 8 treatments over 2 weeks.

An ultrasound image may be taken of the pelvis each day to determine if the prostate is in the proper position for treatment, as it may shift slightly.

Three-dimensional conformal radiation therapy uses special computers to precisely map the location of your prostate. Men undergoing this treatment are fitted with a plastic mold resembling a pelvic cast to keep them in a single position and minimize any movements during actual treatments. Radiation beams are then aimed from several directions.

Each week, special films are taken to ensure doctors are treating the exact areas intended.

After treatment, patients will be asked to return to their doctor every 3 to 6 months to check prostate-specific antigen (PSA) levels and to evaluate any residual side effects from the treatment.

WHEN MAY EXTERNAL BEAM RADIATION THERAPY BE APPROPRIATE?

External beam radiation therapy is an appropriate option as a primary treatment for men considered to have low-risk or early stage prostate cancer (PSA under 10, Gleason score of 6 or less, and T2 stage disease). Men at greater risk of advanced cancer may be offered combination therapy, for example, hormone therapy and EBRT or a combination of EBRT with a permanent or temporary brachytherapy seed implant (see page 209).

External beam radiation can also be used to help relieve bone pain where the cancer has spread to a specific area of bone (see chapter 29 for more information).

The effect of radiation on prostatic intraepithelial neoplasia (PIN) is unknown. Radiation is not used to treat PIN, but a man with PIN may undergo radiation therapy as a treatment for prostate cancer.

ADVANTAGES OF EXTERNAL BEAM RADIATION THERAPY

External beam radiation therapy is appropriate for men in varied situations. Patients with varied prognostic factors and pretreatment symptom status may choose EBRT. EBRT is essentially non-invasive, carries no anesthesia risk, and is available to many patients who are unable to tolerate either prostatectomy or brachytherapy. It also has other advantages, outlined here.

RISKS OF BOWEL AND RECTAL PROBLEMS ARE LOW

The use of 3DCRT has allowed higher doses of radiation to be delivered to the prostate by minimizing exposure of surrounding areas, such as rectal or bowel tissue. IMRT has allowed doctors to further tailor treatment, reducing the potential of rectal problems (in general, to less than 5 percent), even from the low levels that accompany three-dimensional conformal techniques. Facilities may use sequential CT scans, placement of intraprostatic (non-radioactive) seeds (see page 245), daily ultrasound, or even the daily placement of a rectal balloon to detect or prevent prostate motion during radiation therapy. This guards against inadvertently exposing the rectum or bowels to radiation.

ERECTILE FUNCTIONING IS OFTEN PRESERVED

Levels of erectile functioning after external beam radiotherapy are much higher than those of non-nerve-sparing prostatectomy and are similar to or slightly higher than with nerve-sparing prostatectomy. Although neurovascular bundles receive radiation, the nerves are not physically manipulated or severed as in a prostatectomy. Over the last several years, the introduction of medications such as sildenafil (Viagra) have improved assisted erectile functioning in a significant percentage of men undergoing EBRT.

MEN OFTEN ENJOY GOOD QUALITY OF LIFE

Quality-of-life parameters have been assessed in many different ways for prostate cancer patients. In general, men undergoing either radical prostatectomy or radiation have been reported to have similar overall quality of life scores. However, a recent study indicated that patients who underwent radical prostatectomy were more likely to report problems with sexual function and urinary incontinence than men undergoing EBRT. This is true although men undergoing EBRT are often older than those undergoing prostatectomy and have other health issues.

POTENTIAL CONSEQUENCES OF EXTERNAL BEAM RADIATION THERAPY

PROSTATE TISSUE IS NOT STUDIED

Because radiation doesn't remove the prostate, the treatment doesn't allow doctors to obtain information about the extent of cancer in the gland, as is possible through prostatectomy.

EBRT AFFECTS LATER TREATMENT OPTIONS

Having initial radiation therapy affects treatment options for men who need further treatment for cancer. If the cancer appears confined to the prostate, treatment options include hormone-blocking therapy, cryosurgery, or prostatectomy. However, performing a prostatectomy after radiation therapy is more difficult than performing a prostatectomy on a patient who has not had radiation therapy, and patients being considered for prostatectomy after radiation therapy should be certain that their urologist has had experience in this setting.

TREATMENT SIDE EFFECTS

The side effects of radiation treatment are caused by the effects of radiation on the normal tissues surrounding the tumor being targeted (with prostate cancer, these are usually the bladder and the lower intestines or rectum). Additionally, the nerves and blood vessels controlling erectile function pass along the outside of the prostate and receive a high dose of radiation during the course of treatment. Note that radiation should have no direct effect on sexual desire, but some patients find that the psychological stress of a diagnosis of cancer can have an indirect effect.

Early side effects of radiation are the typically mildly bothersome symptoms experienced by patients during the course of treatment, such as urinary side effects. They usually subside within a few weeks after the completion of treatment. Late effects, on the other hand, can develop weeks or months after the completion of treatment. Late effects usually result from the slow, ongoing process of scar tissue formation and other healing responses in normal tissues.

The most common early effects of radiotherapy for prostate cancer include fatigue, discomfort during urination and an increase in the frequency of urination, and diarrhea. Late effects can occur weeks or months after treatment is completed and may include bleeding from the bladder or rectum and erectile dysfunction.

Tissue damage. Modern radiation treatment technology allows a radiation oncologist to visualize and target the prostate precisely, limiting the amount of radiation received by the surrounding normal tissue. Nevertheless, a certain amount of radiation exposure to the normal tissues is unavoidable because the prostate is positioned so closely to the bladder and rectum. Fortunately, in the vast majority of patients, the surrounding normal tissues withstand the temporary inflammation caused by radiation and repair themselves successfully. It is very uncommon for a patient to experience serious permanent side effects in the bladder or rectum.

Fatigue. Fatigue probably results from the extra energy used in the body's response to the radiation, in particular the energy used to repair normal tissue. For most patients, fatigue is modest, perhaps enough to warrant an occasional extra nap during the day or some extra sleep at night for a few weeks after the completion of treatment. Patients are encouraged to maintain their ordinary activities and even to become more active if they are ordinarily inactive, because mild to moderate exercise during the course of treatment probably helps minimize the tiring effects.

Changes in urination. Radiation can irritate the inside lining of a portion of the bladder near the prostate and the urethra (the tube that carries urine from the bladder through the prostate). Pain medications usually relieve any discomfort. Approximately a third of patients experience changes in urination that resemble the symptoms of a bladder infection (such as pain or burning when you urinate and feeling the frequent need to urinate but urinating a small amount), and some of these patients do develop mild bladder infections that require antibiotics.

> ### Combating Fatigue
>
> Both the clinical trial vaccination treatment and my radiation treatment caused fatigue. Although I didn't always feel like exercising, I found that by walking 1 to 3 miles on a treadmill at about 3 miles per hour after each vaccination or radiation treatment I was able to pursue a near-normal level of activity and reduced fatigue so that I didn't miss a day of work.
>
> — *Philip*

Although low-grade urinary side effects occur frequently during external-beam radiation therapy, some severe urinary side effects are less frequent than in men who undergo prostatectomy or brachytherapy. In particular, the incontinence rate is lower than that for prostatectomy, and the urinary retention rate (the inability to urinate, which can be addressed through insertion of a temporary catheter) is lower than that for brachytherapy.

Uncommon but potential side effects of EBRT include increased urgency (the sense of needing to urinate), an increase in the frequency of urination, and waking up at night with the need to urinate, which can often be managed well with medication. Fortunately, urinary side effects are not experienced all the time, and a majority of men have symptoms that disappear over time.

Patients who have symptoms of urinary obstruction from benign prostatic hyperplasia (BPH) before the diagnosis of cancer often have a temporary worsening of these symptoms during their external beam radiation therapy. (If a brachytherapy implant is used, the side effects on urination are usually more noticeable.) Symptoms generally resolve within a few weeks of treatment.

Changes in bowel function. Changes in bowel pattern during radiation therapy are generally proportional to the amount of nearby intestines that receive radiation.

For more advanced cancers, it is usually best to give radiation not only to the prostate itself but also to the nearby lymph nodes that might contain small deposits of cancer. Because treatment to the lymph nodes involves giving radiation to a larger area of the intestines, a patient would likely have more diarrhea than a man who does not require treatment to lymph nodes. These problems can most often be controlled with non-prescription anti-diarrhea medicine for the few weeks they are present.

Bleeding in the rectum or bladder. As the inner surface linings of the bladder and rectum gradually continue to recover from the effects of radiation, these tissues create new blood vessels. The new blood vessels develop close to the surface and are often somewhat fragile until the healing process is complete. A small percentage of patients experience bleeding from these blood vessels and notice blood in the urine or in bowel movements. These symptoms usually resolve without treatment. In severe cases, the problem can almost always be well treated through medications or laser treatments to the blood vessels. It is extremely rare for a patient to require surgery to correct this type of problem.

Erectile dysfunction. One special concern with radiation treatment for prostate cancer is the chance of impairing a man's ability to have an unassisted erection.

Radiation impairs erectile function, probably because it narrows or blocks some of the small blood vessels that supply blood to the penis and cause an erection. Nerves in the body are usually able to tolerate high doses of radiation without noticeable injury, so it is unlikely that radiation therapy would injure the nerves involved in controlling erections.

After radiation, men generally retain sensitivity to touch in the genital area and also the ability to achieve the sensation of orgasm. Some physicians encourage patients to sustain or even increase their frequency of sexual activity throughout their course of treatment to maximize their chances of maintaining erectile function. See chapter 30 for information about medications, pump devices, injections, and implants that may address erectile dysfunction.

Prostate cancer is most commonly diagnosed in older men, and many patients with prostate cancer already have a limited ability to develop erections as a result of high blood pressure, diabetes, or another medical condition. Men who have a normal capacity for erections before radiation therapy have a significant chance of experiencing difficulty in achieving the same degree of erections after treatment. An estimated 30 to 50 percent of men undergoing radiation experience erectile dysfunction (the rates are the same with external beam treatment and brachytherapy; it is possible that combining the treatments might increase the rate of problems). For more advanced cancers, radiation treatment is often combined with therapy that suppresses the production of male hormones (and decreases sexual desire).

EXPECTED OUTCOMES

A recent comparison of surgery to external radiation therapy showed that what is generally considered the minimum effective radiation dose of 72 Gray (Gy; the effects of higher doses are being explored) to be as effective as surgery and permanent seed brachytherapy. PSA levels during the 10 years following radiation therapy are about the same as with surgical options, and the effect of radiation therapy on PSA appears to be comparable to the effect of radical prostatectomy on PSA. (Generally, when cancer is present, the higher the PSA level is, the larger the prostate cancer is and the more likely it is to have spread beyond the prostate.)

Although the three-dimensional conformal radiation therapy procedure is relatively new, the short-term results suggest that it is at least as effective as EBRT. As with three-dimensional conformal radiation, preliminary results of conformal proton beam radiation therapy are promising, but a long-term advantage over standard external beam radiation has not yet been proven. Also, proton beam radiation is expensive, and there are very few proton beam devices in the United States at this time.

Treatment success depends heavily on large clinical experiences; a treatment center with high-dose conformal radiation therapy should have available data about outcomes to compare to other published results.

What Is Brachytherapy?

Brachytherapy is a cancer treatment that uses ionizing radiation to destroy cancer cells. The radioactive material is placed either directly into a malignant tumor or very close to it, thus the term brachytherapy, which means *short therapy* in Greek. Radiation (including external beam radiation) kills the tumor by destroying the deoxyribonucleic acid (DNA, which holds genetic information on cell growth, division, and function) within the cancer cell. When the cancer cell attempts to divide and reproduce itself, it is unable to do so because the DNA is no longer intact and as a result, the cell dies.

Doctors used brachytherapy to treat cancer as long ago as the early 1900s. Over the past twenty years, technology has resulted in dramatic advancements in prostate brachytherapy. Improved ultrasound equipment used to visualize the prostate and precisely guide the placement of radioactive seeds allows for the delivery of a very high dose of radiation to the prostate while minimizing the dose of radiation to the surrounding normal body organs such as the bladder and rectum. The development of computer systems has allowed even more precise brachytherapy. As a result, brachytherapy has become very popular as a treatment option for patients diagnosed with early stage prostate cancer. In 1994, only 8 percent of urologists polled were familiar with the current form of brachytherapy; today more than 90 percent are actively involved with this procedure.

There are 2 common types of prostate brachytherapy: permanent low dose rate (LDR) and temporary high dose rate (HDR). During LDR, also called a permanent seed implant, radioactive materials in the form of "seeds," which are each about the size and shape of a grain of rice, are deposited in the prostate and left in place indefinitely. HDR brachytherapy involves placing radioactive materials in the prostate for a specified period of time and then removing them. Prostate brachytherapy can be performed using either a permanent implant or a temporary implant, but never both.

The total amount of radiation the prostate will receive depends upon the amount of radiation in each seed and the total number of seeds deposited. A typical implant usually requires 60 to 100 seeds, depending on the size and shape of a patient's prostate gland.

WHAT IS INVOLVED?

PREPARATION

Ultrasound images allow the doctors to determine the exact shape and size of the prostate. This is not unlike having a suit made; the tailor must first measure your chest, arm length, and inseam so that he can make the material to custom-fit your body. The ultrasound takes approximately 15 to 30 minutes. Outlining the area of the prostate where the cancer was identified on biopsy also assists doctors in treatment planning. These pictures are then reconstructed on a three-dimensional treatment planning computer, which allows the physician to determine exactly how many seeds are needed and where they should be placed within the prostate gland and in relation to the urethra, bladder, and rectum.

THE PROCEDURE

Typically, patients arrive 1 hour before the procedure. A clear liquid diet is advised the day before and nothing should be eaten after midnight before the procedure. (These recommendations minimize gas and allow better visualization of the prostate.)

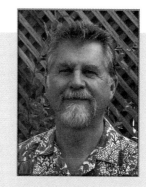

A Proton Beam Therapy Experience

After a lot of research into treatments and side effects I decided proton beam therapy was right for me and my situation. I was able to exercise and enjoy life throughout treatment. Each of my 40 treatments over a 9-week period lasted only 45 seconds, and the side effects were minor. Three months after treatment my PSA was down from 14.9 to .07.

– *Allen*

Conformal Beam Radiation

I monitored my rising PSA for 3 or 4 years. After a biopsy showed 3 areas of cancer with 3 different Gleason scores, I underwent three-dimensional conformal radiation plus hormone blockade. Since 1996 my PSA has held to 1.5 to 2.0 with negative scans and lymph node biopsies.

– *Melvin*

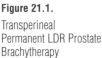

Figure 21.1.
Transperineal
Permanent LDR Prostate
Brachytherapy

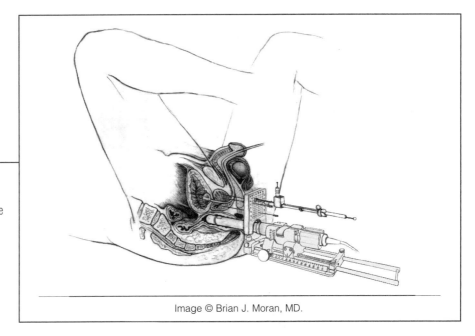

Image © Brian J. Moran, MD.

In the operating room, a fluoroscope (a type of x-ray machine) is positioned over the patient's pelvis to visualize certain parts of the procedure. The placement of needles that contain the radioactive seeds is guided by the use of ultrasound and fluoroscopy. The implant needles are no wider in diameter than those typically used to draw blood and are directed into predetermined areas of the prostate. However, these needles are longer (as long as 8 inches) so they may reach the prostate through the perineum. The needles are inserted through the perineum into the prostate and are then withdrawn, leaving the radioactive materials within the prostate gland.

Typically, men do not experience pain, either during or after the procedure, because either general or spinal anesthesia is given. After the procedure, patients may complain of a dull ache in the area; however, pain requiring anything more than a regular-strength acetaminophen (Tylenol) is extremely unusual. Patients who have general anesthesia can expect 1 to 2 hours of anesthesia and are usually up and walking within a half hour after the procedure. Patients who receive a spinal anesthesia are usually mobile within 2 to 3 hours. Medications given upon discharge from the treatment center usually include antibiotics, anti-inflammatories such as ibuprofen (Advil and Motrin, for example), and alpha-blockers (drugs that allow easier urination).

In an outpatient procedure setting, a man is able to go home approximately 1½ to 2 hours after the implant. Hospitalization after discharge is rare. Some

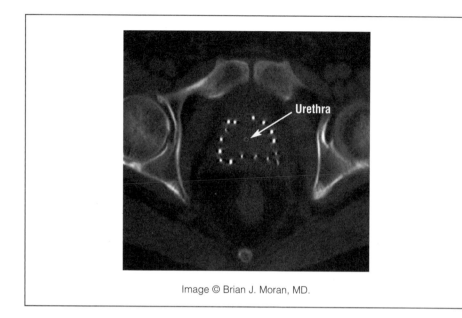

Urethra

Figure 21.2.

CT Scan Showing Implants Around the Urethra

Image © Brian J. Moran, MD.

institutions, however, prefer to have their patients stay in the hospital overnight to be observed.

After the implant has been performed, it is important to know exactly where the radioactive seeds are located. A CT scan of the prostate identifies the prostate gland and the seeds within it. These images are then entered into a computer, and the actual distribution of radiation in and around the prostate is determined. This information is valuable for future follow-up care. For patient convenience, most institutions will perform the CT scan on the same day of the prostate implant.

THE TREATMENT PLAN

Each implant is individually planned to determine the optimal distribution of radiation. Your radiation oncologist and a team of medical physicists are specially trained to understand the best dose of radiation to give to the prostate while also protecting the rectum and bladder from radiation.

Controversy exists among experts as to the best way to design the actual prostate implant, the exact number of seeds, and their arrangement within the prostate gland (see Table 21.1). Many institutions recommend a preplanned approach, while others believe it is better to determine the plan at the time of implant in a "real-time" approach. Neither approach has clearly been proven superior. Others recommend a combination of both philosophies—for example, a prostate volume study 2 weeks before the actual implant and any necessary adjustments in the operating room just prior to the implant. This approach may offer the patient every option to achieve the best outcome.

Table 21.1. COMPARING PRETREATMENT PLANNING AND INTRAOPERATIVE "REAL-TIME" PLANNING

	Pretreatment Planning	Intraoperative Planning
Timing	• Performed days/weeks prior to procedure, shortly after volume study	• Performed on day of procedure, after patient is anesthetized and just prior to implant
Potential Advantages	• Allows for comprehensive review of plan, consultation with colleagues on difficult cases	• Limits variation in prostate and patient positions between planning session and implant
	• Enables staff to calculate and order correct number of seeds	• Minimizes changes in prostate volume between planning session and implant
Potential Consequences	• Patient discomfort may lead to inadequate visualization of gland during volume study	• Greater risk of ordering inaccurate number of seeds
	• Patient position may vary between planning session and implant	• Requires greater skill on part of implant team
	• Prostate volume and position may vary between planning session and implant	• Increases operation room time and cost of procedure

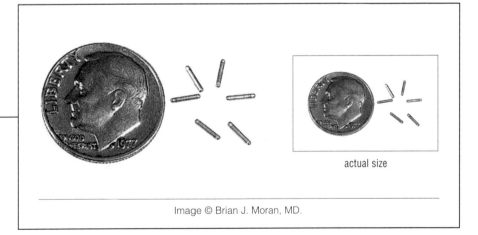

Figure 21.3.

Radioactive Seeds
Next to a Dime

actual size

Image © Brian J. Moran, MD.

WHAT ARE HALF-LIVES?

Iodine has a half-life of 60 days, meaning that in 60 days, 50 percent of the radiation in iodine will be released (with brachytherapy, it is released into the prostate tumor). In another 60 days, half of that 50 percent will be gone, leaving 25 percent of the original amount of radiation after 120 days. Palladium has a half-life of 17 days, and therefore releases radiation more quickly. As a general rule, almost the entire amount of an implant's radiation is given out after a time of 5 half-lives. Patients who receive iodine will have minimal, if any, radiation left within their body after 300 days, while those with palladium will no longer have radiation in their bodies after 85 days. (While radiation is present, it is limited to the prostate and surrounding tissue within 1 centimeter of the gland.)

PERMANENT LOW DOSE BRACHYTHERAPY

A permanent prostate implant (also known as LDR) is performed using either radioactive iodine (I^{125}) or palladium (Pd^{103}) in the form of small radioactive seeds.

Either iodine or palladium is chosen for each implant, never both, because if these seeds were mixed, measuring the radiation precisely would be impossible.

There is believed to be no outcome benefit of using one type of seed versus the other. Iodine tends to cause fewer intense urinary side effects, but they may last many more months than the more intense, shorter duration of urinary side effects of palladium.

By being located close to or within the cancer, the radioactive seeds can deliver a very large amount of radiation in an area no larger than a centimeter while the adjacent area receives minimal, if any, radiation. A physician can therefore implant high doses of radiation into the prostate while avoiding normal critical structures such as the bladder and rectum.

HIGH DOSE RATE BRACHYTHERAPY

Temporary brachytherapy, also known as high dose rate (HDR) brachytherapy, requires the use of a different radioactive isotope, usually iridium-192 (Ir^{192}). Treatment using HDR brachytherapy is similar to permanent prostate brachytherapy in the way it is performed; however, needles placed into the prostate gland are then replaced with nylon tubes called catheters. The HDR machine is attached to the catheters and is programmed by a computer to temporarily position the high-activity source of iridium for specific amounts of time at each location within each catheter.

The total radiation dose given with this type of implant is usually divided into 3 to 4 treatments (or fractions) over a 2-day period while the patient is kept in the hospital. Between each treatment, the patient is disconnected from the HDR machine and returns to his room. After the final treatment fraction, the nylon catheters are removed from the patient and he is discharged. This type of implant is usually performed in combination with a 5-week course of external beam radiation therapy to the prostate. HDR brachytherapy is rarely, if ever, given without supplemental external beam radiation.

WHEN MAY BRACHYTHERAPY BE APPROPRIATE?

Typically, the best candidate for brachytherapy is someone with a small prostate tumor confined to the prostate gland and a very low risk of spreading to other parts of the body.

Brachytherapy alone is not appropriate for patients whose cancer has already spread beyond the prostate and into other areas of the body. Patients who have had a transurethral resection of the prostate (TURP) may have brachytherapy; however, they will need to meet certain criteria. A person with a large prostate or a prostate that is inaccessible to visualize with ultrasound (such as if the anus or rectum has been previously removed) may not be suited for brachytherapy and may be treated instead with EBRT or surgery. For men with large prostate glands, a short course of hormone therapy may be given first to reduce the overall size of the gland.

ADVANTAGES OF BRACHYTHERAPY

Because brachytherapy is an outpatient procedure, a patient usually walks out only hours after the procedure. Furthermore, the seed implant is complete in a single visit, while external beam radiation takes several weeks. Blood loss during a brachytherapy implant is minimal when compared to surgery, and pain is typically negligible. Incontinence rates are usually less than 1 percent. Erectile medications and other aids have proven to be very effective for men who do experience erectile dysfunction (see page 212) after brachytherapy. Perhaps most importantly, cure rates with brachytherapy in men with low-risk disease are essentially equal to other treatment options, including surgery and external beam radiation therapy.

HOW MUCH RADIATION IS ENOUGH?

The amount of radiation delivered to the edge of the prostate is fairly standard for patients: 145 Gy (gray, a unit of radiation) for iodine, between 115 and 120 Gy for palladium. The American Brachytherapy Society provides suggested doses if no prior radiation has been given to the prostate gland. Doses delivered to deep within the prostate can be much higher, reaching up to twice that at the edge of the gland. Most experts recommend a peripherally loaded implant—that is, placing the seeds in the edge of the prostate, away from the urethra.

The extent of treatment a patient requires depends on the likelihood that the cancer is confined to the prostate. As a rule, low-risk patients require one treatment, such as permanent seed implant.

It is often recommended that men at intermediate risk for cancer that has spread undergo more aggressive treatment. At a minimum, this means a combination of hormone therapy plus an implant, or could involve more aggressive measures, such as adding 5 weeks of EBRT to an implant. The purpose of the additional EBRT is to kill any cancer cells that may have escaped the prostate and are in the tissue around the prostate.

High-risk patients may also benefit from brachytherapy, but this is usually done in combination with EBRT and hormone therapy. Unfortunately, in this group of patients, there is still a significant risk of cancer metastasizing (spreading) to other parts of the body. If the cancer is not controlled and is allowed to grow, patients may experience significant urinary bleeding and pain.

POTENTIAL CONSEQUENCES OF BRACHYTHERAPY

URINARY SIDE EFFECTS

Typical side effects of prostate brachytherapy are primarily urinary; patients may feel the urge to urinate more frequently for approximately 3 months. Some patients may actually be unable to urinate because of prostate swelling after the implant. However, it is very rare that patients require the use of a catheter for longer than 1 week.

Brachytherapy is very unlikely to result in total urinary incontinence. The risk of any level of urinary incontinence after brachytherapy of the prostate is negligible. As a result of improved technology, avoiding unnecessary radiation to the muscles that control urine and preventing urinary leakage is possible. Most experts today would say that the likelihood of developing total incontinence (requiring a diaper) is less than 1 percent.

SEXUAL SIDE EFFECTS

Due to the variations in how erectile dysfunction is defined and measured, it is difficult to quote an exact impotency rate. Impotency (defined in this case as some degree of erectile dysfunction but not necessarily complete inability to have an erection) rate estimates following brachytherapy range from 6 to 50 percent. Because nerves are still intact after brachytherapy, sildenafil (Viagra) has been extremely helpful in providing assisted erections for patients who experience some erectile dysfunction. Newer drugs may also have similar benefits (see chapter 30 for more information). As technology evolves and brachytherapy continues to improve, lower erectile dysfunction rates are anticipated.

Patients can have sex after an implant, however, waiting approximately 2 weeks before doing so is recommended.

Patients may experience some sexual side effects after their seed implant. A painful orgasm may be experienced the first few times, but this is very unusual and will go away. Blood in the ejaculate is very uncommon but can occur temporarily and may last up to 2 weeks. After a few months, it is normal for patients to experience a dry ejaculate. This means that a person can have an orgasm but there will be little, if any, semen.

The prostate is essential for reproduction. After prostate brachytherapy, doctors believe a man is no longer fertile because the prostate gland has been destroyed. Therefore, if a patient is going to have brachytherapy but may want to father children in the future, he is strongly encouraged to bank sperm prior to radiation therapy.

RECTAL PROBLEMS

Rectal problems after brachytherapy are very unusual and most often take the form of an irritation that causes a sudden urge to have bowel movements—and, less commonly, causes pain or bleeding.

A more serious potential complication is that of rectal injury. Rectal injury rarely occurs, especially if the implant has been properly performed. Typically, patients with rectal injury complain of pain, blood in the stool, and bowel irritability (a rare and temporary irregular pattern of bowel activity and increased frequency of bowel movements due to radiation). Serious rectal injuries may include a rectal ulcer (damaged tissue in the rectum), the result of too much radiation.

Do I Pose a Radiation Risk to My Family, Pets, or the Public?

When it comes to radiation safety, no one will know a patient has received implants unless he says so. The seed implant or any of the potential side effects will not temporarily or permanently change one's appearance. Permanent seeds will remain within the prostate gland for the remainder of the patient's life but are not a threat to the patient's health during their lifetime. The seeds typically lose their radioactivity over the course of several months. (Patients receiving high dose rate brachytherapy do not leave the treatment center with any radioactivity in them.)

Furthermore, studies show that there is no need to worry about exposing others to radiation. The seeds are placed into the prostate so radiation only affects the prostate and does not affect surrounding tissues. A more recent study states that radiation exposure to family members from a patient receiving a permanent prostate brachytherapy implant with radioactive iodine or palladium is very low and well below the limits recommended by the U.S. Nuclear Regulatory Commission. It states that radiation exposure to members of a patient's family or to the public should not be a deterrent to undergoing this procedure.

Still, as a precaution, your doctor may recommend that you do not come into close contact with small children or pregnant women for a time, especially right after the procedure. Your doctor may also suggest using a condom during sex for a certain period of time.

When traveling, patients with prostate seed implants can indeed walk through metal detectors at the airport without setting off the alarm. Today, however, people are also screened for radiation, and even though the majority of the radiation is confined deep within the body, these very sensitive detectors can pick up even the smallest amount of radiation. As a result, patients who have had brachytherapy should ask for a wallet-sized card listing radioactive information as well as an emergency number if the authorities need more information. This situation would be uncommon, but could possibly occur.

OTHER POTENTIAL SIDE EFFECTS

Radioactive seeds, on rare occasions, can migrate out of the prostate gland. Your doctor may ask that you strain your urine for a week or so after the procedure to capture any seeds in the urine. Seeds can also rarely enter the bloodstream and be deposited in one of the lungs, although this has not been known to cause any ill effects. Fortunately, this is very uncommon and with newer techniques including the use of seeds that are attached to each other, migration is no longer an issue.

EXPECTED OUTCOMES

Results for prostate brachytherapy are available for patients treated over 10 years ago and show outcomes equal to those of radical prostatectomy and EBRT. Approximately 80 to 85 percent of low-risk patients are successfully treated, as are two thirds of men at intermediate risk, and a third of high-risk patients. For an aggressive cancer, a combination of radiation seeds and external beam radiation is recommended and is more likely to achieve better success rates.

While the physical properties of radioactive isotopes will remain the same, prostate brachytherapy will only improve as technology evolves. Furthermore, as clinical studies mature and the data is analyzed, physicians in the field will be better prepared to more precisely identify the specific criteria that will allow even better patient selection for this procedure.

CHAPTER 22

HORMONAL THERAPY (ANDROGEN DEPRIVATION THERAPY)

Christopher L. Amling, MD
Judd W. Moul, MD

A HORMONE IS A PROTEIN PRODUCED BY ONE OF THE BODY'S MANY GLANDS or organs that causes or controls a bodily function. The human body makes many hormones to help our bodies grow and carry out their many activities.

How Hormones Affect Prostate Cancer

Male hormones, called androgens, are produced mainly in the testicles. A small amount is also made in the adrenal glands, which are small glands that sit on top of each kidney.

Androgens, especially testosterone, are responsible for many uniquely male features that appear after puberty, including lower voice, male hair patterns, and the male libido, or sex drive. They are also responsible for the growth and development of the normal prostate gland. Prostate cells, both normal and cancerous, have receptors on their surfaces that allow them to grow when testosterone is present. (This is why removing this hormone can be an effective form of treatment.)

Testosterone levels in the body are tightly controlled by other hormones produced in the brain. A small area of the brain called the hypothalamus acts like a thermostat, sensing when testosterone levels are too high or too low. If more testosterone is needed, the hypothalamus secretes *luteinizing hormone-releasing hormone (LHRH)*, which causes the pituitary gland at the base of the brain to release another hormone called *luteinizing hormone (LH)*. LH then travels through the bloodstream to the testicles, where it stimulates them to make testosterone. The testosterone can then travel to other parts of the body, including the prostate. There it attaches to receptors on the surface of prostate cells, which encourages them to grow.

What Is Hormonal Therapy?

Hormonal therapy is any type of treatment that somehow affects prostate cancer cells' ability to use testosterone to grow. Because there are several steps involved in getting testosterone to the prostate cells, there are different ways to affect the use of testosterone. Hormonal therapy may either stop the body's *production* of hormones, or it may stop cancer cells from *using* hormones.

The goal of hormonal therapy is to make prostate cancers shrink or grow more slowly, but hormone therapy alone will not usually completely rid the body of cancer. Unlike surgery or radiation therapy, hormonal therapy has the advantage of reaching all parts of the body, so it can affect prostate cancer cells even if they've spread to other areas and can't be seen.

Traditionally, hormonal therapy has most often been used in men with metastatic prostate cancer, but doctors are now exploring its use earlier in the course of the disease. It is now often used to shrink tumors before or during (and sometimes continuing after) other treatment, such as surgery or radiation.

The main hormonal therapy options discussed in this chapter are listed here:

- **LHRH agonists:** medications that cause the testicles to stop producing testosterone
- **orchiectomy:** surgical removal of the testicles (also known as castration)
- **antiandrogens:** medications that block prostate cells from using testosterone made by the testicles and the adrenal glands
- **combination hormonal therapy:** an LHRH agonist or an orchiectomy plus daily antiandrogens

Several other types of hormonal therapy, including LHRH antagonists, estrogens (female hormones), and drugs that affect the adrenal glands (ketoconazole and aminoglutethamide) are also used at times (see chapter 29 for more information about estrogens and adrenal inhibitors). They are usually reserved for men whose cancers are no longer responding to initial hormonal treatments.

WHAT IS INVOLVED?

After the discovery in the early 1940s that prostate cancer growth was influenced by testosterone, orchiectomy (see page 224 for more information) became

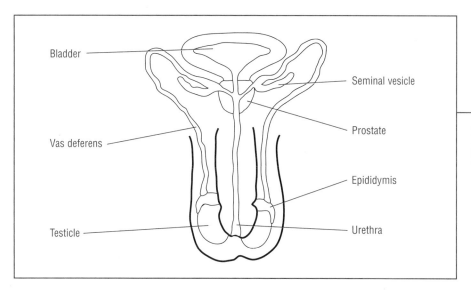

Bladder

Seminal vesicle

Prostate

Vas deferens

Epididymis

Testicle

Urethra

Figure 22.1.
Male Genitals and
Urinary Organs

the mainstay of treatment for metastatic prostate cancer. At the time, doctors thought all testosterone was produced by a man's testicles.

About 20 years ago, doctors realized that the body's adrenal glands also produce male hormones. The adrenal glands are small, crescent-shaped organs that are located above both kidneys and produce 5 to 10 percent of a man's testosterone. A theory was offered that this source of androgens could contribute to prostate cancer growth. Although these glands are responsible for a relatively small amount of testosterone, many doctors believe that it is important to block or eliminate this source of hormones as well.

WHEN MAY HORMONAL THERAPY BE APPROPRIATE?

Patients who may be treated with hormonal therapy include men with metastatic prostate cancer, men with locally spread prostate cancer, and men with early recurrence of prostate cancer after initial treatments such as surgery or radiation. Hormonal therapy can also be very effective for elderly men with early stage prostate cancer or for men in poor overall health who are not candidates for surgery or radiation.

TO ALLEVIATE SYMPTOMS OF METASTATIC CANCER

When prostate cancer is thought to be confined to the prostate gland itself, treatment usually focuses on trying to treat the cancer through surgery (see chapter 20), external beam radiation, brachytherapy (seed implant radiation; see chapter 21), or other treatments such as cryotherapy (see chapter 24) to eradicate the cancer locally. Traditionally, hormonal therapy has been used to treat men with metastatic prostate cancer (cancer that has spread) to alleviate symptoms of cancer rather than to attempt to cure the cancer.

WITH EARLIER STAGE CANCERS AND INTERMITTENT USE

Orchiectomy was once the only hormonal therapy option, and because it was irreversible, it was reserved for patients with advanced metastatic disease. Now, because of the availability of reversible LHRH agonist injections and antiandrogen pills, hormonal therapy may be used on earlier stage cancers. It has also become more common to use intermittent hormonal therapy (alternating periods of therapy with periods of no treatment; see page 225).

WITH OTHER CANCER TREATMENT

Hormonal therapy may also be used as an *adjuvant* (additional) treatment for some early stage prostate cancers. For example, it may be given along with radiation in an attempt to make the radiation more effective, and it may kill cancer cells that could have escaped the prostate prior to or during other treatments.

BEFORE OTHER CANCER TREATMENT

Neoadjuvant hormonal therapy is treatment used before primary treatment— for example, before surgery or before and during radiation treatments—to shrink the prostate gland or the prostate tumor. Men who choose brachytherapy may have neoadjuvant hormonal therapy to shrink the prostate gland and allow for proper seed radiation placement. For men with larger prostate glands (larger than 40 or 50 cubic centimeters, typically; average prostates are closer to 20 to 30 cubic centimeters), neoadjuvant hormonal therapy is usually recommended for a period of months before brachytherapy. (Shrinking the prostate with hormonal therapy is usually not necessary before surgery or external beam radiation.)

LUTEINIZING HORMONE-RELEASING HORMONE (LHRH) AGONISTS

Years ago, estrogen (female hormone) pills were used to block the effects of testosterone. These are now rarely used as initial hormonal therapy because they can cause side effects such as heart attacks and strokes. The medicines currently used are injections called LHRH agonists, which do not have these side effects.

LHRH agonists (also known as LHRH analogs) are medications that cause the testicles to stop making testosterone. Some people refer to these medicines as a

Table 22.1. HORMONAL THERAPY OPTIONS

Hormonal Therapy	How It Is Given	How It Works	Factors to Consider
LHRH agonists	Usually given by injection, either into a muscle or underneath the skin. A small implantable rod is another option.	Disrupt signals to the pituitary gland, causing the testicles to stop producing testosterone	• Require repeated visits and may be expensive, but allow men to avoid the removal of the testicles • Allow for temporary or intermittent hormone therapy • May be given alone or with an antiandrogen in combination hormonal therapy
Orchiectomy	Surgical removal of the testicles	Eliminates the source of most of the body's testosterone production	• Simple and effective • One time procedure that is less expensive than other options, but is permanent • Men may have difficulty accepting the removal of the testicles
Combination hormonal therapy	LHRH agonist or an orchiectomy plus daily antiandrogens	(See individual hormonal options for details)	(See individual hormonal options for details)
Antiandrogens	Pills taken daily or several times a day	Block prostate cells from using androgens	• Used with LHRH agonists or orchiectomy in combined hormonal therapy • Being tested for use alone and with other oral medications
LHRH antagonists	Given by injection into a muscle	Disrupt signals to the pituitary gland, causing the testicles to stop producing testosterone	• May cause an allergic reaction • Approved for use only in men with serious symptoms from advanced prostate cancer and who cannot or refuse to take other forms of hormonal therapy

Table 22.2. LHRH AGONISTS

LHRH agonists are listed on the left; dosage and delivery options and factors to consider related to side effects for all LHRH agonists are also listed.

LHRH Agonists	Options for Delivery and Dosage Frequency	Potential Side Effects Include
leuprolide acetate (Lupron or Eligard)	• Injection every month, 3 months, 4 months, or 6 months • Implant every year • Intramuscular injection (Lupron) or subcutaneous injection (given under the skin; Eligard)	• Hot flashes, tumor flare, bone pain, constipation, decreased sex drive, impotence, dizziness, breast swelling or tenderness, long-term bone thinning (osteoporosis)
leuprolide acetate (Viadur)	• Titanium implant releases medication for 1 year	
goserelin acetate (Zoladex)	• Subcutaneous injection every month or every 3 months	
triptorelin (Trelstar)	• Intramuscular injection every month	

"medical orchiectomy," a "medical castration," or a "chemical castration" because they are equivalent to the effect produced by orchiectomy surgery.

The LHRH agonists work by stopping the pituitary gland from releasing luteinizing hormone (LH), the main hormone that causes the testicles to produce testosterone. When the LHRH agonists eliminate the supply of LH, the testicles stop producing testosterone.

WHAT IS INVOLVED?

LHRH agonists are most often given by injection, either into a muscle (usually in the buttocks) or underneath the skin. It is important that men get treated on schedule and not skip any treatments unless directed by their doctor. LHRH agonists may be given alone or with an antiandrogen in combination hormonal therapy (also called combined androgen blockade).

The LHRH agonists available in the United States are leuprolide acetate (Lupron or Eligard), goserelin acetate (Zoladex), and triptorelin (Trelstar). Leuprolide acetate is available as an injection in doses lasting 1, 3, 4 or 6 months. Goserelin acetate implant is available as a 1-month and 3-month injection, and triptorelin is an injection given once a month. A 1-year leuprolide acetate implant (Viadur) is also available. It is a small titanium rod that is implanted in the upper arm and releases medication for a year.

ADVANTAGES OF LHRH AGONISTS

Most men choose LHRH agonists over surgical orchiectomy. LHRH agonists eliminate the need for the removal of the testicles.

Some men taking LHRH agonists find the need for periodic visits to their doctor an advantage because they get to check in regularly and feel they are under more active surveillance. (Other men find the same visits a disadvantage because of time or schedule requirements.)

Unlike orchiectomy, the use of LHRH agonists is reversible—that is, the medication can be stopped if needed because of side effects or if a man is on an intermittent hormonal therapy schedule.

POSSIBLE CONSEQUENCES OF LHRH AGONISTS

Please see page 228 of this chapter, *Possible Consequences for Any Hormonal Treatment*, for side effects and other factors common to the 3 main hormonal treatments discussed in this chapter. The issues outlined here are more specific to LHRH agonists.

Tumor flare. When beginning LHRH agonist therapy, men may experience an increase or surge in testosterone levels as a result of increased testosterone production by the testicles. This is called tumor flare. Tumor flare may cause bone pain or, rarely, more serious complications if the tumor is in an important location, such as the spine. Giving short-term antiandrogen therapy (see page 222) before LHRH agonist treatment helps prevent this flare.

Access and cost. Treatment with LHRH agonists is more expensive than orchiectomy, and the costs continue as long as a man is on treatment.

In 2004 the Medicare program lowered the reimbursement rate doctors receive for administering LHRH agonists. This rate change may make it more difficult for some men to receive LHRH agonists or may increase out-of-pocket costs, and may change again in the future.

Long-term treatment. LHRH agonists, like antiandrogens, require men to take either periodic or constant dosages to prevent androgen production. Therefore hormonal treatment is generally a long-term treatment.

LHRH ANTAGONISTS

A newer drug, abarelix (Plenaxis), is an LHRH *antagonist*, another type of medicine that lowers testosterone levels in the blood. It is thought to work in a similar way to LHRH agonists, but it appears to lower testosterone levels more quickly and does not cause tumor flare like LHRH agonists do.

However, in clinical trials, a small percentage of men (fewer than 5 percent) had serious allergic reactions to the drug. Because of this, it is approved for use only in men who have serious symptoms from advanced prostate cancer and who cannot or refuse to take other forms of hormonal therapy.

Abarelix is given only in qualified doctors' offices. It is injected into the buttocks every 2 weeks for the first month, then every 4 weeks. Men taking abarelix are asked to remain in the office for 30 minutes after the injection to make sure they are not having an allergic reaction.

Bone thinning (osteoporosis). Recent studies have shown that long-term use of LHRH agonists can lead to significant losses in bone density, which can place a man at risk for bone fractures. Some doctors are now recommending that men have their bone density monitored while on treatment.

EXPECTED OUTCOMES

The expected outcomes of LHRH agonists are the same as those of orchiectomy; see page 229 for information about these outcomes.

ANTIANDROGEN THERAPY

Recall that LHRH agonists work by stopping the pituitary gland from releasing luteinizing hormone, which in turn causes the testicles to stop production of testosterone. Antiandrogens, in contrast, stop prostate cancer cells from using testosterone that has already been produced by the testicles or the adrenal glands.

WHAT IS INVOLVED?

Antiandrogens, which are taken daily in pill form, include drugs such as bicalutamide (Casodex), flutamide (Eulexin), and nilutamide (Nilandron).

Your doctor may prescribe an LHRH agonist or an orchiectomy along with an antiandrogen. This combination hormonal therapy may provide a small survival advantage for men with metastatic prostate cancer over an LHRH agonist or orchiectomy alone.

Table 22.3. ANTIANDROGENS

The following table outlines important facts about antiandrogens.

Antiandrogens	Potential Side Effects and Other Information
bicalutamide (Casodex)	• 50 mg given once daily as part of complete hormonal therapy with an LHRH agonist • low level of gastrointestinal side effects
flutamide (Eulexin)	• 250 mg given 3 times daily • some patients may experience diarrhea, and in rare cases patients may experience liver dysfunction • first FDA-approved antiandrogen as part of combined hormonal therapy
nilutamide (Nilandron)	• 300 mg given daily for a month, then 150 mg given daily thereafter • used least often because of unusual but possible side effects of alcohol intolerance and delayed visual adaptation to light changes

Antiandrogens are also being tested for their effectiveness when used alone or in combination with other oral drugs, such as 5-alpha reductase inhibitors (medications that prevent testosterone from being converted to a more active hormone), for earlier stages of prostate cancer.

ADVANTAGES OF ANTIANDROGEN THERAPY

Antiandrogen therapy may be used as part of combined hormonal therapy or alone. Adding antiandrogens to LHRH agonist treatment may provide a small survival advantage for men with metastatic prostate cancer. Antiandrogens are not currently approved for use without another hormonal therapy, but antiandrogens alone may not cause some of the side effects that may accompany LHRH agonists, such as decreased sex drive. The use of antiandrogens without other hormonal treatment is being studied in clinical trials.

POSSIBLE CONSEQUENCES OF ANTIANDROGEN THERAPY

See page 228, *Possible Consequences for Any Hormonal Treatment*, for side effects and other factors common to the hormonal treatments discussed in this chapter. Factors to consider that are more specific to antiandrogens may include:

Cost. Antiandrogens are generally expensive and may be a burden for men whose insurance does not cover oral cancer treatment medicines. Antiandrogen manufacturers have programs for needy patients. Flutamide is now available as a generic drug so it may be less expensive, although it must be taken 3 times per day. (To learn about pharmaceutical patient assistance programs for hormonal treatment and instructions for finding out if you may qualify, see page 126 of chapter 14.)

Dosage frequency. The frequency of doses is a potential disadvantage of taking antiandrogens; some must be taken several times per day, and men may forget to take all the needed medicine. Like LHRH agonists, antiandrogens must be taken at least intermittently for the rest of a man's life in order to prevent prostate cancer cells from using these hormones.

Side effects. Overall, antiandrogens are very safe, and all of the potential problems listed here are rare or uncommon. In rare cases, antiandrogens may cause liver dysfunction. Typically your doctor will monitor your liver with blood tests periodically and will discontinue the antiandrogen if significant liver abnormalities occur. Liver problems due to antiandrogen use are almost always reversible upon discontinuation of the drug. Men with known liver disease may not be good candidates for treatment.

The antiandrogen flutamide may cause diarrhea in 10 to 15 percent of men. Taking a lower dose or switching to another antiandrogen may eliminate the problem.

Nilutamide may cause a delayed adaptation to darkness, which may affect nighttime driving, and it may also cause alcohol intolerance. In rare cases nilutamide may cause pulmonary fibrosis, scarring in the lungs that may result in temporary or permanent breathing problems, which is reversible.

In rare cases, bicalutamide causes heart problems.

EXPECTED OUTCOMES

Antiandrogen therapy is prescribed along with LHRH agonists or orchiectomy. The use of antiandrogens without another hormonal therapy is not approved by the Food and Drug Administration.

ORCHIECTOMY

Orchiectomy involves removing the testicles from the scrotum. Some men mistakenly believe that in an orchiectomy the surgeon removes the testicles *and* the sac of skin covering them (the scrotum), or even these plus the penis. An orchiectomy only removes the testicles from the scrotum.

Intermittent Hormonal Therapy

Nearly all prostate cancers treated with androgen deprivation therapy become resistant to hormonal treatment after months or years. Some doctors believe that constant androgen suppression may not be necessary, so they recommend intermittent (on-again, off-again) treatment.

In one form of intermittent therapy, hormonal therapy is stopped when a man's blood prostate-specific antigen (PSA) level drops to a very low level. If his PSA level begins to rise, the drugs are started again. Another form of intermittent therapy involves using androgen suppression for fixed periods of time—for example, 6 months on followed by 6 months off.

Clinical trials of intermittent hormonal therapy are in progress, and it is too early to compare the effectiveness of this new approach to continuous hormonal therapy. However, one advantage of intermittent treatment is that for a while some men are able to avoid the side effects of hormonal therapy such as impotence, hot flashes, and loss of sex drive.

Orchiectomy is the oldest treatment for prostate cancer and is the gold standard for treating advanced cancer. Despite the more recent and widespread use of other forms of hormonal therapy, such as LHRH agonists, orchiectomy remains the standard by which other forms of hormonal therapy are measured. Like LHRH agonist therapy, orchiectomy nearly eliminates circulating blood levels of testosterone, removing the 90 to 95 percent of circulating testosterone that originates in the testicles.

WHAT IS INVOLVED?

Orchiectomy is performed at a hospital or outpatient surgical facility. A man undergoing the operation usually returns home the same day.

This relatively simple operation is usually performed by a urologist and takes approximately 30 minutes to complete. The operation can be performed using general anesthesia (you are completely asleep for the entire operation), a spinal anesthetic (you are awake but numb from the waist down), or a local anesthetic (you are awake but the area around the testicles is numbed), often with an intravenous (IV) sedative.

The testicles are removed from the scrotum through a 1- to 2-inch incision on the front side of the scrotal sac. The spermatic cords, which supply the nerves and blood supply to the testicles, are cut. The scrotal incision is then closed with a stitch that will dissolve on its own, and a sterile dressing is applied.

While some men are not psychologically bothered by removal of the testicles, others are disturbed in part because of the appearance of an empty scrotum. There are some ways around this, however. Subcapsular orchiectomy is an option that maintains a relatively normal appearance and avoids leaving behind an empty scrotum. In this procedure, the inside glandular tissue of the testicles is removed, but the outer shells of the testicles are left in place. This procedure has been criticized because of the possibility of leaving some of the functional testicular tissue behind. However, studies have shown that this risk is minimal when the operation is performed correctly. Another option is to have testicular prostheses implanted. These are sacs filled with saline (salt water) that look and feel like normal testicles.

Significant pain, swelling, or discomfort with orchiectomy is unusual. Some men have mild aching or soreness for several days. However, most men have minimal or no discomfort. Applying ice packs to the scrotum helps keep the swelling down, as does avoiding significant physical activity, including heavy lifting and straining, for a period of 1 to 2 weeks.

ADVANTAGES OF ORCHIECTOMY

Both LHRH agonist therapy and orchiectomy lower circulating testosterone levels. However, orchiectomy is a one-time procedure that provides complete and permanent lowering of the blood testosterone levels. There is therefore no need for repeated shots or injections, which are required with LHRH agonists. The permanence of orchiectomy also eliminates the possibility that therapy might be missed or delayed.

Almost all of the body's testosterone is gone within hours of orchiectomy. (In contrast, it may take several weeks after LHRH agonist therapy for testosterone levels to drop dramatically). This fast reduction in testosterone quickly and effectively reduces pain in men with metastatic prostate cancer. (However, most men do not require this rapid lowering of testosterone and are treated instead by LHRH agonist therapy.)

Since there is no increase or surge in testosterone levels (as may occur with LHRH agonist therapy unless short-term antiandrogen therapy is also used), even temporarily, there is no potential for flare in symptoms such as bone pain.

As noted earlier, the surgical procedure is simple for a urologist to perform and can be done on an outpatient basis.

The procedure is also relatively inexpensive and is one of the most cost-effective forms of hormonal therapy, particularly for men who are committed to long-term courses of treatment.

POSSIBLE CONSEQUENCES OF ORCHIECTOMY

Orchiectomy is associated with the common and well-known side effects possible with any form of hormonal therapy: decreased sexual desire, hot flashes, anemia, decreased muscle strength, weight gain, and osteoporosis (see page 229 for more information). Other potential consequences are listed here:

Surgery. The primary disadvantage of orchiectomy as compared to other antiandrogen therapies is that it requires a surgical procedure. As with any surgical procedure, although relatively uncommon, bleeding, infection, and wound problems may result. Rarely, significant bleeding after the procedure requires surgical exploration of the scrotum and drainage of blood swelling the scrotum. Limiting activity for at least 48 hours after orchiectomy minimizes the risk of this bleeding. Wound infection is a potential complication of orchiectomy, but is quite rare.

Psychological challenge. For some men, the psychological consequences of not having testicles can be a challenge. After orchiectomy, scarring within the scrotum usually results in what looks like some testicular tissue. The cosmetic result is acceptable to most men and the psychological effect is limited. If a man is disturbed about having an empty scrotum after orchiectomy, a subcapsular orchiectomy (see previous page) can be performed or testicular prostheses can be surgically implanted. Made of silicone and filled with saline, they simulate the consistency, size, and shape of testicular tissue.

Permanence. Orchiectomy permanently lowers testosterone levels. This is the goal of any hormonal treatment for prostate cancer. In some settings, when hormonal therapy is given in conjunction with radical prostatectomy or radiation therapy, shorter courses of hormonal therapy are sometimes used. But because orchiectomy is permanent hormonal therapy, it does not allow a limited course of therapy.

The permanence of orchiectomy does not allow reversal of therapy if troublesome adverse effects, such as hot flashes, erectile dysfunction, or mood changes develop. This is unlike LHRH agonist therapy, which can be stopped if a man experiences significant side effects.

EXPECTED OUTCOMES

The expected outcomes for orchiectomy are identical to those of LHRH agonists and depend upon the prostate cancer stage when treatment is begun. Although this procedure is performed less commonly than in the past, it is a viable and effective option for some men. Removing both testicles is equally effective as LHRH agonist therapy in treating all stages of advanced prostate cancer. It simply offers another option for men who need hormonal therapy.

POSSIBLE CONSEQUENCES FOR ANY HORMONAL TREATMENT

Like all treatments for prostate cancer, hormonal therapies have side effects. They are usually not life-threatening, but they may detract from a man's quality of life.

Men are often concerned that hormonal therapy will affect their other male sexual characteristics such as deepness of their voice or hair growth. Fortunately, these side effects are uncommon. Men are not likely to notice a change in their voice or an alteration in hair growth.

DECREASED SEXUAL DESIRE

The most prominent side effect of hormones is their effect on sexual desire, or libido. Most men lose their desire for sexual relations and may lose the ability to obtain or maintain an unassisted erection. However, men do maintain their ability to foster loving and nurturing relationships with their spouses or significant others.

ERECTILE DYSFUNCTION

Most men will have trouble achieving erections while on hormonal therapy. However, it's important to note that orgasms can be experienced even without an erection. Your doctor can also suggest treatments that may help restore your ability to have an erection that is satisfactory for sexual intercourse. Studies are underway testing lower-dose hormonal therapies, such as antiandrogen pills alone, which may not affect sexual function as much as traditional hormonal therapy does.

HOT FLASHES

Most men also experience "hot flashes" (also called hot flushes) from time to time. These are sudden rushes of body heat that cause reddening and sweating.

> ### Relating to Women Through Hot Flashes
>
> I had 3 months of hormone therapy and handled the side effects, one of which is hot flushes. I can talk to any menopausal group of women now with some degree of authority, and I have a lot of fun with that.
>
> — Ron

For the majority of men, these are a minor nuisance and do not interfere significantly with their quality of life, although for some men they may be very bothersome. Medical literature has not shown that soy alleviates hot flashes, but some men may take soy in an attempt to reduce the intensity or frequency of hot flashes. Doctors can suggest medications (such as some antidepressants) that lessen or eliminate the symptoms for men who do experience frequent or bothersome hot flashes. Be sure to ask your doctor if these are bothering you. Further studies of low-dose antiandrogen therapy, as noted above, may demonstrate that they are less likely to cause hot flashes.

BREAST ENLARGEMENT OR NIPPLE TENDERNESS

Although in the past estrogen pills often caused breast enlargement and tenderness, current hormonal therapies (orchiectomy and LHRH agonists) do not commonly cause this side effect. However, antiandrogens used alone or with other oral drugs such as finasteride (Proscar) may cause breast enlargement or nipple tenderness, which may be prevented by small doses of radiation to the breast before treatment starts.

OSTEOPOROSIS AND OTHER SIDE EFFECTS

Long-term hormonal therapy with LHRH agonists or orchiectomy may result in mild anemia (low red blood cells), decreased muscle mass and strength, and can even accelerate the loss of bone mineral density, leading to osteoporosis (bone thinning and weakness).

Studies are underway to determine how common and severe these side effects are. Some doctors are now recommending measuring a man's bone mineral density before he begins therapy. Intermittent hormonal therapy use may lessen or eliminate these side effects. Bisphosphonates are medications that treat weakened bones and may be used to help prevent osteoporosis (see chapter 29).

WEIGHT GAIN

Some men notice weight gain, particularly around the midsection of the body. Men on hormonal therapy may benefit from regular exercise, a balanced diet, and regular evaluation of any side effects.

EXPECTED OUTCOMES FOR ANY HORMONAL THERAPY

Ridding the body of testosterone commonly results in decreased symptoms from prostate cancer. Ideally, it also causes the prostate cancer to go into long-term remission.

For men who choose radiation as their primary treatment, using hormonal therapy during and after the treatment has resulted in improved survival rates.

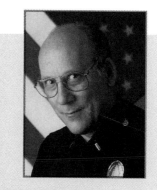

Spending Time Together When Sexual Desire Is Decreased

Hormone injections depressed my testosterone levels and therefore my sex drive, and I didn't like it. But I spent more time with my wife doing household tasks and I was more cuddly and affectionate, even if it didn't lead to sex. I asked my wife if I had become a better husband, and she said yes, almost tearing up.

– Kent

The Balance of Treatment Effectiveness and Side Effects

After prostate cancer was found to have spread to my bones, I began taking daily hormonal pills and quarterly hormonal shots. My PSA dropped from 78 to .04 in 3 months. I couldn't believe it (my doctors could). My side effects include tiredness, constipation, and a little less mental agility, but as Maurice Chevalier said about old age, "[It] isn't so bad, considering the alternative."

– Edward

Hormonal therapy may be begun several months prior to radiation and continued during radiation for many men with clinical stage T3 disease. After radiation, hormonal treatment may continue, depending on the characteristics of the cancer, such as grade and PSA level. Medical studies have shown that combination therapy of hormones and external beam radiation improves the outcomes in stage T3 prostate cancer.

A recent study suggests that men with advanced prostate cancer who begin hormonal therapy at the time of diagnosis may not only experience reduced symptoms from prostate cancer but may also live longer than men who began hormonal therapy later, after they had already developed symptoms. However, more research is needed to confirm this finding.

Studies have shown that having hormonal therapy for 3 months prior to local treatment will shrink the prostate gland by about one third. Doing this prior to radical prostatectomy results in a lower risk that cancer cells will be found in the surgical margins (outer edges) of the removed prostate gland. It therefore lowers the chance that cancer cells will evade prostatectomy and continue to grow. So far, however, neoadjuvant hormonal therapy before prostatectomy has not resulted in better long-term outcomes.

Soy and Hot Flashes

Since beginning quarterly hormonal injections 2½ years ago I've been drinking a soy protein powder drink every day and my hot flashes have been minimal. I'm not sure how much that's connected to my soy intake, but I drink my daily soy protein powder drink blended with fruit just in case.

— *Craig*

CHAPTER 23

WATCHFUL WAITING (EXPECTANT MANAGEMENT)

Rekha N. Attigere, MBBS
L. Michael Glode, MD

WATCHING AND WAITING MAY BE RECOMMENDED if your cancer is not causing any symptoms, is expected to grow very slowly, and is small and contained within 1 area of the prostate. Because prostate cancer often spreads very slowly, if you are older or have other serious health problems, you may never need active treatment for your prostate cancer. Some men choose watchful waiting because they feel the side effects of aggressive treatment outweigh its benefits.

What Is Watchful Waiting?

Watchful waiting sounds passive, but choosing not to have active treatment does not mean that you will not receive medical care or follow-up care. While your cancer will not be treated with surgery or radiation, for example, your condition will be carefully observed and monitored, usually through a prostate-specific antigen (PSA) blood test and digital rectal examination (DRE) every 6 months and possibly through a yearly transrectal ultrasound-guided biopsy of the prostate. Watchful waiting need not be a permanent choice. If you develop bothersome symptoms or your cancer begins to grow more quickly, you can consider active treatment.

It can be difficult for a man with prostate cancer to decide on watchful waiting. The process of discovering that cancer is present is time-consuming and emotionally draining for most men. Once the presence of cancer is determined, it may be a challenge for a man to accept a plan to monitor the cancer rather than remove it.

WHEN MAY WATCHFUL WAITING BE APPROPRIATE?

If the Gleason score and staging information show that cancer has not spread beyond the prostate, the man with prostate cancer and his health care team may decide to pursue watchful waiting—undergoing close monitoring instead of active treatment. Watchful waiting might be a reasonable choice for an older man with a small tumor that might grow very slowly, for example.

In some cases, a decision is made even before the prostate is biopsied to observe and not treat any cancer that is found. For example, a man with severe medical problems might, along with his doctor, evaluate the threat of prostate cancer to his health and feel that other health issues are more important to address, and, in fact, are more likely to eventually cause death.

Nomograms (computer-based tools; see chapter 17 and Figure 23.1) may help both doctor and patient better understand if the patient's cancer is likely to be indolent (pose a minimal threat; a total tumor volume of less than 0.5 cubic centimeters cancer confined to the prostate, and not Gleason pattern 4 or 5) and therefore make him a candidate for watchful waiting. Nomograms are simplified estimates of prognoses and are not a prediction of any particular individual's outcome. Watchful waiting should be discussed with the doctor along with other treatment options.

WHAT IS INVOLVED?

There are no tests that can really tell us when or if a cancer has changed its behavior. Aside from the Gleason score and PSA at the time of diagnosis, only a regular physical exam, perhaps on a semi-annual basis, and PSA testing can follow the progress of the cancer. Most experts agree that even the slowest-growing cancers will eventually cause problems, potentially metastasizing (spreading) beyond the prostate gland to other areas of the body (although this may take many years).

However, if during a digital rectal exam (DRE) a cancer cannot be felt by the doctor or is found to be very small, and if the PSA is staying the same or rising very slowly (for example, if the doubling time—the time it takes the PSA to go from 2 to 4, or from 4 to 8, and so on—is greater than a year), it is not likely to pose an immediate threat.

WHEN ACTIVE TREATMENT MIGHT BE DISCUSSED

The patient and his doctor may agree in advance about what changes in PSA or DRE might trigger a discussion about pursuing active treatment. Alternatively,

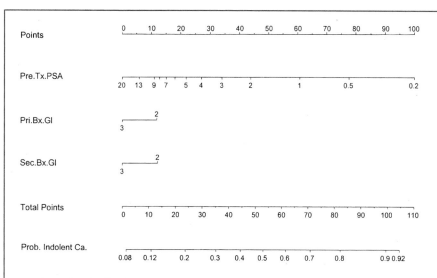

| Points | 0 | 10 | 20 | 30 | 40 | 50 | 60 | 70 | 80 | 90 | 100 |

Pre.Tx.PSA   20   13   9   7   5   4   3   2   1   0.5   0.2

Pri.Bx.Gl   2   3

Sec.Bx.Gl   2   3

Total Points   0   10   20   30   40   50   60   70   80   90   100   110

Prob. Indolent Ca.   0.08   0.12   0.2   0.3   0.4   0.5   0.6   0.7   0.8   0.9 0.92

Figure 23.1.

Nomogram for Predicting Cancer Behavior

Instructions for Physician: Locate the patient's PSA on the **PreTx PSA** axis. Draw a line straight upwards to the **Points** axis to determine how many points towards having an indolent cancer the patient receives for his PSA. Repeat this process for the remaining axes, each time drawing straight upward to the **Points** axis. Sum the points achieved for each predictor and locate this sum on the **Total Points** axis. Draw a line straight down to find the patient's probability of having indolent cancer.

Instruction to Patient: "Mr. X, if we had 100 men exactly like you, we would expect <predicted probability from nomogram * 100 > to have indolent cancer."

You may use factors such as PSA level and Gleason score to estimate your prognosis and evaluate how appropriate watchful waiting may be for you.

In the above nomogram the patient's pre-treatment (pre-TX) PSA level is marked on the **Pre-TX PSA** axis. A straight line is drawn upward to the **Points** axis and shows how many points that PSA score warrants. (For example, if the patient has a pre-treatment PSA level of 9 ng/ml, a straight line drawn to the Points axis indicates about 11 points.) Straight lines are also drawn upward from the primary and secondary biopsy Gleason scores. (Note that the axes for Gleason scores only show 2 and 3. A man with a 4 or 5 Gleason score may not be a good candidate for watchful waiting.)

The points are added and the total score is marked on the **Total Points** axis. A straight line is drawn down from Total Points to the **Probable Indolent Cancer** axis to indicate the patient's probability of having indolent, or minimally threatening, cancer. The more complex versions of this nomogram provide more detailed predictions.

The higher your score is, the more likely it is that your cancer will be minimally threatening. For example, if your total is about 30 points, there appears to be only a 25 percent chance your cancer will be minimally threatening, and you would be more likely to consider active treatment. On the other hand, if your score totals 100 points, there would be a 90 percent chance that your cancer will be minimally threatening.

Key: *Pre-Tx PSA:* Pre-treatment PSA; *Pri.Bx.Gl.:* Primary biopsy Gleason score; *Sec.Bx.Gl.:* Secondary biopsy Gleason score; *Prob.indolent.Ca.:* Probability of indolent cancer.

Kattan MW, Eastham JA, Wheeler TM et al. Counseling men with prostate cancer: a nomogram for predicting the presence of small, moderately differentiated, confined tumors. *J Urol.* 2003 Nov; 170 (5):1792–7.

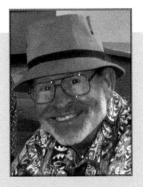

Taking Time to Consider Future Steps

I have been monitoring my PSA in the 4 years since my diagnosis of prostate cancer. Watchful waiting has allowed me to take time to decide on more aggressive treatment options for the future. Because I am in control of my treatment decisions, I am confident that I will be able to deal with whatever outcomes result from treatment.

— Dave M.

a man with severe health problems and a shorter life expectancy might reasonably choose never to have another DRE or PSA and simply live his life to the fullest extent while assuming that one of his other illnesses will be more likely to end his life.

ADVANTAGES OF WATCHFUL WAITING

Men who choose to have their situation observed unless a "trigger" such as a specific PSA level or specific DRE finding occurs avoid experiencing the side effects of active therapy. Therapy may later become warranted, but in the meantime these men have delayed the possibility of treatment-related impotence and/or incontinence, for example.

For a man with significant medical illnesses, doing nothing at all, not even further PSA testing, provides the psychological freedom of not worrying about prostate cancer along with the other problems he must face on a daily basis.

POTENTIAL CONSEQUENCES OF WATCHFUL WAITING

There are several potential consequences of watchful waiting. While postponing treatment allows men to also postpone the side effects of treatment, it can cause men to be treated at an older age, when treatment may be more difficult to tolerate.

CANCER MAY BE MORE ADVANCED THAN IT APPEARS

A man opting for watchful waiting may worry at length about the accuracy of the biopsy results. He might wonder if the tumor might be larger or more aggressive than is thought. Some men may not like the idea of living with a cancer without getting treated.

Approximately 15 to 25 percent of prostate cancer cases produce a smaller amount of PSA than they are expected to, giving a false indication that cancer is in the early stage when it is actually more advanced. Biopsies, even when many are taken, cannot perfectly predict a Gleason score. Thus there could be a more aggressive component of the cancer (for example, containing some Gleason pattern 4 or 5) "hiding" in an unbiopsied portion of the tumor. Therefore the Gleason score from the biopsy sample may be lower than it would be if the entire prostate was removed (via prostatectomy) and examined.

CANCER IS GROWING

The biggest potential downside of watchful waiting is decreasing the chance to control the disease before it spreads. It is possible that the window of opportunity to cure cancer while it is small and treatable will close while active treatment is delayed.

Even if a patient is followed closely, there is a possibility that his cancer may grow rapidly and spread quickly between visits. Sometimes small, slow-growing tumors grow rapidly if left untreated. Thus interventional treatment may be unintentionally delayed longer than it should be.

All of these factors must be weighed against the advantages of avoiding therapy side effects and dying of some other cause. Talk to your doctor about your thoughts, your concerns, and your priorities. A support group such as the American Cancer Society Man to Man group in your area may help you further consider the options.

EXPECTED OUTCOMES

In general, watchful waiting allows prostate cancer to slowly progress. If the rate of progression is slow enough, a man will most likely die of other causes. This is why any other conditions you have, such as heart disease, emphysema, diabetes, or high blood pressure, are relevant to your treatment discussion with your doctor. Many conditions have the potential to cause an earlier death than prostate cancer would.

The level of urinary symptoms experienced by men who chose treatment seems to be approximately similar to that of men who chose watchful waiting. More untreated men may develop urinary obstructive symptoms (weak stream) than treated men, while more treated men have problems with erections or urinary leaking.

On the other hand, there doesn't appear to be much difference in overall survival between men with low-risk cancers choosing watchful waiting versus radical prostatectomy. While the death rate from prostate cancer is lower for men who are treated, on average, other causes of death result in treated men living only about as long as untreated men. In other words, you are just as likely to die in a car accident if you are monitoring your cancer as you are if you had treated the cancer. Thus only a crystal ball could offer absolute advice about whether choosing active treatment would prolong an individual's life.

Studies are now in progress to address this topic in more detail. A large study sponsored by the National Cancer Institute and the Veterans Affairs Cooperative Studies Program is looking into how active treatment affects survival and quality of life of prostate cancer patients of different ages. The PIVOT (Prostatic Intervention Versus Observation Trial; see chapter 32) is still in progress.

QUESTIONS TO ASK YOUR MEDICAL TEAM ABOUT WATCHFUL WAITING

- Given my overall health status and the stage and grade of my tumor, what do you think the chances are that prostate cancer, if left untreated, will either cause my death or significantly impact my life?
- If I were to opt for watchful waiting, what are the odds that I might have to seek treatment due to the progression of my cancer?
- What tests would you recommend doing during the watchful waiting phase of my prostate cancer? How often will I be tested for the rate of progression of my cancer?
- Are there any medications I could take or other things I could do that could slow down the progression of my cancer?
- Do I need to change my lifestyle to incorporate watchful waiting as an option?
- If the cancer is found to be growing, should we then consider active treatment? What would trigger this revisiting of treatment options (PSA level, symptoms, etc.)? What treatment would you recommend?
- What percentage of your patients with prostate cancer have opted for watchful waiting and how many of them have died from prostate cancer? How many have died from other causes?

CHAPTER 24

OTHER THERAPIES IN USE

Brian D. Kavanagh, MD, MPH
Daniel P. Petrylak, MD
James Clifton Vestal, MD

MOST MEN WITH PROSTATE CANCER pursue treatment options such as prostatectomy, radiation, hormonal therapy, or watchful waiting. Several other treatments may also be used for prostate cancer, although they are not as widely used as those mentioned above. In this chapter we explore cryotherapy, chemotherapy, and hyperthermia and outline situations in which these therapies might be appropriate for a man with prostate cancer.

What Is Cryotherapy?

Cryotherapy (also called cryosurgery or cryoablation) is the destruction of a tumor through freezing temperatures. We have known for a long time that freezing tissue can potentially damage or kill tissue or organs; frostbite is one example of tissue damage caused by cold temperatures. Applying cooling temperatures to abnormal tissues was first described in the mid 1800s. Cryotherapy was used in an attempt to treat prostate cancer in the past, but problems controlling the amount of tissue frozen originally made side effects a problem. Newer techniques now allow for more precise use of this technique.

WHAT IS INVOLVED?

Cryotherapy is commonly performed in an operating room under general or spinal anesthesia.

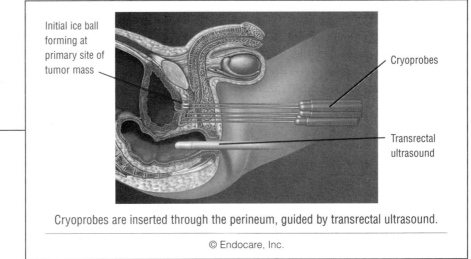

Initial ice ball forming at primary site of tumor mass

Cryoprobes

Transrectal ultrasound

Figure 24.1.
Transperineal Prostate Cryosurgery

Cryoprobes are inserted through the perineum, guided by transrectal ultrasound.

© Endocare, Inc.

A cryoprobe is the instrument that comes into contact with the prostate to freeze it with argon gas, while helium gas is used to warm nearby tissues to prevent them from freezing. Six to 8 cryoprobes are inserted into the body through the perineum (the area between the scrotum and the anus), and directed into place by transrectal ultrasound (see chapter 8 for more information).

Thermocouples are inserted through the perineum. These are devices that measure the temperature at critical areas within the prostate to ensure that a temperature of –40 degrees Celsius is reached for tumor cells and to prevent freezing in areas of normal tissue that should not get cold.

A urethral warming device, inserted through the penis into the bladder, decreases potential complications associated with freezing the urethra.

A suprapubic catheter (a tube that drains urine from the bladder outside of the body through a hole in the skin of the lower abdomen) is usually inserted before cryotherapy. This is because the prostate swells up after the freezing, much like frostbitten tissue, and may obstruct the urethra and prevent normal urination.

Doctors use transrectal ultrasound to guide the probe to the prostate, freezing it and preserving healthy nearby tissue, such as the rectal wall. The prostate is then allowed to thaw completely prior to a second freeze, after which the probes and thermocouples are removed. The small incisions on the perineum where the devices were inserted are either closed with an absorbable suture (threads used to close wounds; they dissolve over time) or pressure is applied to prevent bleeding. The patient may be taken to the recovery room with or without the urethral warmer in place.

The procedure can range from 1 to 2 hours. Typically men undergoing cryotherapy of the prostate can go home the same day. Patients often urinate on their own after 10 to 15 days, and the catheter is removed when a man is able to urinate and empty his bladder. Men may experience fatigue for approximately a week following treatment, as well as discharge, swelling of the scrotum, pain or burning during urination, and increased urination frequency or urgency.

WHEN MAY CRYOTHERAPY BE APPROPRIATE?

In reality most men with prostate cancer might be candidates for cryotherapy, from men with low-grade disease to those with more advanced cancers. At this time, however, there is not a lot of data on the long-term effectiveness of the procedure.

As with all treatment options, the surgeon and the patient consider the overall condition of the patient before making any decisions. Men with high-risk disease (such as cancer that has not responded to radiation therapy), high-volume cancer, high Gleason score tumors, and possibly those with cancer that has spread but has not been detected may be good candidates for cryotherapy. Cryotherapy may not be appropriate in cases where cancer is likely to have spread beyond the prostate.

ADVANTAGES OF CRYOTHERAPY

As noted above, cryotherapy may be appropriate for men with a range of stages and grades of prostate cancer. Other advantages of cryotherapy include:

- Cryotherapy is not as invasive as radical prostatectomy. This allows for less bleeding and pain, and avoids the potential complications of a more invasive surgical procedure.

- Because of the precise methods used to destroy cancer cells in cryotherapy, healthy tissue is preserved.

- Cryotherapy may be used if necessary after standard treatments such as brachytherapy and external beam radiation and can be performed repeatedly if necessary.

Cryotherapy results are comparable to and in some instances are better than other forms of therapy (see *Expected Outcomes* on page 240).

POTENTIAL CONSEQUENCES OF CRYOTHERAPY

As with all surgical procedures there is the possibility that problems may develop after the procedure.

Erectile dysfunction is very common after cryotherapy of the prostate. Up to 80 percent of men undergoing the procedure may experience impotence. Some surgeons are now performing nerve-sparing cryotherapy in men with lower grade tumors and are able to preserve erectile function in about 50 percent of the men treated.

A rare (occurring 4 percent of the time) potential complication of cryotherapy is the "prostatic slough," which occurs if the section of the urethra that runs through the prostate is damaged by the freezing process. This is treated through prolonged catheter drainage or, more commonly, transurethral resection of the prostate (see page 196 for more information).

The inability to urinate following cryotherapy sometimes occurs when the prostate swells after freezing and blocks the urinary channel. (Most surgeons place a tube in the bladder to bypass the obstruction; see page 177). A man with this situation will typically be able to urinate normally within 1 to 2 weeks, and the tube is removed in a painless procedure.

Permanent urinary leakage or incontinence occurs less than 1 percent of the time with cryotherapy. Urinary leakage that occurs because of an urge to urinate is very common following cryoablation but usually resolves spontaneously several months after the procedure.

Fewer than 1 percent of men experience an extremely rare but serious potential complication of cryoablation of the prostate: a urethro-rectal fistula. This is a hole that is created between the rectum and the urethra if tissue next to the rectum is frozen accidentally. An experienced doctor may produce fewer fistulas than doctors who have performed fewer procedures. These holes will usually heal. However, if a patient who has undergone radiation develops a fistula, more aggressive surgical management will be required.

Other potential consequences following cryoablation of the prostate include swelling of the genitalia, discomfort in the rectal area, bruising, penile numbness, and incomplete voiding of the bladder. Most of these problems will disappear soon after the procedure.

EXPECTED OUTCOMES

Very little information has historically been available about long-term results of targeted cryotherapy of the prostate. However, some outcome information about modern cryotherapy techniques is now available. After 8 years, patients with low-grade tumors have a 92 percent chance of showing no evidence of disease. Those with slightly more aggressive cancers have an 80 percent chance of no evidence of disease. More impressively, those with the most aggressive cancers have a 65 percent chance of no evidence of disease after eight years.

Anywhere from 85 to 95 percent of the biopsies taken after cryotherapy are negative for malignancy, regardless of the original nature of the cancer.

THE FUTURE OF CRYOTHERAPY

Advances in technique and equipment such as newer computerized methods of freezing the prostate are in development, and are likely to become useful in planning and performing cryotherapy. A more standardized form of cryotherapy called focal ablation of the prostate could be used to treat low-risk disease, thus sparing normal prostate tissue. This could also possibly be used with cryotherapy to improve survival in men with advanced disease; early outcomes appear positive, but more testing is needed to compare outcomes with standard therapies.

What Is Chemotherapy?

Chemotherapy is a type of treatment that uses medications—either injected or swallowed in pill form—to kill cancer cells. The drugs travel in the bloodstream and move throughout the body, which makes them useful against cancers that may have spread to distant parts of the body.

Chemotherapy drugs interfere with a cell's process of growth, division, and repair. Doctors give chemotherapy in cycles so chemotherapy can act on cells during different times of their growth and division activity. Chemotherapy affects both normal and cancerous cells. However, cancer cells are less proficient at repairing themselves than normal cells, so they are more strongly affected by chemotherapy drugs.

About 10 different drugs can be used for men with prostate cancer (see Table 24.1). Oncologists generally prescribe 1 or 2 drugs in combination. These may include pills along with an intravenous injection. Many more drugs are currently being tested in clinical trials.

Chemotherapy medicines vary widely in their composition, how they are taken, their usefulness in treating specific forms of cancer, and their side effects.

WHEN MAY CHEMOTHERAPY BE APPROPRIATE?

Chemotherapy is not used to cure prostate cancer and is not recommended as a treatment for men with early prostate cancer. It is most often used to reduce bone pain, lower PSA levels, and shrink tumors for men with metastatic prostate cancer that is no longer responding to hormonal therapy. New evidence indicates that chemotherapy also prolongs the lives of men with metastatic disease by several months.

Table 24.1. CHEMOTHERAPY DRUGS USED FOR PROSTATE CANCER

Drug Name	Dosage Route and Frequency	Potential Side Effects and Complications
cyclophosphamide (Cytoxan)	taken orally for 21 out of 28 days	nausea, vomiting, decrease in white blood cells, which fight infection
doxorubicin (Adriamycin)	taken intravenously on days 1 and 8 every 4 weeks	heart muscle damage, decrease in white blood cells, fevers
epirubicin (Ellence)	intravenously every 3 weeks	a decrease in white blood cells, inflammation of the mucus membrane in the mouth and throat, heart muscle damage
mitoxantrone (Novantrone)	intravenously in combination with prednisone (Deltasone), which is given twice a day	decrease in white blood cells, hair loss, heart muscle damage, constipation, nausea and vomiting, diarrhea
docetaxel (Taxotere)	intravenously every week or every 3 weeks, in combination with either estramustine taken by mouth three times a day or prednisone twice a day	fatigue, decrease in white blood cells, nausea, diarrhea, numbness or tingling in hands or feet, nail changes, fluid retention, constipation, hair loss
paclitaxel (Taxol)	intravenously weekly either alone or with estramustine	weakness, pain, numbness or tingling in the hands or feet, hair loss, nausea and vomiting, diarrhea
vinblastine (Velban)	intravenously in combination with daily estramustine	weakness, pain, numbness or tingling in the hands or feet, nausea and vomiting, decrease in white blood cells
vinorelbine (Navelbine)	intravenously once a week either alone or with daily estramustine	decrease in white blood cell cells, nausea, vomiting, loss of appetite, mouth sores, diarrhea or constipation
estramustine (Emcyt)	3 oral doses a day	nausea, diarrhea, blood clots in the legs
etoposide, VP-16 (VePesid)	intravenously in combination with estramustine or carboplatin	fatigue, decrease in white blood cells, fevers
carboplatin (Paraplatin)	intravenously alone or in combination with VP-16	decrease in white blood cells, nausea, vomiting, loss of appetite, diarrhea or constipation, numbness and tingling in the hands or feet, tiredness

Some newer clinical trials are evaluating the use of chemotherapy to reduce the risk of the cancer returning after prostatectomy or radiation therapy; however, this approach is still experimental.

If you are considering chemotherapy, you may want to ask your doctor about side effects, how often you will receive treatments and for how long, if the treatments can be interrupted if you wish to travel or have other plans, and how the doctor will assess whether the treatment is working.

ADVANTAGES OF CHEMOTHERAPY

Chemotherapy may offer men with prostate cancer the following advantages:

- reduced bone pain
- reduced soft tissue masses
- longer survival
- reduced PSA

POTENTIAL CONSEQUENCES OF CHEMOTHERAPY

Chemotherapy, like most other cancer treatments, may cause side effects. Each person's response to chemotherapy is different, and the medications used to control side effects such as nausea and vomiting are much improved over the medications used for the same purpose years ago.

As mentioned before, chemotherapy drugs act on cells that divide rapidly, especially cancerous cells. But other normal cells in your body divide rapidly too—those in your bone marrow, your digestive tract, the reproductive system, and your hair follicles, for example—and they can be affected by chemotherapy. However, many people go through chemotherapy without significant side effects.

Drugs such as mitoxantrone (Novantrone) or docetaxel (Taxotere) administered every 3 weeks can cause a drop in the white blood cell count, which makes a patient more susceptible to infection. Therefore if a patient develops a fever while on chemotherapy he must call his doctor immediately.

Drugs such as docetaxel or paclitaxel (Taxol) administered on a weekly basis have different side effects. Drops in white blood cell counts are less common, and tearing of the eyes as well as nail bed changes are more prevalent. Numbness of fingers and toes can also result. Docetaxel can also cause fluid retention, and your doctor may prescribe medications to reduce fluid accumulation.

Any asymmetrical swelling of the legs can be a sign of a blood clot and requires immediate evaluation, because blood clots can travel to the lungs. Blood clots can occur in approximately 10 percent of patients treated with estramustine (Emcyt).

Studies are now underway evaluating the outcomes of using chemotherapy after local therapy for men who are at high risk for recurrence. However, these studies will take years to complete.

The focus in treating metastatic prostate cancer is to improve upon the current agents. Studies are looking at the effectiveness of combining chemotherapy with drugs that attack blood vessels, with vitamin D, or with gene blockers.

Mitoxantrone can also reduce the pumping efficiency of the heart, and your doctor should periodically check whether the heart continues to pump efficiently.

Most side effects disappear once treatment stops. Remedies exist for many temporary chemotherapy side effects. For example, drugs can prevent or reduce nausea and vomiting. Other drugs boost blood cell counts.

EXPECTED OUTCOMES

For men with metastatic cancer, as noted above, chemotherapy may reduce bone pain and reduce the size of soft tissue masses. The chemotherapy drug docetaxel (Taxotere) has recently been shown to prolong the life of men with metastatic cancer by several months.

Studies are being performed to evaluate the outcomes for adjuvant chemotherapy (a treatment used along with another main treatment) used to treat prostate cancer. While adjuvant chemotherapy is the standard of care for some other cancers, such as high-risk breast cancer, using early chemotherapy to treat prostate cancer is experimental. Many breast cancer adjuvant studies were started many years ago and have demonstrated a positive effect on survival, but prostate cancer studies will take years to complete and analyze. Men for whom chemotherapy may be an adjuvant treatment option are encouraged to enter clinical trials to determine if this use of chemotherapy may help men with prostate cancer.

What Is Hyperthermia?

Hyperthermia, also called heat therapy, is the application of heat in treating diseases, including cancer. There are many different ways to apply heat to specific areas. For example, transurethral microwave thermotherapy (TUMT) is a type of hyperthermia often used in treating of benign prostatic hypertrophy (BPH).

Hyperthermia is not usually used against cancer by itself. Instead, it is often used to try to improve the effectiveness of radiation therapy or chemotherapy. This is usually done by raising the temperature of a certain part of the body (such as the abdomen). Although the results of treatments involving a combination of hyperthermia plus radiation therapy or chemotherapy have been promising for a variety of cancers other than prostate cancer, hyperthermia is not currently established as a standard part of prostate cancer treatment.

The benefit of types of hyperthermia without other treatments has not been scientifically proven, and hyperthermia used alone is considered an experimental treatment.

WHAT IS INVOLVED?

Several different techniques are being studied to provide hyperthermia for cancer treatment:

- External microwave-based systems can be used for tumors on the surface of the body but do not provide deeply penetrating heat useful for prostate cancer.

- Interstitial radiofrequency (RF) methods require the insertion of small catheters (tubes) directly into the prostate gland, typically guided into place by a needle. Wire-like RF probes placed inside the catheters contain electrodes through which electromagnetic energy heats the prostate tissue. Non-invasive devices using similar electronic technology have also been developed to provide regional hyperthermia to structures deep within the body, including the prostate gland.

- High frequency sound waves (ultrasound) can also be used to heat tumors. (This technique is described in the next chapter.)

- A transrectal approach has also been evaluated and found to be feasible (Figure 24.2).

- A relatively new technique for providing interstitial hyperthermia for prostate cancer is through implanting so-called "thermoseeds," non-radioactive metallic pellets, directly into the prostate. The thermoseeds generate heat when placed into a magnetic field, providing hyperthermia inside the prostate tumor.

It is quite difficult to raise the temperature within a particular part of the body. The body's automatic self-control responses work against the temperature change by increasing blood flow to the area and creating a cooling effect. For this reason it is always necessary to monitor the tumor temperature at numerous points within the tumor. Some hyperthermia delivery systems automatically adjust the intensity of the heat applied in response to measured tissue temperatures.

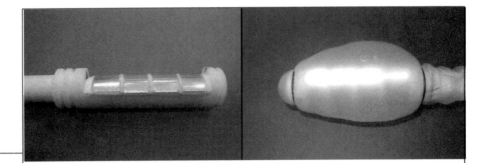

Figure 24.2.

TRUS Applicator and Cooling Balloon

Left, a transrectal ultrasound applicator that delivers ultrasound energy to heat the tumor. When the applicator is in place, water is circulated through a balloon (shown on right) next to the rectal wall to provide a cooling effect.

Figure 1(a) & (b) from "Feasibility and patient tolerance of a novel transrecatl ultrasound hyperthermia system for treatment of prostate cancer" by MD Hurwitz, et al. *International Journal of Hyperthermia.* 2001:17(1):31-37. Available at: http://www.tandf.co.uk/journals

Because of the variability of temperature changes that are routinely measured within an individual patient's tumor, it has been difficult to determine exactly what constitutes a "dose" of hyperthermia. Is it the minimum temperature elevation above normal achieved, the maximum temperature, or the average temperature? Or is it simply necessary to raise the temperature in a certain percent of the tumor to a certain level for a certain length of time? Experts are not certain.

ADVANTAGES OF HYPERTHERMIA

Because there remains opportunity for improvement in treatment outcomes for patients who receive radiation therapy for prostate cancer, hyperthermia remains a field of active clinical research. The addition of hyperthermia to radiation treatment for prostate cancer is worth studying for at least 2 reasons. Hyperthermia is a "local" treatment, meaning that all side effects should be limited to the location of the heat treatment given. And, at least in laboratory conditions, hyperthermia can sometimes have a particularly strong effect on cancer cells that are not as easily destroyed by radiation, particularly cancer cells in areas of the tumor with low levels of oxygen. However, at this time the amount of information available for long-term patient follow up after hyperthermia treatment is limited, and all results are considered preliminary.

THE FUTURE OF HYPERTHERMIA

One new application under investigation for prostate treatment relates to hyperthermia and chemotherapy drug delivery. It is possible to contain chemotherapy drug molecules within a small protective coating called a liposome and to construct the liposome from a material that disintegrates when heated above a certain temperature. In an ongoing early clinical trial, the chemotherapeutic agent doxorubicin (Adriamycin) is encapsulated in a heat-sensitive liposome and then administered to patients. Hyperthermia is then applied to the prostate with the intention of releasing the doxorubicin directly into tumor tissue but not into other parts of the body.

POTENTIAL CONSEQUENCES OF HYPERTHERMIA

Heat therapy can cause injury to the normal tissues surrounding the cancer. Ulceration of the lining of the rectum or bladder is possible, and scarring of the urethra can occur. Fortunately, results reported to date suggest that heat therapy adds few if any side effects when used in combination with radiation, but heat therapy should be administered only under careful supervision by qualified physicians.

EXPECTED OUTCOMES

Expected outcomes have not been established, and more studies are needed into the potential benefit of hyperthermia as a treatment for men with prostate cancer.

In laboratory studies hyperthermia has been observed to cause greater improvement in the response to radiation in prostate cancer cells than in the other types of cancer cells tested. The precise mechanism for this effect is not completely understood. Unfortunately, it is not yet possible to know with certainty whether the favorable effects observed in laboratory studies will translate into beneficial effects in prostate cancer patients, since there have been no prospective randomized comparisons of radiation therapy with or without hyperthermia for prostate cancer.

There have been several prospective randomized studies of radiation therapy and hyperthermia for a variety of other cancers, however. Perhaps most encouraging for the potential use of hyperthermia for prostate cancer is the improved outcome observed when hyperthermia was added to radiation therapy for uterine cervical cancer. While there are many differences in the expected behavior of cervical and prostate cancer, heating a tumor deep within the pelvis appears potentially effective.

CHAPTER 25

INVESTIGATIONAL TREATMENT: HIGH-INTENSITY FOCUSED ULTRASOUND

John H. Lynch, MD

THE MANY POTENTIAL SIDE EFFECTS of standard prostate cancer treatments have led researchers to study new forms of therapy for early stage prostate cancer. A promising treatment known as high-intensity focused ultrasound (HIFU) is an investigational procedure currently used in Europe but not yet available in the United States. We will explain how HIFU works and discuss its advantages and potential consequences in this chapter. (For more information about early research and potential future methods of prostate cancer treatment, see chapters 31 and 32.)

What Is High-Intensity Focused Ultrasound (HIFU)?

Using various energy sources to treat disease by destroying tissue is not new. In fact, high-intensity *unfocused* ultrasound was first introduced as early as 1927, and high-intensity focused ultrasound was used as early as 1955. HIFU destroys cancer cells by heating them with highly focused beams.

The high-intensity sound energy used in HIFU is channeled through a small probe that can be inserted into the rectum to destroy cancerous tissue. The probe also allows doctors to view the prostate area through an ultrasound image. In theory, any part of the body accessible by diagnostic ultrasound could eventually be treated by HIFU.

WHAT IS INVOLVED?

A man undergoing HIFU, which can be an outpatient procedure, is given anesthesia and is positioned on his left side on the treatment table with his knees pulled to his chest. The probe is inserted into the rectum and a rectal balloon is generally inserted and filled with cooled circulating fluid. This is done to cool the rectal wall and reduce the risk of rectal injury from the heat. The doctor views the prostate through ultrasound images to plan exactly where to deliver the heat, then withdraws the probe and replaces the viewing head with the firing head. This is what will send ultrasound waves to heat and destroy cancerous tissue while preserving the tissue around it.

Treatment can take several hours. Computer software is used to detect where the rectum is, and software allows shots of ultrasound energy to be lined up along the bottom of the prostate, allowing the rectal wall to remain unaffected and undamaged. Each shot lasts several seconds and there is a delay of several seconds in between shots. The treatment is continued layer by layer until the entire target area has been treated. The balloon is then deflated and the firing head is removed.

Patients have fast recovery times but very frequently go home with temporary catheters unless they have undergone a transurethral resection of the prostate (see page 196) at the same time.

WHEN MAY HIFU BE APPROPRIATE?

Although it is not yet well-proven, HIFU could be used instead of radical prostatectomy or radiation, or it could be used after external beam radiation therapy to treat a recurrence of cancer in the prostate. Men who are not good candidates for prostatectomy because of advanced age or other health issues and whose cancer has not spread from the prostate may be candidates for HIFU.

Men with large prostate glands may not be able to undergo HIFU; the distance between the rectal wall and the top of a large prostate may be too great for HIFU to be effective.

ADVANTAGES OF HIFU

High-intensity focused ultrasound is a promising option for men who may not be able to tolerate other treatments. HIFU can also be repeated without complications if cancer recurs. Recovery time is quite short; most men return home within a day of treatment.

High-intensity focused ultrasound has the capability of eliminating cancer in the prostate gland while preserving the rest of the prostate. This would minimize the potential of treatment side effects. However, until more advanced imaging devices can show doctors precisely where cancer exists within the prostate, the entire prostate must be treated.

POTENTIAL CONSEQUENCES OF HIFU

Technical refinements in HIFU have led to decreased rates of major side effects. However, as with all prostate cancer treatments, complications may occur. Complications can include urinary retention or difficulty urinating, which can be managed with temporary catheter placement, a high rate of urinary tract infections, and bleeding. Incontinence can also occur; the frequency of this side effect is very much dependent upon the experience of the operator of the HIFU device.

One serious but rare potential complication is a recto-urethral fistula, a hole burned through the prostate to the urethra.

Impotence occurs in approximately one half to two thirds of patients.

EXPECTED OUTCOMES

More research is needed into long-term effects and minimizing side effects. The HIFU device is currently investigational in the United States, and only small or early studies have been done on patients here to determine its potential. There has not been enough study to compare HIFU outcomes to those of prostatectomy, which is still the gold standard in treatment.

In Europe the experience is much broader, and European clinical results have been very promising, generally showing that no cancer is present in 85 to 90 percent of biopsies performed after the procedure. Five years after the procedure, over two thirds of men remain disease free. Less than a quarter of patients need additional treatment, such as external radiation treatment or hormones. PSA levels drop to very low levels in the majority of men treated with HIFU.

CHAPTER 26

CLINICAL TRIALS

Samira Syed, MD
Ian M. Thompson, MD
Anthony W. Tolcher, MD

EXPERTS KNOW THAT THERE IS MUCH MORE left to discover about prostate cancer that could help predict, diagnose, treat, and improve the quality and longevity of life for men with prostate cancer. Potential developments in cancer care are explored and established through studies called clinical trials. Using clinical trials, researchers try to answer certain questions about a new treatment, such as:

- Is the treatment helpful?
- How does this new type of treatment work?
- Does it work better than other treatment currently available?
- What side effects does the treatment cause?
- Are the side effects greater or less than the standard treatment?
- Do the benefits outweigh the side effects?
- In which patients is the treatment most likely to be helpful?

Your doctor or medical team may suggest that you look into a clinical trial focused on prostate cancer. This doesn't mean that your case is hopeless. It means that your doctor believes you may benefit from the treatment being studied.

WHAT TOPICS ARE STUDIED IN CLINICAL TRIALS?

Clinical research studies for cancer are developed to answer a myriad of questions about how to reduce the impact of cancer on men and women. Clinical trials may be investigations into:

- prevention
- screening
- diagnosis
- treatment
- supportive care
- patient comfort (pain control)
- psychological impact of the disease
- effective rehabilitation methods after treatment

What Is a Clinical Trial?

Clinical trials are research studies in people. They take place after studies on cells or animals suggest that a treatment or method of prevention is likely to be safe and effective in people. Doctors' recommendations for their patients are often based on what has been learned from the experiences of groups of patients in clinical trials.

Many advances in medicine are achieved through clinical trials. Findings from clinical trials allow scientists to continually change the way cancer is managed and improve the health of the population. Thousands of people are helped each year because they decided to take part in a clinical trial, and millions more have benefited from others' participation in clinical trials.

The decision to participate in a clinical trial is a very personal one. It depends on many factors, including the benefits and risks of the study, what a person hopes to achieve by taking part, and other personal preferences.

WHAT MAKES A STUDY A CLINICAL TRIAL?

Despite the wide variety in types of studies, each clinical trial has a number of common factors. These factors determine if a person may be eligible for or interested in the study and if he or she may benefit from participating.

THE STUDY IS DESIGNED TO ANSWER ONE PRIMARY QUESTION

A study may examine a number of questions or issues, but it generally seeks to answer 1 specific question or meet 1 objective. For example, a study of 2 chemotherapy drugs may ask the question: "Does new drug A help men with prostate cancer live longer than standard drug B?"

THE STUDY EXAMINES A GROUP OF PATIENTS WHO MEET SPECIFIC CRITERIA

Eligibility criteria determine who may participate in a study by specifying circumstances that must be true for all participants. These criteria ensure that doctors can evaluate a factor's effects on a group of people with similar health factors and more clearly evaluate the implications of those effects. For example, a study of a new prostate cancer screening test will only enroll men old enough to be at risk for prostate cancer, and will almost certainly require that men who enroll not have a previous diagnosis of prostate cancer.

THE STUDY INVOLVES AN INTERVENTION OR EVALUATION

For most clinical trials, a specific change (called an intervention) or set of interventions is part of the study. A patient in a study examining a new treatment for prostate cancer may undergo a new type of operation or radiation therapy, for example.

Participants in a prevention or screening study may go about their regular lives but be regularly evaluated in some way. For example, a prostate cancer screening study may require participants only to have periodic blood tests.

ENOUGH PARTICIPANTS ARE TESTED TO ANSWER THE PRIMARY QUESTION

Assumptions about the treatment or intervention being tested help determine how many patients should to be studied to answer the primary question. For example, if a new treatment shows tremendous promise in the treatment of men with advanced prostate cancer, fewer than 100 men may be required to answer the primary question of whether or not the treatment is effective. Other studies may require 10,000 or 20,000 men to answer a primary question. Studies that do not include enough participants run 2 risks: (1) no effect may be noted with the intervention although an effect did exist or (2) an effect may be noted with the intervention but it was really only due to chance.

THE STUDY HAS POTENTIAL RISKS AND BENEFITS

The risks and benefits of a study depend upon the type of question being answered and are generally related to how the patient's cancer risk may be affected by the study's interventions. For example, a study of a promising new treatment for men with aggressive prostate cancer has a potential for both risks (the cancer is not successfully treated or serious side effects are noted) and benefits (the cancer is successfully treated). Although researchers who design studies of cancer prevention would not intentionally include an intervention that increases cancer risk, in rare cases interventions that were expected to reduce risk turn out to slightly increase risk.

CLINICAL TRIAL PHASES

For cancer *treatment* studies, physicians and scientists generally refer to 3 phases of study development. These are some of the most common types of studies in which men with prostate cancer participate.

PHASE I: IS THE TREATMENT SAFE?

Phase I clinical trials are intensive and closely-monitored studies that are conducted at a limited number of institutions in the United States. The primary purpose of a phase I study is to determine if the new treatment is safe, and to establish the highest dose that can be given safely. These studies are often offered to patients whose cancer has not been cured by standard treatments and who want to try a promising investigational treatment.

PHASE II: DOES IT WORK?

A medication or treatment that passes phase I testing with an acceptable level of safety can then examine the response of cancer to the new treatment. In phase II studies, all participants, who are patients with cancer, receive a standard dose of treatment (determined from the phase I study) and are repeatedly examined to determine if the cancer responds.

PHASE III: IS IT BETTER THAN WHAT IS ALREADY AVAILABLE?

If a treatment has been demonstrated to affect cancer and benefit patients, its effects are compared against the "standard" treatment (such as prostatectomy or radiation). Phase III studies are often randomized trials, studies in which eligible patients who enroll are randomly assigned to one treatment or another. Generally, hundreds of patients and several institutions are involved in a phase III clinical trial. Phase III studies have the potential to change the standard of care for cancer treatment and prevention.

WHO RUNS AND FUNDS CLINICAL TRIALS?

Clinical trials are generally conducted at an academic medical center (for example, a cancer center or a university medical school clinical program), Veterans Affairs

THE PLACEBO EFFECT

A placebo is a substance or other kind of treatment that seems therapeutic but is actually inactive. Although placebos lack chemical or other value in and of themselves, they have a very real effect in some patients. This is called the placebo effect. The placebo effect is real and has been the object of many careful scientific tests.

Placebos may be used in clinical trials to test new medications or other new treatments. The placebo looks, tastes, or feels as much like the actual treatment as possible.

Placebos are used only when there is no effective standard therapy. If there is already a treatment known to be helpful, it will not be withheld from patients. In such situations, clinical trials will often randomly assign patients to either the standard treatment or the new treatment. In other cases, the new treatment may designed to be added to the standard one. These trials randomly assign patients to receive either the current standard of care plus the new treatment, or the current standard of care plus a placebo. In a "double-blind controlled study," neither the subjects nor the investigators know who receives which treatment. The use of placebos allows studies to be conducted while avoiding patient—or doctor—biases and expectations of treatment results.

Because people usually do not know when they are taking a placebo, and because they believe in the treatment and in their doctor, some people will react to the placebo as though it were the active treatment. In these cases, the patient's mind influences other physiologic systems in the body to bring about helpful results. Their pain will lessen, or they will feel better generally. Because placebos often have an effect, even if it is temporary, some people think that the placebo contributed to a "cure." But placebos cannot cure.

Medical Center, military medical center, within a network of community hospitals, or at a physicians' practice.

Clinical trials are monitored by a group of scientists and community representatives who ensure that the trial is properly designed and conducted. They also ensure patients' rights are protected. Often, in addition to a principal investigator (who administers the study and is most often a physician), a clinical research associate interacts with patients, ensures that testing is scheduled and completed in accordance with the trial's requirements, and often serves as the patient's first contact for medical or other issues related to their cancer.

Large clinical trials may involve hundreds or even thousands of patients and may require follow up for as many as 10 years or more. These studies are generally funded by either private or government organizations, such as the National Institutes of Health's National Cancer Institute (NCI). They may be overseen by a network of cooperative groups, investigators, and institutions from around North America who pool efforts and resources to design and conduct large-scale clinical trials. Cooperative groups allow for the highest level of scientific review and support to ensure that important questions are being asked, patient safety is assured, and that when the study is complete, the results are reported accurately.

Some studies are funded and administered locally. Support may be provided by the organization that has a stake in the study. A pharmaceutical company producing a medication for advanced prostate cancer might design a study of the medication's effectiveness, ensure that the design is acceptable to regulatory authorities, recruit institutions and investigators, and provide the support and oversight as the study is conducted.

Why Would a Man Participate in a Clinical Trial?

Ultimately it is the men and women who participate in clinical trials who allow scientists to change and improve how cancer is managed. Without people willing to take part, clinical trials and the many advancements they allow simply would not exist.

Some clinical trials involve study sponsors that pay for part or all of participants' medical care during the study. However, this is not the case with all clinical trials, so be sure that you are aware of any costs for participation.

ACCESS TO NEW TREATMENTS

Men often participate in clinical trials for prostate cancer in the hope that it may benefit them personally. Through clinical trials, they may have access to treatments that are not available to the general public, including new drugs or treatments.

PERSONALIZED ATTENTION

Men who participate in these rigorously designed studies will often be encouraged by the personalized and frequent attention they receive. In many institutions, specific research nurses are assigned to a man's case to ensure that all study tests and follow-up exams are performed on the schedule pre-specified by the study. A partnership may develop between the patient and members of the research staff. Because the primary goal of the research team is to provide the very best care and best outcomes for the patient, patients often report that they feel their level of care is excellent when they are in a clinical trial.

HELPING OTHERS

Men who participate in clinical trials for prostate cancer also often have a desire to advance the field of care and to help others. This is especially important to many men with prostate cancer because of the very high association of family history and prostate cancer. A man with a father, brother, or son with prostate cancer has approximately double the risk of developing prostate cancer as other men. If he has more than 1 relative with the disease, the risk can go up as much as tenfold. Many men are not only helping men in general, but members of their own family.

Potential Disadvantages of Participating in a Clinical Trial

Participating in a clinical trial may require a man to undergo more frequent or invasive tests than those required for standard care, face the inconvenience of traveling to a participating institution, and possibly incur expenses not covered by some insurance plans. (Be sure to talk to your insurance provider about costs and coverage before you decide to participate in a clinical trial.)

Other potential drawbacks are that the doctor and patient may not be able to select the treatment received, and additional or unknown side effects may result from the treatment.

There are risks involved in having any medical test, procedure, or taking any drug. Risks may be greater in a clinical trial than in undergoing standard treatment because some aspects of any new treatment are unknown. This is especially true of earlier phase clinical trials. People with cancer are often willing to accept a certain amount of risk for a chance to benefit from a treatment, but it is always important to have a realistic idea about expected results.

Ask questions about how a clinical trial treatment differs from standard treatments, and make sure you understand the difference in risks, benefits, and procedures of the clinical trial and standard treatment.

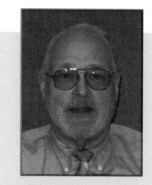

Giving Back Through Participating in a Clinical Trial

I was fortunate to have qualified and be selected for a clinical trial vaccination to develop a natural immunity to prostate cancer. In conjunction with the vaccinations I received external beam radiation. If you are so inclined, please consider being part of a clinical trial. It is one thing to deal with cancer of any kind, but to be involved with the potential to find a solution that might help others is priceless!

– Philip

QUESTIONS TO ASK YOURSELF ABOUT CLINICAL TRIALS

Should you take part in a clinical trial? There is no right or wrong answer to this tough question. Some of the questions below may not have clear-cut answers, but they should help you start thinking about some important issues. Each person's situation is unique, and each person's reasons for wanting or not wanting to participate may be different.

When trying to decide the best route for you, first ask yourself some basic questions:

- Why do I want to take part in a clinical trial?
- What are my goals and expectations if I decide to participate? How realistic are these?
- How sure are my doctors about what my future holds if I decide to participate? If I decide not to participate?
- Have I considered:
  - potential benefits versus potential risk?
  - other factors, such as time and money?
  - other possible treatment options?

How to Find Out About Clinical Trials

Men with prostate cancer or who are at risk of prostate cancer may want to keep themselves abreast of new advances in the field and opportunities to participate in clinical trials. Much of this information can be obtained from a person's doctor and other members of the health care team, but because of the extraordinary volume of research in this area, it is almost impossible for all medical professionals to know the full range of research opportunities.

Fortunately, there are some excellent sources of information for men who are interested in checking on the availability of clinical trials for prostate cancer. The following is a partial list of these sources. See the *Resources* section in the back of this book for more information and for information about organizations such as Prostate Cancer Foundation and Us TOO that support research and may have additional information. Chapter 32 also outlines research studies that may be of interest to men at risk of prostate cancer as well as men with prostate cancer.

CANCER ORGANIZATIONS

THE AMERICAN CANCER SOCIETY

The American Cancer Society offers a clinical trial information and matching service (800-ACS-2345 or http://www.cancer.org; click on "Find a Clinical Trial" to go to "American Cancer Society/EmergingMed Clinical Trials Matching Service"). Patients who enter information about their cancer type and stage, their prior treatments, general health, and personal preference will receive a list of relevant trials they can discuss with their doctor. The American Cancer Society also sponsors a prostate cancer support group called Man to Man, led by prostate cancer patients. Guest speakers often include individuals who can help guide men with prostate cancer to opportunities for clinical trials research. Call 800-ACS-2345 or go to http://www.cancer.org for more information.

THE NATIONAL CANCER INSTITUTE CANCER INFORMATION SERVICE

The National Cancer Institute Cancer Information Service is another good source of clinical trial information available in 1 location. The phone is answered by regional centers that help people contact institutions or doctors in their area (800-4-CANCER or http://www.cancer.gov). The clinical trials Web site allows you to enter specifics about your case to find potential cancer screening or prevention studies (http://cancer.gov/search/clinical_trials/search_clinicaltrialsadvanced.aspx).

SPECIALTY MEDICAL ORGANIZATIONS

Organizations often include as members the leaders of clinical trials and research studies available in certain specialties. The following is a partial list for patients seeking to discuss research opportunities:

- American Urological Association: the largest organization of urologists involved in prevention, diagnosis, and treatment of men with prostate cancer (http://www.auanet.org).

- Society of Urologic Oncology: the specialty society of urologists who have special expertise in the management of cancer patients (http://www.societyofurologiconcology.org).

- American Society of Clinical Oncology: the largest oncology organization in the world, which involves physicians of all specialties who treat cancer patients. A specific service of ASCO is the People Living with Cancer Web site, where a number of resources can be found (http://www.peoplelivingwithcancer.org).

- American Society of Therapeutic Radiation Oncology: the professional organization of radiation oncology physicians, doctors who provide all forms of radiation to treat prostate cancer patients (http://www.astro.org).

ACADEMIC MEDICAL CENTERS AND COMMUNITY HOSPITALS

Individual academic medical centers conduct their own small-scale trials. Major discoveries are often the products of these studies. They also participate in larger multi-institution trials sponsored by cooperative groups of pharmaceutical companies.

Community (nonacademic) hospitals and practices may participate in cooperative group trials, which are usually phase III studies and also sometime phase II studies.

These institutions often have their own Web sites and lists of studies and may offer periodic seminars for patients. Men with prostate cancer might therefore want to be aware of any physicians at their nearest medical center or hospital who specialize in prostate cancer.

ASSOCIATION OF COMMUNITY CANCER CENTERS

This is an excellent resource that helps locate cancer centers in your community. Generally these are smaller facilities, and these cancer centers should not be confused with the comprehensive and clinical cancer centers designated by the National Cancer Institute. The association's Web site can be searched by state and used to identify a cancer center closest to you that is a member of the association (http://www.accc-cancer.org).

Every patient with prostate cancer (and those who do not develop prostate cancer due to prevention) benefits enormously from the knowledge developed through clinical research. A man with prostate cancer who demands the highest standards for the care of his cancer will benefit from understanding ongoing research opportunities. Even if you do not participate in the research studies themselves, knowing about the treatments being used allows you to understand the cutting-edge management options for the disease. If you participate in a clinical trial, you will not only receive high-quality care, but you will also endow future generations with better care and outcomes.

CHAPTER 27

ALTERNATIVE TREATMENTS AND SUPPLEMENTS

Mark A. Moyad, MD, MPH

ALTERNATIVE THERAPIES ARE UNPROVEN TREATMENTS sometimes used *instead of* conventional therapy to attempt to prevent, lessen, or cure disease. Some alternative therapies may be harmful in and of themselves or may be dangerous because they are used instead of conventional medicine and thereby delay treatments that are proven to be helpful.

Alternative therapies should not be confused with complementary therapies (such as meditation, yoga, or massage therapy) that are used to complement, or add to, conventional treatments. If you are interested in complementary therapies, ask your doctor for information about therapies that might be appropriate for your situation.

If you are considering using any complementary or alternative treatments, first discuss them openly with your cancer care team.

In this chapter, we'll focus on outlining the risks and purported benefits of alternative treatments—especially dietary supplements people with prostate cancer may read or hear about. As you read the rest of this chapter, remember 2 important things:

1. While many dietary supplements may be touted as cancer cures, to date **there is no evidence that any dietary supplements can cure cancer.**

2. Particularly in the case of people undergoing treatment for cancer, **self-medication with dietary supplements can be risky and harmful.**

Do Your Research

When you're researching any alternative treatment, keep in mind the following tips for finding reliable and helpful information about safety, interactions, and how to make your treatment as effective as possible. See also *Questions to Ask About Alternative Treatments and Supplements* on page 267.

- **Speak with your doctor** or other health care provider about any alternative treatment you are considering. Find information about the product written by recognized medical experts, leading cancer centers, or government agencies. Bring this information to your doctor's attention so you can discuss it together. Your doctor can probably tell you if it poses any risks to your health and if it is safe to pursue along with other medications you may be taking.

- **Be a skeptic.** Be skeptical of sources that make grand claims based on a few people's testimonials or vague references to "scientific proof." Most of what you hear or read about dietary supplements is based on anecdotal evidence—that is, evidence based on people's (even some doctors') personal observations rather than on objective, controlled scientific studies. Instead, rely on materials by experts in dietary supplements or those trained about natural sources of medically beneficial agents, especially plants (pharmacognosists). Keep in mind the saying, "if it sounds too good to be true, it probably is."

- **Rely on a trusted source** such as the Memorial Sloan-Kettering Cancer Center's Herbs and Botanical Information Web site (http://www.mskcc.org/aboutherbs) for reliable information about effectiveness, potential problems, and interactions.

Alternative Treatments for Prostate Cancer

"PROSTATE-HEALTHY" SUPPLEMENTS

Many herbal mixtures labeled "for prostate health" have appeared on the market, some containing herbs similar to those in PC-SPES (see next page). They often include "PC" in their names. Like all "dietary supplements" (and unlike drugs), these mixtures are not required by the US government to undergo testing to prove they are effective, or even safe. Therefore the risks and benefits associated with many of these mixtures have not been studied and are not known. If you are using such a product, tell your doctors.

PC-SPES

PC-SPES ("PC" stands for prostate cancer and "spes" means "hope" in Latin), a mixture of herbs, has been popular among men with advanced prostate cancer over the past few years.

PC-SPES was removed from the US market in February 2002 because some PC-SPES capsules were found to be contaminated with compounds identical to or similar to other prescription drugs that could cause serious health problems, including diethylstilbestrol (DES), a synthetic estrogen; indomethacin (Indocin), a potent anti-inflammatory drug; and warfarin (Coumadin), a powerful blood thinner. It is not known whether PC-SPES will be available again.

While PC-SPES lowered prostate-specific antigen (PSA) levels in clinical trials (it did not show evidence of shrinking prostate tumors or extending survival), these results are now in question. The supplement may have been effective not because it contained active herbal extracts, but because it contained a form of the female hormone estrogen. Another complicating factor is that the ingredients of PC-SPES varied over time and in concentration. It therefore may not be possible to accurately compare studies of PC-SPES.

OTHER SUPPLEMENTS AND ALTERNATIVE MEDICINES

There is no evidence that many supplements presented as beneficial for prostate health actually provide a health benefit. Talk to your doctor before trying any supplements, including those below:

SUPPLEMENTS WITH POTENTIAL BENEFITS

Selenium. A few clinical trials indicate that this antioxidant may reduce the risk of prostate cancer. Studies into its potential benefits are underway (see *SELECT: the Selenium and Vitamin E Cancer Prevention Trial* on page 330).

Vitamin E. This antioxidant is being evaluated for its potential to lower men's risk of prostate cancer (see *SELECT: the Selenium and Vitamin E Cancer Prevention Trial* on page 330).

Lycopene. This antioxidant may reduce prostate cancer risk; more study is needed. It is not clear if lycopene supplements provide the same benefits as lycopene in tomatoes and tomato products.

Flaxseed. In one study, flaxseed powder (ground from flaxseeds) along with a low-fat diet slowed the growth rate of prostate cancer cells, increased the death rate of prostate cancer cells, and lowered PSA levels in men without aggressive tumors. Further study is needed. Flaxseed oil supplements have not been clinically tested.

Garlic. There is no evidence that garlic is effective in treating cancer. Limited data suggest that garlic consumption *may* be associated with lowered risk of some cancers. However, using garlic supplements for less than 3 to 5 years was not associated with decreased risks of cancer.

SUPPLEMENTS WITH UNKNOWN OR INCONCLUSIVE EFFECTS

Saw palmetto. There is no published scientific evidence that saw palmetto has any value in the treatment of prostate cancer. Some research has found that saw palmetto extract may reduce symptoms of benign prostatic hyperplasia, BPH.

Mushroom (supplements). Shiitake mushroom supplements have not been shown to be effective in treating prostate cancer.

Shark cartilage. There have been only a few human studies of cartilage as a treatment for cancer, and the results are inconclusive. Additional clinical trials of cartilage as a treatment for cancer are now being conducted. The FDA has not approved the use of cartilage as a treatment for cancer or any other medical condition.

Soy (supplements). Taking large amounts of soy protein, as found in most soy pills or powders, could have effects on cancer risk that are not yet certain. Soy-derived substances are being tested in men with early prostate cancer as well as men who look like they have a high risk of developing the disease.

Black cohosh. This herb may have estrogen-like effects. Some proponents claim that it reduces prostate cancer risk. No clinical trials addressing this issue have been conducted.

Zinc. There is no clinical evidence to support the use of zinc supplements to affect the growth or spread of cancer. Zinc supplements have been associated with some protective effects against prostate cancer risk. However, taking more than 100 mg daily of this mineral may increase a man's prostate cancer risk.

SUPPLEMENTS THAT MAY BE HARMFUL

Dehydroepiandrosterone (DHEA). There is no scientific evidence that this steroid hormone is safe or effective. Some researchers believe DHEA may increase prostate cancer risk and promote the growth of prostate cancer. It should not be used for treating cancer.

Laetrile. Laetrile is a compound produced from amygdalin, a naturally occurring substance found in the pits of many fruits. There is no scientific evidence that Laetrile is effective in treating cancer or any other disease. It contains a small percentage of cyanide, and several cases of cyanide poisoning have been linked to its use. Laetrile use is illegal in the United States.

Questions to Ask About Alternative Treatments and Supplements

If you hear of a treatment option that seems promising, research it and talk to your health care team about it. Make sure you understand study results and the potential side effects, applying the same standards for treatment that you do for prescription drugs.

- Has the treatment been shown effective in clinical trials?
- Are there known potential side effects?
- Are there interactions with drugs?
- What are the costs associated with use?

Licorice (supplements). There is no evidence that supplements made of the licorice plant are effective in treating cancer. Licorice supplements are occasionally associated with side effects that can cause serious problems.

St. John's wort. This herb may be used to treat mild or moderate depression. It has been shown to diminish the effects of chemotherapy and some other drugs.

Carry a list of *all* of the medicines, vitamins, and supplements you are taking every time you visit your doctor and make sure that your doctor knows about them. Many supplements could reduce the effectiveness of a prescription medication.

Talk to your doctor about the latest advances. Some of the largest dietary supplement trials in medical history are ongoing, including those testing the potentially positive effects of selenium and vitamin E, so consult with your doctor. (See chapter 32 for more information about ongoing studies.)

LIFE AFTER TREATMENT: WHAT NOW?

NOW THAT YOU'VE UNDERGONE TREATMENT, YOU MAY BE facing temporary or long-term side effects and learning how to cope with and address them. You may also have concerns about having to deal with cancer all over again if it recurs. Be alert to changes in your body. Some men with prostate cancer will experience recurrence, so adhering to a follow-up plan is essential to finding recurrent cancer early and managing it.

In chapters 28 and 29 we outline the elements of a follow-up plan and your options for treating recurrence if it does arise. Chapter 30 explores issues related to possible changes in your life following treatment, particularly relating to intimate aspects such as erectile dysfunction and incontinence. You should expect to main a high quality of life after treatment. There are measures that can help you deal with the side effects you may be experiencing. Try to be open to new ideas, and be willing to communicate fully with your partner about your needs and how you might find satisfaction in your personal and sexual lives together. Both you and your partner may find Chapter 30 valuable to read.

Be Alert to Changes in Your Body

Some men with prostate cancer will experience recurrence, so adhering to a follow-up plan is essential to finding recurrent cancer early and managing it.

CHAPTER 28

FOLLOW UP

Paul H. Lange, MD
Bruce Montgomery, MD

AFTER YOU HAVE COMPLETED YOUR TREATMENT for prostate cancer, your health care team will want to carefully and regularly monitor your health. Remember that your body is as unique as your personality and your fingerprints. Although your cancer's stage and the effectiveness of your treatment options can help predict the outcomes and challenges you may face, no one can say precisely how you will respond to cancer or its treatment.

What Is the Likelihood My Cancer Will Come Back?

Your doctor will usually talk to you about the likelihood that the treatment that you receive will successfully treat your cancer. The risk of cancer not being completely eradicated varies substantially depending on prognostic factors (discussed in chapter 17) and the type of treatment you decided to receive. The level of prostate-specific antigen (PSA) at the time of diagnosis and treatment, the Gleason grade of the tumor at biopsy or prostatectomy, and the extent of the tumor all significantly affect the risk of recurrence.

Although doctors and patients often talk about cancer "coming back," when we say cancer has "recurred," we really mean that it never really left—it wasn't completely destroyed for any of a number of reasons. For example, the cancer may have spread outside of the area that was treated with radiation or surgery, the cancer may not have been completely killed by radiation or other treatment, or some cancer may have been left behind after surgery because it was difficult to remove all of it at the time of the operation.

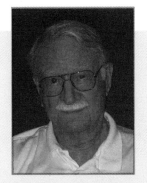

Follow Up Is Essential

My diagnosis of prostate cancer made me think of what we infantrymen used to say in World War II, "You don't hear it until it hits you." At my first follow-up visit after hormone shots and radiation, my doctor told me I had a prostate that felt flat and like a 20 year old's.

— *William M.*

You aren't through with prostate cancer after treatment. We go back every 4 months for a blood test, or every 6 months for a PSA, or every 8 months for a PSA and a digital rectal exam. When you have a toothache, the dentist pulls the tooth out and you don't deal with it anymore. But with prostate cancer, we need checkups.

— *Dennis*

When doctors talk about the cancer growing again, the greatest risk occurs within the first 5 years after treatment, although it is possible to have a recurrence 15 years or more after treatment.

The Follow-Up Plan

Men who have been treated for prostate cancer require close follow up, and some men will require regular follow up for the rest of their lives. Follow up helps your health care team monitor your health and progress. The plan usually includes regular doctor's visits, PSA blood tests, and digital rectal examinations (DREs). X-rays or other imaging tests may also be done, depending on your medical situation. The health care team will evaluate any new symptoms or side effects and be sensitive to the possibility of local recurrence (recurrent cancer in the area of the prostate gland) or metastatic recurrence (recurrent cancer in a distant part of the body). In some situations, detecting a recurrence early provides time for additional therapy to give men a second chance for cure.

CHECKING FOR A CHANGE IN STATUS OR NEW SYMPTOMS

A doctor's visit will include a review of any new symptoms that might suggest problems with the prostate or problems in an area where cancer may have spread. Any new symptoms indicating a prostate problem would likely be very similar to those your doctor asked you about when you were first being evaluated for a diagnosis of cancer (see chapter 5). These might include changes in your ability to urinate, pain in the groin or the bones, bleeding or blood in the urine, fatigue, or weight loss.

A digital rectal examination may also be performed to feel for any changes in the prostate gland (or in the prostate area, if you have had a prostatectomy). In addition, your PSA will often be checked.

A man may have a low PSA reading during or immediately after hormone treatment, but this low level may not be a true measure of the amount of prostate tissue in the body. If you are receiving hormone therapy, ask your doctor if you should wait a few months after completing hormone treatment before having a PSA test.

EVALUATING LONG-TERM TREATMENT SIDE EFFECTS

Most men who are treated for prostate cancer are concerned with immediate challenges, including incontinence, impotence, and proctitis (damage to the colon and rectum causing diarrhea and bleeding). Some of these problems may be permanent. However, these and other treatment-related side effects may develop 1 or 2 years after treatment and are referred to as delayed side effects, or late effects. It can be important for your doctor to detect any side effects of treatment early. These include:

- bleeding and spasms of the rectum, which can occur in up to 15 percent of patients treated with radiation to the prostate
- bleeding, abnormal urinary habits, or narrowing of the urethra, which makes it more difficult to urinate; occasionally radiation reaches the bladder and causes these symptoms
- bladder cancer, which may very rarely develop after radiation

When some of these symptoms appear, they may seem to be caused by cancer. Many are actually benign and can be treated effectively once they are recognized.

FREQUENCY OF FOLLOW-UP VISITS

Many urologists and radiation oncologists schedule follow-up appointments with patients every 3 to 6 months for the first several years after treatment. In many cases, after a few years, visits become less frequent and usually occur yearly. Some of the factors discussed above, including PSA, Gleason score, and how much cancer was thought to be present before therapy will have an impact on how frequently your doctor will perform these examinations.

The timing of follow-up visits will depend in part on what sort of treatment you have received. Different prostate cancer therapies carry different expectations about how quickly PSA levels and prostate status may change in response to the treatment:

- If you were treated with **radical prostatectomy**, the purpose was to remove all of the cancer and normal prostate tissue (which also creates some PSA). Therefore PSA should be essentially undetectable (usually considered to be below 0.2 ng/ml) within a few months after prostatectomy. If the PSA does not drop to an extremely low level, cancer may still be present, and additional studies may be necessary.
- After **radiation therapy** (external beam or brachytherapy) the prostate gland is still present, and some level of PSA is usually detectable even many years after treatment. It usually takes between 6 months and 2 years for the PSA to reach its lowest level, which should be below 1 ng/ml.

- For men treated with **hormonal therapy**, PSA levels will usually drop below 5 to 10 ng/ml within 3 months.
- When a man decides on the **"watchful waiting"** approach, the PSA will generally not decline and will usually increase to some degree over time.

WATCHFUL WAITING CHECKUPS

Because prostate cancer generally grows slowly and treatment often causes side effects that negatively affect quality of life, some men opt not to have active treatment but to have their cancer and their health monitored. Men who pursue "watchful waiting" rather than undergoing treatment may choose to treat prostate cancer if it causes symptoms or if it spreads. (See chapter 23 for more information.)

These men should have PSA tests every 3 to 6 months and should undergo thorough medical examinations for symptoms of growth or spread. Serious complications can occur if cancer is left unchecked; if you are pursuing watchful waiting, stay on your doctor's follow-up plan and monitor your own health for any changes. Discuss these with your health care team.

HOW IMPORTANT IS PSA TESTING DURING FOLLOW UP?

Because PSA provides the most sensitive method of following potential prostate cancer development, following PSA levels has become a standard part of follow up after treatment. The level of PSA is generally a reflection of the amount of normal prostate tissue or prostate cancer that is present in a man's body.

However, despite the sensitivity of PSA, it is not perfect, and changes in PSA do not always reflect growth of prostate cancer. Small increases in PSA, such as a rise from 0.1 to 0.2 ng/ml, may reflect normal variations in the body or a laboratory error, instead of a potential recurrence. Therefore, your doctor will probably recommend another PSA test to confirm any increase that is noted.

There are also unusual prostate cancers that make low levels of PSA, such as small cell cancer (a cancer found in the lungs and, less often, in several other organs; named for the way the cancer cells look), for example, and PSA does not do a good job of detecting these cancers.

Coping With Concerns About Follow Up

I have a PSA test every year; my surgery was 7 years ago. In a discussion at our support group we all pretty much agreed that once the PSA test is over, the thought of cancer goes into the back of our minds and doesn't resurface until the following year when it's PSA test time again.

– Dave R.

I'm not really a worrier about follow-up tests. I was in Korea and when I heard the shelling, I figured I'd never return from there. And I've had other health issues. Right now I'm having breathing problems. These are all just parts of life and I don't worry about one more than the other. In fact, I don't really worry about them at all, it's just another thing to deal with along the way. Otherwise I would have been worrying all these decades since the Korean War.

– Peter

The PSA "Bounce"

After radiation therapy, PSA drops slowly, and after treatment there is the possibility of a phenomenon known as the "PSA bounce." This means that at some time between 6 months and 2 years after radiation therapy, the PSA begins to rise, but on subsequent tests it is shown to have come back down. This bounce in PSA level is thought to be due to inflammation of the prostate gland from the radiation; the inflammation eventually resolves on its own, and the PSA drops.

The PSA will be monitored closely during this time. If a man's PSA level falls below the initial level, he has no greater risk of recurrent prostate cancer than men who do not have this bounce.

WHEN PSA RISES

Regardless of the treatment you may have received, if the PSA rises and remains elevated after therapy, it suggests—but does not definitively indicate—that prostate cancer is present. In many cases a rise in PSA reflects a very small amount of cancer, too small to be causing symptoms.

Although a rising PSA can be frightening, the fact that PSA is elevated does not mean the same thing for all men. Several studies have shown that even when men have a consistently elevated PSA after prostatectomy or radiation, it can take some time before they develop problems related to their cancer. If a man's PSA rises after prostatectomy, it takes an average of 8 more years before he develops symptoms from his cancer. A rapidly rising PSA suggests that symptoms may develop sooner than this, but for some men, the fact that their prostate cancer is growing again does not impact the duration or quality of their lives. (See chapter 23 for more information about situations in which cancer may be monitored and may not impact a man's daily life.)

When the PSA rises, many doctors will do tests to try to determine where any cancer is located. These tests may include bone scans, CT scans, MRI, or tests such as ProstaScint studies, in addition to a physical examination and digital rectal examination (see chapter 15 for more information about imaging studies). Some doctors will recommend a biopsy of the prostate area to determine if there is evidence that the prostate cancer might still be in the area where it was originally treated.

In some situations, additional therapy such as radiation, cryotherapy, hormone treatment, or surgery may be possible to treat recurrent cancer. The details of these treatments and when they might be pursued is discussed in more detail in chapter 29.

QUESTIONS TO ASK YOUR DOCTOR ABOUT RECURRENCE

Not everyone wants to know the same amount of information about possible recurrence. Discussing follow up and recurrence with your doctor will help you understand the testing that goes on after treatment and the decisions you may make with your doctor regarding monitoring and therapy. Questions you may want to pose after your treatment is complete may include:

- What are the risks that my cancer will come back?
- Was there any evidence that surgery or radiation did not remove or destroy all of the cancer?
- Are there additional treatments such as hormone therapy or radiation available that might reduce my risk of recurrence?
- How often will you see me and what tests will you do?
- What symptoms might suggest that my cancer has returned and what should I do if they develop?

If your PSA is elevated after prostatectomy:

- Might radiation therapy to my prostate area and/or hormonal therapy be appropriate?
- Can you tell how quickly the PSA is rising?
- Have any research studies been done on therapy that could treat my cancer?

If your PSA is elevated after radiation:

- How likely is it that the elevated PSA is related to the "bounce"?
- Should we consider a biopsy of the prostate?
- What further treatment options might be appropriate?

CHECKING IN WITH YOUR HEALTH CARE TEAM

It is important to continue communicating with your health care team after treatment. Some men keep symptoms to themselves or prefer to avoid thinking about the cancer coming back rather than seeing their doctor on a regular basis. Share any concerns with your health care team. Finding out that everything is going well can be a load off of your mind. Knowing where things stand with any recurrent cancer allows you to explore available treatments before a delay might limit your options. Problems related to treatment side effects are important to evaluate and address early as well. In many ways, close monitoring is just as important as the original treatment.

CHAPTER 29

RECURRENCE

Nancy A. Dawson, MD
Rafael V. Miguel, MD
William K. Oh, MD
Fred Saad, MD, FRCSC
Miah-Hiang Tay, MD

RECURRENT CANCER IS CANCER THAT WAS NOT DESTROYED during your earlier treatment. The cancer is not necessarily where it started. It might have spread to other parts of your body. If the cancer is discovered after treatment, it will still be considered prostate cancer no matter what part of the body it is found in. This is because the cancer cells themselves are still prostate cancer cells; they have just moved to another part of the body. The primary site, the place where cancer began, always remains the same.

Unfortunately, it is estimated that up to 40 percent of men treated initially for localized prostate cancer (cancer that has not spread beyond the prostate) will later learn that additional prostate cancer has been discovered. Because of the possibility of recurrence, it may be more accurate to think of cancer as a chronic life-long disease that needs to be monitored and cared for throughout your life, rather than a one-time illness that can be cured by a short period of treatment.

Understanding recurrence allows you to partner with your health care team, both in monitoring your health after treatment and if you eventually do need to decide how to handle a cancer recurrence. As you saw in chapter 28, follow-up PSA testing and other care is essential for men who have undergone treatment for prostate cancer. After treatment ends, it is especially important to be alert to changes in your body and to report any unusual symptoms to your doctor.

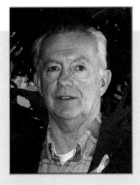

Having a Plan B

There is no definitive treatment for prostate cancer. Our support group emphasizes "What if..." What happens if your cancer returns? How do you handle it and how do you deal with it? Having a plan B in effect seems to be working very well, reducing a lot of stress. I know if prostate cancer returns, I just fall into plan B and go on my merry life. Our motto is "Knowledge Equals Survival." The more knowledge you have about your disease, the better your chances of survival, especially if you have a recurrence.

— *Dennis*

Facing the Possibility of Recurrence

You may have a recurrence. I accepted that fact, pursue follow-up visits, which are very important, and try to face the future with a positive attitude.

— *Wilson*

How Does Cancer Recur?

Cancer recurs because prostate cancer cells survived treatment—in the prostate area after prostatectomy, in the prostate gland after radiation, or in other places in the body where cancer cells spread but were not detected at the time of primary treatment. These prostate cancer cells will produce prostate-specific antigen (PSA) that can be detected in the blood and will signal to a man's health care team that cancer may be present.

After the initial diagnosis, if no evidence shows that cancer has spread beyond the prostate, a man may undergo prostatectomy to remove the gland—and the cancer. But whether all of the cancer was truly confined to the prostate gland can't be determined until after the prostate is removed and examined. Unfortunately, if the cancer had already spread, there is a good chance that some of the cancer cells were left behind when the prostate was removed or had traveled into other parts of the body before surgery. Sometimes no matter what type of treatment is used, a few cancer cells can survive and eventually grow into tumors.

So recurrent cancer is really "residual cancer," cancer left over after treatment because it wasn't killed or removed, or because it had already spread beyond the prostate. Most likely, the residual cancer involved only a small number of cancer cells, too few to produce enough PSA to be detected—until they had enough time and nourishment to grow.

Fear of Recurrence

It is normal to fear the recurrence of cancer. Some men prefer not to think about the possibility; others want to learn about and talk about recurrence in order to cope with their fears. Many of the organizations listed in the *Resources* section of this book provide support and helpful information, including support groups such as Us TOO and Man-to-Man. These groups educate and allow men to share experiences, emotions, and knowledge.

QUESTIONS TO ASK YOUR MEDICAL TEAM ABOUT POTENTIAL RECURRENCE

- Am I at high risk for recurrence?
- How will I be monitored for possible recurrence?
- Is there anything I can do to decrease my chance of recurrence?
- What are symptoms of recurrence?
- Where can I find information about prostate cancer recurrence?

A recurrence of cancer does not mean cancer has beaten you. It does not mean you will die. It does not mean you will experience unchecked pain and suffering. *Recurrence may not affect the length or quality of your life.*

Coping with a diagnosis of cancer and fear of recurrence—as well as actual cancer recurrence—can cause considerable stress. Although you cannot predict the future or magically alter your health, you can take control of how you respond to your cancer and the fear and upheaval it can cause. This might include seeking help and guidance from a mental health professional who has helped others through similar situations, which may allow you to enjoy your life more, rather than letting fear and worry diminish your happiness.

Types of Recurrence

The treatment that is most appropriate for recurrent cancer depends upon where in the body it occurs and if it responds to hormone therapy.

LOCATION OF RECURRENCE

The type of cancer recurrence is classified in part by the location of the recurrence:

- **apparently local recurrence:** cancer that *seems* to have recurred only in the prostate, or in the prostate bed (within the original location of the prostate) if the prostate has been removed; although we cannot know with certainty that cancer has not spread beyond local recurrence.
- **PSA-only recurrence (also called "biological recurrence"):** based on a rise in the PSA level, the cancer has recurred, but imaging studies show no evidence of prostate cancer The PSA is likely coming from microscopic areas around the body that are too small to be seen on imaging tests.

- **metastatic disease:** the cancer has spread to more distant tissues or organs in the body (prostate cancer most commonly spreads to bone, lymph nodes, and the lungs); metastatic cancer can be detected by imaging studies.

RESPONSE TO HORMONE THERAPY

Recurrence may also be classified based on if and how the cancer responds to hormone therapy. This designation is important in determining which systemic treatment options (treatments that reach and affect cells throughout the body) may best treat the cancer, such as second-line hormone treatment (a different hormonal therapy than initially used) or chemotherapy. Therefore, metastatic or PSA-only cancers may be further classified as hormone naive, hormone sensitive, or hormone refractory.

HORMONE-NAIVE OR HORMONE-SENSITIVE RECURRENCE

Recurrent cancer is considered hormone naive if the patient has never been treated with hormone therapy. Recurrent cancer is referred to as hormone sensitive if the cancer responded to hormonal therapy. A response to the hormone treatment is usually evident if there is a drop in PSA level. Men whose cancer no longer responds to the first hormonal treatment may also respond to another (second-line) hormonal treatment, although the chance of a response is much lower (see page 285).

HORMONE-REFRACTORY RECURRENCE

Hormone-refractory recurrent cancer is also called androgen-independent or hormone-independent disease. This is when the PSA rises while the patient is being treated with hormone therapy. In other words, the cancer is able to grow although levels of male hormones in the body have been reduced.

Current therapy for hormone-refractory prostate cancer is palliative, which means the goal is prolonging a positive quality of life rather than curing cancer.

HOW IS THE TYPE OF RECURRENCE DETERMINED?

Some men with recurrence may want to know if their PSA levels may reveal important information about their type of recurrence. PSA is only part of the equation. PSA level has different meaning for each man and depends in large part upon prior treatments. However, very high PSA levels indicate that advanced or metastatic disease is more likely. Over time, the implications of PSA level may change for a particular man. The man's PSA, symptoms, and imaging studies are evaluated; they are essential elements of the doctor's assessment.

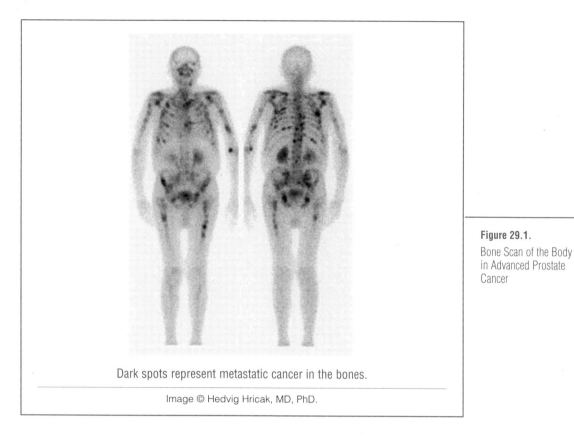

Figure 29.1.
Bone Scan of the Body in Advanced Prostate Cancer

Dark spots represent metastatic cancer in the bones.

Image © Hedvig Hricak, MD, PhD.

IMAGING TESTS

The exact location of the recurrence cannot always be determined with certainty. If the cancer has spread, imaging tests are routinely done to try to detect the disease. A bone scan is often done first to try to detect any cancer spread to the bones, the most common place prostate cancer spreads. A computerized tomography (CT) scan of the chest, pelvis, and abdomen may detect recurrence within the pelvis, lymph nodes, lungs, or other organs.

A ProstaScint scan (see chapter 15) can detect the spread of prostate cancer to lymph nodes and other soft (non-bone) parts of the body and can distinguish prostate cancer from other cancers and benign disorders. The test is able to find about 90 percent of cancers, but it also has a high rate of false positives, meaning it shows an abnormality (often in the prostate bed) when in fact there is no cancer there. The scan can help determine if a man may be effectively treated with local therapy, such as radiation. If the ProstaScint scan shows an abnormality outside the pelvis, there is a high chance that radiation treatment to the area will not cure the cancer.

The Risk of Recurrence

Cancer recurs because there are residual cancer cells that survive treatment, grow, and possibly spread throughout the body. Therapy to reduce the risk of recurrence is aimed at killing this small number of cells.

CAN A MAN LOWER HIS RISK?

Many men want to know what they might do to affect their risk of recurrence. Researchers are exploring drugs and dietary factors that might play a role in preventing recurrence and helping men live healthy lives after treatment.

MEDICATIONS

Researchers are exploring ways recurrence might be prevented in men who have been treated for prostate cancer. Potential approaches involve the use of drugs such as finasteride (Proscar, which prevents an enzyme in prostate cells from converting testosterone to a more active hormone called dihydrotestosterone, DHT), flutamide (Eulexin, an antiandrogen), and LHRH agents (manmade hormones).

DIET AND A HEALTHY WEIGHT

Researchers also are investigating whether healthy diets or dietary components that may help prevent prostate cancer might also help prevent a recurrence. Some studies have suggested that decreasing saturated fat and increasing mono-unsaturated fat *may* help reduce the risk of recurrence. Studies into soy's potential effects for men who have been treated for prostate cancer are underway. One small study indicated that flaxseed could have potentially beneficial effects on PSA levels in prostate cancer survivors, but any implications for men's prognoses are not clear. While vitamin E and selenium may reduce the risk of developing initial prostate cancer, a positive effect has not been proven for men after prostate cancer treatment. Studies are now underway to address this.

A direct link has not been found between either physical activity or being overweight and risk of recurrence. However, studies indicate that being physically active and maintaining a healthy weight prevents other serious diseases and may improve the overall survival of men who have had prostate cancer.

While eating a low-fat diet that includes 5 or more servings of vegetables and fruits each day and being physically active have not been shown to lower the risk of prostate cancer recurrence, these steps will prevent other health problems such as heart disease, a major cause of death for men who have had prostate cancer.

QUESTIONS TO ASK YOUR MEDICAL TEAM
IF YOU ARE DIAGNOSED WITH A RECURRENCE

- What type of recurrence do I have?
- What tests will I need to have?
- What treatment(s) do you recommend?
- Do I have different treatment options?
- Have any new treatments been introduced since my initial diagnosis that could benefit me?
- How much time can I reasonably take to choose my treatment?
- How long will the different treatment options last?
- What treatment side effects should I be aware of?
- What is the chance that the different treatment options will put my cancer in remission?
- Are the treatment options and tests for recurrence covered by my insurance company?
- Am I eligible for clinical trials?
- If the treatment is effective, what is my risk for subsequent recurrence?
- What support groups are available to me?

WHO IS AT RISK FOR RECURRENCE
AFTER SURGERY OR RADIATION?

As discussed in chapter 18, it is possible to distinguish cases of prostate cancer that are at high risk for recurrence even before initial treatment. Factors that indicate a high risk of recurrence include cancer that involves both sides of the prostate gland or extends outside the prostate *or* a PSA level greater than 20 ng/ml *or* a Gleason score greater than 7. Over 70 percent of cancers with any one of these features will recur within 5 years of initial treatment.

Treatment Options

For men who develop metastatic cancer and who have not been on hormonal therapy, the "gold standard" is hormonal therapy. In other words, there is general agreement among doctors that hormonal therapy best treats cancer in these situations.

Table 29.1. TREATMENT OPTIONS FOR RECURRENT CANCER

Localized Recurrence*

If Initial Treatment Was	Options Now Include
Radical prostatectomy (RP)	External beam radiation therapy (EBRT) with or without hormonal therapy, hormonal therapy, or watchful waiting
EBRT or brachytherapy	Hormonal therapy, watchful waiting, surgery in selected cases, cryotherapy, or investigational local therapies as part of a clinical trial

Distant Recurrence

If Initial Treatment Was	Options Now Include
RP	Hormonal therapy or watchful waiting
EBRT or brachytherapy	Hormonal therapy or watchful waiting

Progression on Hormone Therapy

Initial Treatment	Second Line Therapy	Third Line Therapy
Orchiectomy or LHRH agent	Add antiandrogen	Other hormonal therapies chemotherapy, bisphosphonates, and/or radiopharmaceuticals
LHRH agent plus antiandrogen	Stop antiandrogen	Other hormonal therapies, chemotherapy, bisphosphonates, and/or radiopharmaceuticals
Antiandrogen alone	Stop antiandrogen, start LHRH agent or orchiectomy	Other hormonal therapies, chemotherapy, bisphosphonates, and/or radiopharmaceuticals

*Recurrence believed to be local

Note: Investigational therapies as part of a clinical trial are an option for men with prostate cancer at any stage.

Based on *Prostate Cancer Treatment Guidelines for Patients, Version IV/August 2004,* the American Cancer Society and National Comprehensive Cancer Network.

In all other situations, however, there is not necessarily a standard treatment, and there are many treatment options for any stage of recurrence. Clinical trials have not established one treatment as superior over others, and different doctors may recommend different treatments.

Although the most common treatment is hormonal therapy, men with recurrence often receive varied types of treatments over a period of years. As with primary cancer treatment, the treatment you and your doctor choose may depend on several factors, such as your general health, treatment side effects, and cost. It is important for you to understand the options and to have a clear understanding of the side effects and how the treatment may affect your quality of life.

Many more treatments are available to men with recurrence at any stage than a decade ago, and new treatments are currently under evaluation in clinical trials. For more information about clinical trials and research into prostate cancer, see chapters 26, 31, and 32. The field of treatment for prostate cancer is changing rapidly. If your doctor is not aware of the range of treatment options for your stage of prostate cancer, ask to be referred to a specialist who is knowledgeable about newer advances in prostate cancer.

HORMONAL THERAPY

As outlined in chapter 22, the male hormone testosterone stimulates prostate cancer growth. Therefore hormonal treatments aim to decrease testosterone levels in the body or prevent cancer cells from using what testosterone is there. LHRH agents, orchiectomy, or combination hormonal therapy may be used to treat metastatic cancer.

Although hormonal treatment is very effective against prostate cancer, cancer will almost always begin to grow again eventually. The length of time initial hormonal therapy will work varies from patient to patient, but the average is about 2 years in men who have metastatic disease. For those who have PSA-only recurrence (no evidence of disease on imaging tests or exams), the average length of response to hormonal therapy is often much longer. Patients whose cancer grows after hormonal therapy have what is called hormone-refractory prostate cancer (see page 280 of this chapter).

A rising PSA blood test is the most common indication that the disease is no longer responding to treatment. Other indications include the development or worsening of symptoms such as bone pain or weight loss. It is imperative to monitor PSA levels regularly, for example, every 3 months, during hormone treatments.

SECOND-LINE HORMONAL THERAPY

A rise in PSA when the testosterone level is already low (due to hormonal therapy) indicates that some prostate cancer cells have learned to grow in the absence of testosterone. The doctor will usually recommend that a man in this situation remain on the original hormonal treatment because some of the cancer cells could reactivate if the testosterone level rises. But "second-line" hormonal treatments may now be considered.

Table 29.2: COMMON HORMONAL AGENTS USED FOR HORMONE-REFRACTORY PROSTATE CANCER

Class of Hormones	Names of Medications	Potential Side Effects and Complications
Antiandrogens	bicalutamide (Casodex) flutamide (Eulexin) nilutamide (Nilandron)	Breast swelling and tenderness, liver inflammation, diarrhea, visual impairment (nilutamide), abnormal liver function
Adrenal Inhibitors	ketoconazole (Nizoral) aminogluthemide (Cytadren)	An unusual lack of energy, skin rash, headache, nausea and vomiting, yellowing of the eyes or skin, muscle ache
Estrogen	Diethylstilbestrol	Blood clotting, breast swelling, abdominal bloating, yellowing of the eyes or skin

While LHRH analogs and orchiectomy stop the testicles' production of testosterone, prostate cancer may still progress in part because of hormones produced by the adrenal glands. In most men, this source of testosterone only creates about 5 to 10 percent of total male hormones. However, even this small amount provides sustenance to prostate cancer cells, so treatment to decrease the adrenal gland's production of androgens or prevent its activity can further control the disease.

The most commonly used drugs in this situation are antiandrogens, which block the effects of androgens on any remaining cancer cells. These drugs are usually the first to be added when hormonal therapy (LHRH agents or orchiectomy) no longer seems to be effective.

For men whose PSA continues to rise while on an antiandrogen, doctors have noticed that stopping the antiandrogen ("antiandrogen withdrawal") may lower PSA levels for a time. It is not clear why this occurs.

For men whose cancer no longer responds to these forms of therapy, other hormonal therapy options include ketoconazole (Nizoral), diethylstilbestrol (DES), and aminoglutethamide (Cytadren). Both ketoconazole and aminoglutethamide decrease the adrenal glands' production of male hormones. DES is a female hormone (similar to estrogen) that has been used for decades to treat prostate cancer. Each of these drugs has its own unique side effects; ask your health care team about their effects if you are going to receive one of these drugs.

RADIATION THERAPY

As noted in chapter 21, radiation delivers local therapy to treat a specific area. Men previously treated with a prostatectomy with rising PSA who appear to have local recurrence may be candidates for radiation therapy, which is aimed at the "prostate bed" to kill microscopic cancer that is present. The more favorable the conditions before radiation (i.e., the longer the doubling time of the PSA level or the lower the PSA level), the more likely the radiation will control the cancer.

Radiation therapy is generally not an option for men who had radiation as initial therapy to treat their cancer—that is, it cannot be repeated. This is because body tissues can only withstand a certain cumulative dose of radiation, and higher doses would likely lead to serious side effects.

External beam radiation therapy can be used not only to cure cancer that has recurred locally, but also to shrink tumors and reduce pain in men with metastatic prostate cancer. Radiation can be aimed specifically at metastatic tumors, and is usually very effective in controlling pain from prostate cancer that has spread to the bone. (See page 290 for more information about pain control.)

CRYOSURGERY

When prostate cancer recurs after initial treatment with radiation or prostatectomy, some men may opt for cryosurgery (see chapter 24). Studies suggest that while the procedure can be very effective, cryosurgery is likely to be most effective soon after cancer recurrence is detected—that is, when the PSA has started to rise but when the cancer has not spread beyond the prostate.

Men with PSA levels of 5 ng/ml or lower may be the best candidates for cryosurgery, and cryosurgery may not be as effective against cancer that has recurred after radiation treatment plus hormone therapy. More study is needed to measure outcomes and more clearly establish how well cryosurgery treats recurrent cancer.

CHEMOTHERAPY

Until less than a decade ago, prostate cancer was considered to be a chemotherapy-resistant disease. Great advances have been made in this area, and doctors now routinely offer chemotherapy treatments for advanced stages of prostate cancer. Many physicians are already recommending drugs like paclitaxel (Taxol) to manage advanced prostate cancer. The Food and Drug Administration (FDA) has approved docetaxel (Taxotere) injection in combination with prednisone (Deltasone, a steroid) for patients with advanced metastatic cancer. A randomized clinical trial of 1,000 men showed that patients lived an average of 2½ months longer with this treatment.

Table 29.3: COMMON CHEMOTHERAPY AGENTS USED FOR HORMONE-REFRACTORY PROSTATE CANCER

Chemotherapy Drugs	Potential Side Effects and Complications
Paclitaxel (Taxol)	Nausea and vomiting, low blood counts, numbness or tingling in hands or feet, muscle aches, hair loss, diarrhea
Docetaxel (Taxotere)	Fluid retention, mouth sores, diarrhea, low blood counts, nail changes, numbness or tingling in hands or feet, hair loss, tiredness
Mitoxantrone (Novantrone)	Depressed heart function, hair loss, nausea and vomiting, diarrhea, constipation
Estramustine phosphate (Emcyt)	Blood clots, nausea, diarrhea, fluid retention
Vinblastine (Velban) Vinorelbine (Navelbine)	Numbness or tingling in hands or feet, low blood counts, pain, weakness, nausea and vomiting
Carboplatin (Paraplatin)	Low blood count, nausea and vomiting, numbness or tingling in hands or feet, tiredness, diarrhea, constipation, loss of appetite

The chemotherapy drug mitoxantrone (Novantrone) has been approved by the FDA to treat hormone-refractory prostate cancer. That means it may be sold legally in the United States for this purpose.

The goal of any cancer treatment is to either maintain or improve quality of life. You and your doctor will need to weigh the potential positive effects of the treatment against potential negative effects, such as side effects, on your quality of life. Combining chemotherapy drugs has shown positive effects with levels of side effects that most patients can tolerate.

Chemotherapy's impact has been measured in some clinical trials through effects on pain levels and on quality of life. Men with metastatic prostate cancer receiving chemotherapy had better pain control and seemed to have longer disease control than other patients. Recently, chemotherapy regimens that include the drug docetaxel (Taxotere) have been shown to prolong life by several months.

Research is now focusing on improving current treatments by adding another drug or combining chemotherapy with second-line hormonal therapy.

BISPHOSPHONATES

Bisphosphonates are well-known medications that treat weakened bones. Over time, men with prostate cancer may develop bone weakness, whether from low levels of vitamin D and calcium in the blood that lead to osteoporosis; cancer invading the bones; or as a side effect of long-term hormonal treatment for cancer, which can accelerate the loss of bone mineral density.

Weakened bones are more likely to break, causing pain and affecting mobility. The spread of cancer to the bones may cause serious complications, including bone fractures and spinal cord compression (see chapter 3 for more information).

Bisphosphonates maintain bone health by slowing down the action of bone-eating cells called osteoclasts, thereby slowing the destructive effect due to the spread of cancer in the bones. They can provide several positive effects in men with prostate cancer, including preserving bone strength during hormonal therapy, providing relief from bone pain, and preventing bone damage in patients with cancer that has spread to the bone. By reducing the occurrence of bone complications, it is hoped that bisphosphonates will help prevent hospitalizations, prevent or reduce pain, and improve quality of life and mobility for men with prostate cancer.

Bisphosphonates come in pill and intravenous (IV) form. Only the form given intravenously has been shown to be effective in men with prostate cancer. Intravenous bisphosphonates such as zoledronic acid (Zometa) are given through an infusion in the vein (similar to an IV antibiotic) in a doctor's office or clinic. This process is not painful and lasts between 15 minutes and 2 hours, depending on the drug chosen.

Bisphosphonates generally cause few potential side effects, but may cause flu-like symptoms such as muscle aches, fever, and fatigue in about a quarter of patients. These effects typically occur for a few hours following the first treatment and can usually be relieved with mild pain medications such as acetaminophen (Tylenol) or ibuprofen (Advil or Motrin). Bisphosphonates may affect kidney function; although this is rare, regular blood tests are used to monitor this potential side effect.

Cancer Pain

Recurrent prostate cancer rarely produces severe pain, unless cancer metastasizes (spreads) to bones—most commonly to the spine, causing back pain. With the increasing use of magnetic resonance imaging (MRI) to help with cancer staging, more tumors are now found early, before they cause weakness or paralysis. But for men who are in pain from the spread of their cancer, various pain control options are available, and early and aggressive pain therapy can make men more comfortable.

THINGS TO REMEMBER IF YOU HAVE BEEN DIAGNOSED WITH RECURRENCE

- Continue to play an active role in your medical care. Ask questions, take notes, stay informed, and take part in informed decisions about your care.
- Seek support. Don't be afraid to ask for help from your family, friends, and other supporters to help you get through this difficult time.
- Take it easy on yourself. Allow yourself time to work through your feelings and to find constructive ways to deal with them.
- Focus on healthful behaviors. Before, during, and after treatment, it is important to eat a nutritious diet in order to keep up your strength and energy level and recover and heal as quickly as possible.
- Stay active, both physically and mentally. Try to be physically active on a regular basis if you are able. Keep your mind active with work, play, or other aspects of your life.

IDENTIFYING THE SOURCE OF PAIN

Sometimes patients do not mention pain to doctors because they think it is "the same pain" they've had for years. If your back pain worsens when you lie down or if it awakens you at night, cancer in the bone may be putting pressure on the spinal cord or the nerves coming out of the spinal cord. It is essential that you let your doctor know about your pain, which is treatable with radiation and medication but must be caught early to avoid injury to the spine or nerves.

An examination to identify the source of pain will include an MRI, or a myelogram (an x-ray following an injection of dye into the spinal canal so it may be viewed more clearly) and computed tomography (CT) scan if an MRI is not possible (for example, if a man has claustrophobia or a pacemaker).

MANAGING CANCER PAIN

If you have pain, you can help your doctor treat it effectively by rating the degree of pain you experience on a scale of 0 to 10, 0 being no pain and 10 being the most severe pain you can imagine.

Pain therapy is aimed at preventing pain when possible and controlling pain that occurs, while balancing pain medications' side effects in order to maintain a positive quality of life. Cancer pain can be treated in a variety of ways, including

FEAR OF ADDICTION TO PAIN MEDICATION

People are often hesitant to take opioid medications. Probably the most widespread misconception about cancer pain treatment is that pain medications lead to addiction, or uncontrollable drug craving, drug seeking, and drug use. This worry prevents many people from taking medications prescribed to relieve pain.

People who take cancer pain medicines as prescribed by their health care team rarely become addicted to them. People who take opioids to relieve cancer pain are not addicts. Nor are they at serious risk of becoming addicts, no matter how much of the drug they take or how often they take it.

by treating the cancer itself. But pain-relief medicines are the cornerstone of pain treatment and provide significant relief in most cases.

PAIN-RELIEF MEDICINES

An interdisciplinary approach to pain relief is ideal; treating pain through different methods helps preserve well being and functioning. Oral therapy may consist of the following:

- nonsteroidal anti-inflammatory drugs (NSAIDs): such as aspirin and ibuprofen
- opioids: strong prescription pain relievers, such as morphine (MS Contin) or hydrocodone (Vicodin)
- steroids: prescription drugs such as prednisone (Deltasone) and dexamethasone (Decadron) used to lessen swelling, which often causes pain
- anticonvulsant or antidepressants: adjuvant medications not only used for convulsions or to treat depression, but also used along with a primary cancer pain medicine to control burning and tingling pain, such as pain caused by nerve damage or spinal compression

Pain should be immediately and aggressively treated with analgesic (pain-killing) drugs while the longer-term pain-control options outlined above kick in. For mild pain, non-steroidal drugs such as cyclooxygenase-2 (COX-2) inhibitors can be very effective. (These are a newer type of NSAID with a better safety profile, especially in patients with a history of gastrointestinal ulcers. Medications such as celecoxib [Celebrex] or rofecoxib [Vioxx] can help relieve cancer pain as well as treat arthritis pain, their original application.) For moderate to severe pain, opioid medications are usually used. Opioid medications may be prescribed alone or in conjunction with one of the other medications listed above.

If one medicine or treatment does not work, there is almost always another option. If your medication schedule or the method by which you are taking medicine does not work for you or causes serious side effects, changes can be made. Talk to your health care team about finding the pain medicine or method that works best for you.

RADIOPHARMACEUTICAL THERAPY

Radiopharmaceutical therapy, or the use of radioactive medicines, is usually offered to treat pain due to cancer in the bones if there are too many areas in the skeleton to be safely treated with standard radiation. Injection of radioactive medicines is far more effective than aiming external beam radiation at each affected bone.

Radiopharmaceuticals consist of radioactive substances such as strontium-89 or samarium-153 attached to a bone-seeking drug. They are injected into a vein and settle into the bones, where they deliver radiation to areas of metastases. The radiation emitted by the drug kills cancer cells, thereby relieving pain.

Radiopharmaceuticals can effectively control pain for weeks or months and can be repeated if bone pain returns. In some cases, radiopharmaceuticals are used together with external beam radiation aimed at the most painful bone metastases. Since radiopharmaceutical therapy can cause low blood counts, your doctor may want to delay this therapy until after you have tried chemotherapy. Some patients experience a "flare" or increase in bone pain several days after the injection, which subsides after a few days. Doctors are also investigating combining a radiopharmaceutical with chemotherapy, but this approach is still investigational.

OTHER STRATEGIES

Other methods of relieving pain can be explored with a pain specialist. These strategies usually involve more invasive approaches, such as nerve blocks or administering opioids, alone or with a combination of other drugs, directly into the spine.

In addition, newer surgical techniques that address stabilizing bones in addition to removal of the tumor have allowed for better pain control and even immediate relief from compression of the spinal cord. These techniques are particularly important solutions for patients with spinal instability or whose tumors have progressed despite previous radiation therapy.

Your doctor should refer you to a pain specialist if you are not receiving adequate relief with oral medications.

CHAPTER 30

QUALITY OF LIFE AND RELATIONSHIPS AFTER TREATMENT

Sylvie Aubin, PhD

FINDING OUT YOU HAD PROSTATE CANCER was undoubtedly upsetting. But you may find that a surprising and positive aspect of the otherwise difficult and painful experience of having prostate cancer is that you have emerged from the experience with a new wisdom and strength, and possibly with the resolve to reach out to others.

Survivorship

You may hear the terms *survivor, 5-year survival rate*, and *remission* in reference to you or your cancer, and you may wonder what they mean.

Survivor is not a medical term; it's a word adopted by cancer advocates. It can have several different meanings. Some people use the word to refer to anyone who has been diagnosed with cancer. For example, someone living with cancer may be considered a "survivor." Some people use the term when referring to someone who has completed cancer treatment, and still others call a person a survivor if he or she has lived several years past a cancer diagnosis.

For doctors and scientists, the 5-year survival rate refers to the percentage of people who are alive 5 years after a cancer diagnosis. Five-year and 10-year rates are used as a standard way of discussing the chances that a person might live a certain length of time after being diagnosed with cancer. Medical professionals use survival rates to follow groups of people with similar diagnoses.

Remission is the complete disappearance of the signs and symptoms of cancer in response to treatment. It's the period during which a disease is under control and there is no evidence that the cancer exists. A remission may not be a cure or a permanent disappearance of cancer.

It's impossible to pinpoint a moment when one has "survived" cancer. Living 5 years after diagnosis does not mean that a person is cured or that the cancer will not recur. A person who has had cancer is monitored indefinitely to ensure that if cancer recurs, it is found and treated as soon as possible. This uncertainty is one reason some people with cancer are uncomfortable with the term "survivor" and don't use it. Others simply don't relate to this term for various reasons. Some people with cancer consider being a survivor a state of mind rather than a scientific measure of their life with the disease.

The American Cancer Society believes that each individual has the right to define his own experience with cancer and considers a prostate cancer survivor to be anyone who defines himself this way, from the time of diagnosis through the balance of his life.

A New Outlook on Life Since Diagnosis

At 47, I became a member of a club I did not want to join. I was diagnosed with prostate cancer. I got myself into the best possible shape and had treatment. Now I look at life differently: it's temporary, and now I make the most of every day.

— Joel

Diagnosis Was a Wake-Up Call

This experience reawakened my own spiritual path. My diagnosis was a wake-up call. So it's been more of an opportunity, and in many ways my diagnosis has been a blessing. Not something that I would wish on anybody, of course, but on the other hand, it's been a chance for me to learn more about myself and about humanity.

— Fred

Setting Post-Treatment Life Goals

People who have faced cancer share a unique understanding of time and the desire to make every day count. Before you find yourself immersed in daily commitments and routines, with new resolutions in danger of fading into the background, set down on paper the goals most important to your happiness and satisfaction.

Some men may want to help others going through the challenges of prostate cancer treatment by taking part in Man to Man or another support group, or by raising awareness about prostate cancer screening by talking to relatives and male friends. Others find volunteering with not-for-profit organizations like the American Cancer Society or political action groups who lobby on behalf of increased funding for prostate cancer research a rewarding experience.

Many men see the period after treatment as a time to recapture the satisfying lives they had before cancer's interruption. Setting a goal of returning to normal is also a valid way to cope with cancer. You may want to take this opportunity to take stock of your life, revisit your goals and desires, and resolve to take steps to achieve them, whatever they may be.

Maintaining a High Quality of Life

The period after treatment may be viewed as a time for new beginnings, a chance to make lifestyle improvements or to simply resume the valued aspects of your life. But coping with cancer and treatment side effects also means learning to achieve the best quality of life possible. It means maintaining self-esteem and finding meaning and pleasure in life, being comfortable, and enjoying important relationships in the face of the emotional and physical challenges that can sometimes feel overwhelming.

Because treatment side effects for prostate cancer include incontinence and erectile dysfunction, your sexual response was probably affected by treatment. Therefore this chapter will focus on helping you and your partner cope with changes in your personal relationships, including your sex life, and will encourage you to explore positive changes and growth.

Most men with prostate cancer report significant changes in their sexual response after treatment. For some, problems getting erections interfere with expressing affection and feeling close to a partner. But as you may already be discovering on your own, prostate cancer does not automatically signal the end of your sex life or emotional intimacy in your relationship.

Regardless of the prostate cancer treatment you choose, physical and/or sexual side effects are to be expected. Side effects vary in intensity and duration from one person to another.

MANAGING INCONTINENCE

Incontinence is the inability to control the stream of urine, causing leakage or dribbling. It is often temporary. But it can be demoralizing to lose control over such a basic life function. Some men may feel frustrated at having to modify their work life, social encounters, or physical activities—let alone their sexual encounters—to accommodate incontinence. Incontinence is a common problem, and there are a variety of ways you can address it.

No matter how severe your incontinence problem may be, you have a choice of safe, effective methods to deal with it. Even if the condition cannot be completely corrected, you can learn to cope and maintain your quality of life.

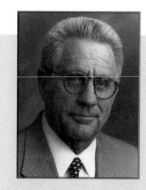

Reaching Out to Others

After I got through denial about my diagnosis, I reached out to others. I lobbied congress for more research support, joined a cancer wellness community, acted as a sounding board for the newly diagnosed, and joined the boards of local and state non-profit organizations that advocate for, educate about, or support prostate cancer in some way.

– *Will C.*

Raising Funds and Awareness

As a man who had been treated for prostate cancer, I was privileged and honored to take part in a fashion show fundraiser for cancer. It was a thrill to be a model for a day and have my "cancer résumé" and activities read to the audience, to a great round of applause. But I took the most pride in the fact that we raised over $65,000 to fight cancer.

– *Robert*

THREE PUFFING MILES

An excerpt of a poem by Tom Morris

In just the past year
I have learned quite a lot.
Some lessons were priceless.
Others, I would not have bought.

I know more about cancer.
I've joined ACS and Us Too.
I've taken some pills
That turn everything blue.

For the first time since high school
I've had a cavity.
Tooth problems are for Susan,
I didn't think they'd happen to me.

I've had lingering infections
That just won't go away.
Three rounds of antibiotics
And the cough seems here to stay.

I'm still easy to tire
Yet I don't get much sleep.
I'm sleeping in spurts,
So it's not very deep.

My stamina's slowly returning,
But a side effect does persist.
I'll just remain patient
Whenever I'm kissed.

I am not back to normal –
Not yet 100 percent.
But compared with a year ago,
I have little to lament.

A year ago today
On exactly this date,
I told my sons I had cancer
And wasn't sure of my fate.

It was only four days earlier
When the doctor told me
Only two strips were benign
On my biopsy.

We didn't know what would happen,
There were many blank pages.
I took a short-course on cancer
In various stages.

Now the cancer is out,
And the margins were clear.
I'll be regularly tested
Four times per year.

So tonight's a birthday dinner,
Just the four of us tonight.
My family is here.
And that's quite a sight.

You may benefit from one or more treatment methods. Talking with your health care team will help guide you in choosing the method most suitable for you. Choose a method you feel comfortable with, one that will allow you to best maintain your lifestyle.

Note that for men with urinary *retention* (an inability to urinate), such as following chemotherapy or HIFU, self-catheterization (inserting a thin tube into the urethra to drain urine and empty the bladder) is usually a very safe and painless procedure that can be done at home.

KEGEL EXERCISES

These simple exercises mainly involve training the pelvic and lower abdominal muscles to contract, which improves muscle tone and strength. Training usually consists of starting and stopping the flow of urine to locate and specifically exercise pelvic muscles. After a person is able to completely stop the urine flow, a series of daily muscle contraction exercises over a couple of months to a year or more if needed will continue to strengthen muscles.

Pelvic muscle training has also been integrated into many treatment programs for arousal and orgasm difficulties that may or may not have been caused by medical conditions. Speak with your doctor about whether or not Kegel exercises might be helpful for you and if so, how best to perform them.

MEDICATIONS

Appropriate medications vary according to the type of incontinence a man is experiencing. Incontinence is sometimes treated with a group of medications called anticholinergic drugs that relax the nerves that cause bladder spasms. Oxybutynin (Ditropan), tolterodine (Detrol), or dicyclomine (Bentyl) may be prescribed. Some patients take oxybutynin on an as-needed basis because it may cause side effects such as dry mouth and constipation. Tricyclic antidepressants, medications used to treat depression, such as imipramine (Tofranil), may also reduce incontinence. Talk to your health care team if you are interested in these options to find out if they are appropriate for you.

Post-Treatment Wisdom

I attend monthly support group meetings, where I picked up some words of advice. (1) Cancer is only a word, not a sentence. (2) If you have a chance to pee, always take it! (3) If you get an erection, make the most of it!
– William M.

Keeping a Positive Attitude Despite Incontinence

I haven't yet gotten the urination situation under control post-treatment, which leads to some embarrassing and uncomfortable situations. I cope with the help of my understanding and patient wife, and I begin each day with the hope that I have regained control and can feel normal again. I still think that day is coming and keep up a positive attitude. Don't let a negative, defeatist, or hopeless attitude take over.

– Barrie

Precautions That May Help Prevent Incontinence Accidents

Incontinence problems may also be dealt with through simple, common-sense precautions that may include:

- emptying your bladder before bedtime or before you engage in strenuous activity or if you plan on participating activities for an extended period of time
- watching your fluid intake, particularly drinks that contain caffeine or alcohol
- losing extra weight; because fat tends to press on your bladder, reducing or maintaining a healthy weight not only improves your bladder control but also your overall quality of life

You may also talk to a dietitian to find out more about healthy eating habits or to help you deal with problems of nausea or stomach upset from your treatments.

COLLAGEN INJECTIONS

Positive treatment results have also been found with injecting collagen into the neck of the bladder to thicken it and thereby improve continence. Because the effects of these injections do not last for long, it is necessary to have repeat injections, which can be expensive. Injections can be done on an outpatient basis under local or general anesthesia or sedation.

SPHINCTER IMPLANT

For severe and persistent incontinence problems, an artificial bladder sphincter (the muscular valve that keeps urine in the bladder) can be surgically implanted. Due to the very special nature of this type of surgery, a surgeon experienced in this type of procedure is recommended. Your health care team should be able to give you more details about whether or not surgery is appropriate for you, what you might expect, and the name of a specialist.

INCONTINENCE PRODUCTS

A wide variety of products are sold at pharmacies and specialty stores to help people cope with incontinence problems. Products include adult pads or undergarments, as well as bed pads or absorbent mattress pads to protect linens and mattresses. Most products are worn under clothing. Undergarments are bulkier than pads but offer more protection. Most products are comfortable, discreet, and do not interfere with mobility or daily activities. Many men report that these simple solutions have helped alleviate their worries about leakage.

SHEATH PRODUCTS

Sheath products, which may include condom catheters and compression devices, are placed on the penis and offer extra support to prevent leakage. Talk to your health care team about these products to see if they may address your incontinence problem.

COPING WITH ERECTILE DYSFUNCTION
UNDERSTANDING ERECTILE DYSFUNCTION (ED)

Erection problems, erectile dysfunction (ED), or impotence are all terms to describe the inability to achieve or maintain an unassisted erection (i.e., without the help of treatment) that allows penetration for intercourse. Unfortunately, erection problems are very common after treatment for prostate cancer. Men who are under age 60 and have prostate cancer treatments designed to spare their ability to have and/or maintain erections may only notice mild changes in the firmness or reliability of their erections, but for most, it is not possible to get an unassisted erection firm enough for intercourse to occur.

Almost all men who have had hormonal therapy notice a loss of desire for sex. Still, with mental and physical sexual excitement, about 20 percent of men report that they can have fairly normal erections. It may take a longer time, and more effort, to reach a climax. Because testosterone controls the body's production of semen, the orgasm may be completely dry, or very little liquid may come out of the penis. There is still much to learn about the unpredictable effects of hormones on sexual desire and erectile functioning.

Aside from the type and intensity of your treatments, the recovery of your erection may be affected by other factors:

- men under 60 have better chances of recovering erections after treatment
- the firmer and more reliable your erections were pre-treatment, the better the chances of a positive erectile response after treatment
- nerve-sparing surgery increases the chances of normal erectile functioning, especially if nerves on both the left and right sides are spared
- your sexual relationship can affect not only your erections, but how easy it is to use a medical treatment to improve them. Couples do better when they can talk openly about lovemaking and work together at resuming or maintaining an active sex life.

Table 30.1. MALE SEXUAL PROBLEMS CAUSED BY CANCER TREATMENT

This table lists sexual issues that may occur after various cancer treatments and describes how common they are. Refer to the treatment chapters in this book for more detail about treatments and their side effects, and talk to your health care team about what to expect after treatment and options for how to cope.

Treatment	Low Sexual Desire	Erection Problems	Lack of Orgasm	Dry Orgasm	Weaker Orgasm	Infertility
Radical prostatectomy	Rarely	Often	Rarely	Always	Sometimes	Always*
Pelvic radiation therapy	Rarely	Often	Rarely	Sometimes	Sometimes	Always
Hormonal therapy	Often	Often	Sometimes	Sometimes	Sometimes	Often
Orchiectomy (removal of both testicles)	Often	Often	Sometimes	Sometimes	Sometimes	Always
Chemotherapy	Sometimes	Rarely	Rarely	Rarely	Rarely	Often

* If a man did not bank sperm and wanted to conceive a child after prostatectomy, sperm cells could be retrieved from his testes and used for in vitro fertilization (IVF) with intracytoplasmic sperm injection (ICSI; eggs are removed from a woman, sperm is injected into an egg, and the egg is placed into the uterus).

Adapted from the American Cancer Society booklet *Sexuality and Cancer: For the Man Who Has Cancer, and His Partner.*

Although your treatments may have lessened your chances of getting or maintaining an erection, your ability to feel pleasurable sensations from genital caressing remains unaffected. With the right kind of caressing, you still should be able to reach a pleasurable orgasm, even if you have no erection and little or no semen comes out of your penis. If you and your partner feel pressured to restore your sex life exactly as it was in the past, however, you may get too anxious or discouraged to get as much arousal and pleasure as remain possible.

Focusing on the negative or non-arousing aspects of sexual encounters, such as worrying about how your penis responds or thinking that you will not be able to satisfy your partner, causes performance anxiety. The vast majority of men with erectile difficulties (whether or not they had prostate cancer) experience

Sexuality: A State of Body and Mind

Most men do not spend a lot of time thinking about what sexuality means to them. If an erection problem or other sexual problem occurs, men may find it important to redefine what is important about their sexual relationships. Although mutual caressing and kissing may be thought of as preparation for intercourse, arousing each other and even reaching orgasm through hand or oral stimulation is an important component of intimacy and a common way to share physical pleasure and emotional closeness. Your sex life should be based on what you and your partner mutually define as sexually satisfying and pleasurable and may or not include penetration.

performance anxiety. These thoughts not only distract you from the pleasurable aspects of your sexual encounters but also make you feel physically tense or nervous. As a result, your chances of getting or keeping your erection are greatly reduced, and you may think that you have lost your ability to have an erection since treatment. Men may not realize that state of mind and anxiety may have prevented them from having erections and that maybe their responses could be different if performance was not an issue.

Performance anxiety. Performance anxiety is a very common cause of erectile dysfunction, for example, mainly because it hinders your sexual arousal and pleasure. Signs of performance anxiety may include:

- erectile dysfunction problems that happen only during certain types of sexual activities (for example, when you are with your partner versus during solitary masturbation)

- erections that are better when you feel relaxed or improve when you are focused on a pleasurable caress

- spontaneous erections that occur outside sexual situations or at specific times such as in the morning or during the night; you may have these sexual responses in your sleep because they are unaffected by your conscious thoughts or mood

If you experience any of the above situations, your sexual changes are more likely to be psychological than physical. An erectile dysfunction problem that is caused by psychological rather than physical factors may be more likely to be temporary.

DECIDING WHETHER TO SEEK TREATMENT FOR ERECTILE DYSFUNCTION

Many men do not undergo treatment for erectile dysfunction. They are satisfied achieving intimacy and building a sex life without intercourse. Other men seek treatment. In the past 20 years, medical treatments for erectile problems have evolved rapidly. These important advancements may be in part explained by the growing demand for new treatments to deal effectively with both men's and women's sexual problems. The release of oral treatments such as sildenafil (Viagra) has caused excitement and focused attention on these issues. Regardless of the cause of problems with erectile dysfunction, there are a wide selection of treatment options with varying degrees of effectiveness and side effects.

There are several factors to consider when choosing a treatment. Make sure to discuss them with your health care team and understand how they affect your options. Although these methods will not interfere with your prostate cancer treatments, we still have limited information as to how effective they are for men with prostate cancer and what factors best predict treatment success. The following factors influence how effective treatment for erectile dysfunction may be for men with prostate cancer:

- your age
- the type of treatment you had (for example, nerve-sparing surgery or external beam radiation)
- your past and current use of luteinizing hormone-releasing hormone (LHRH) agents and anti-androgen medications
- any sexual problems your partner experiences

Fearing Erectile Dysfunction

Most men are very concerned about their sex lives. I was certainly no exception there, and it was a major, major concern. There never seemed to be a fear that I was going to die, but it seemed like death that my sex life was over. Of course, I was exaggerating that in my own mind.

There's nothing to be ashamed of. We are what we are, and we must take full advantage of all the good things that we have. We still have our lives, and there *is* a sex life after prostate cancer.

— *Ron*

ORAL MEDICATIONS

Three oral medications are now available by prescription to treat erectile dysfunction: sildenafil (Viagra), vardenafil (Levitra), and tadalafil (Cialis).

All of these medications work in generally the same way, by increasing blood flow to the penis and by blocking an enzyme that breaks down the substance that helps maintain an erection. The cost of these medications can be upwards of 10 dollars per dose. (Note that drugs obtained from an Internet source may not be as tightly regulated as those available in a pharmacy and may contain only minute amounts of active agents. It is essential to consult your doctor before using any medications to treat erectile dysfunction.)

Side effects may include headaches, flushing, nasal congestion, and blue-tinged vision. Because of possibly serious drug interactions, it is important to speak with your doctor about any other medications you are taking before attempting to use these drugs. For example, when taking any of these medications, it is very important to avoid nitrates (drugs for heart disease). Your doctor will also tell you to avoid certain types of alpha blockers (drugs sometimes used to help men who have difficulty urinating due to benign prostatic hyperplasia—BPH—or other causes) when taking some of these medications. For example, alpha blockers of any type may not be used with vardenafil (Levitra), while one type of alpha blocker called tamsulosin (Flomax) is safe for use with taladafil (Cialis), and you may need to take precautions with your dosage and timing of administration with sildenafil (Viagra).

Effectiveness. All 3 types of oral medications promise a 70-percent to 80-percent success rate with erectile dysfunction caused by either medical or psychological factors. Unfortunately, this rate of success may or may not apply to men treated for prostate cancer by surgery or radiation therapy. In general, oral medications help men who can achieve close to a full erection on their own and need some added firmness for penetration. The pills rarely work well for prostate cancer survivors who achieve only slight swelling of the penis with sexual excitement and stimulation. Oral medications appear to work much better when nerve-sparing prostatectomy has taken place than non-nerve-sparing prostatectomy, particularly if both nerve bundles remain intact.

NONPRESCRIPTION PRODUCTS

The release of medications to treat erectile dysfunction has not only increased society's awareness of sexual problems but also generated a growing number of alternative, over-the-counter medications and/or products available in drugstores that claim to improve a person's sexual responses. These products are considered dietary supplements (as opposed to drugs) and have undergone limited or no scientific testing to verify their safety and efficacy. Therefore little or no proof exists that they will work, despite claims of effectiveness in advertisements or on packaging, and little is known about their side effects or other health risks. Consider the following before trying any of these products:

- Is this product approved by the Food and Drug Administration (FDA)? Most prescription medications are. FDA-approved products have been scientifically proven to be safe and effective.

- Do claims sound too good to be true? They probably are. Watch out for promises of quick, easy, and dramatic changes in a short period of time.

See chapter 27 for more information about alternative treatment and special cautions.

HORMONAL THERAPY

Recent clinical developments have been proposed to preserve sexual desire and erectile functioning of men undergoing hormonal therapy. Interventions include the intermittent use of an androgen blocker, either alone or in combination with finasteride (Proscar). Although still considered experimental, intermittent hormonal therapy, which allows for rest periods between treatments, is associated with improved sexual responses.

PENILE INJECTIONS AND INTRAURETHRAL SUPPOSITORIES

Some methods of managing erectile dysfunction work by delivering chemicals into the penis to increase blood flow and produce an erection.

Penile injections involve injecting a prescription medication into the side of the penis using a small and often painless needle a few minutes before a sexual encounter.

Intraurethral suppositories involve placing a substance in small pellet form into the urethra at the tip of the penis with an applicator.

Because they offer a more direct means of delivery, penile injections are generally more effective than pellets, but they are also more invasive. Although both methods have similar side effects, penile injections have a higher risk of prolonged erections that may pose a medical emergency, scarring in the penile tissue that produces a small lump, and, in severe cases, permanent curvature of erections from repeated injections.

VACUUM PUMPS AND CONSTRICTION DEVICES

Vacuum pumps and constriction devices work to create and/or prevent the loss of an erection.

Vacuum pumps require a man to place a plastic cylinder over his penis, after which air is pumped out of the cylinder. This produces a vacuum around the outside of the penis and draws blood into the spongy tissues of the penis. When the desired erection level is obtained, a stretchy ring is placed around the base of the penis to hold the blood in and maintain the erection, and the pump is removed.

Constriction devices include stretchy rings or other adjustable constriction loops. They may be used with or without the pump to help keep blood from leaving the penis and maintain the erection.

Although generally safer than penile injections or pellets, vacuum pumps may disrupt a sexual encounter. The constriction device may stay on the penis for only 30 minutes, and as a result, the duration of a sexual encounter may need to be shortened. While the erection produced by the pump is usually firm, because the erection is maintained by a constriction ring placed at the base of the penis, the erect penis may twist or swivel at the base, limiting comfort and intercourse positions.

Vacuum pumps and/or constriction devices therefore present an important learning curve and require frequent, open communication between partners as to how these devices can be comfortably integrated into lovemaking.

PENILE IMPLANTS

Since their release in the early 1980s, penile implants have been considered one of the most effective, reliable ways to treat permanent, irreversible erectile dysfunction. They may be recommended after a man has tried less invasive methods of treating erection problems. Penile implants involve surgery to implant silicone rods and/or inflatable devices into the groin area. Implants come in various models, including rigid, semi-rigid, and inflatable implants.

The rigid and semi-rigid models are usually made of silicone rods and are surgically inserted into the spongy tissues of the penis, causing the penis to hang from the body at a 45 degree angle and stay about 80-percent erect. The semi-rigid model is often preferred to a completely rigid one because it is malleable and allows the penis to be bent to conceal the erection during non-sexual activities.

Inflatable implants are self-contained pump systems filled with sterile saline solution and may have 2 or 3 pieces, as well as tubes to connect them. These devices are placed entirely inside the body and offer a man a choice of having an erection or not. They are easily concealed and are associated with fewer lifestyle changes and/or adjustments than other implants. For example, physically active men may be very satisfied with inflatable implants since they generally do not limit physical activities.

How do inflatable penile implants work? An inflatable implant relies on the use of 2 inflatable silicone cylinders that are placed inside the penis. When a man is preparing to have sex, he creates an erection by squeezing a pump (located in the scrotum) several times to fill the cylinders with saltwater and inflate the penis. When the sexual encounter is over, the erection is released by pressing a valve located at the bottom of the pump, causing the cylinders to deflate, the saltwater to return to a chamber or reservoir, and the penis to become soft.

For the self-contained implant, each cylinder contains its own pump system, whereas in the 2-piece implant, the reservoir and pump are unified into the scrotal

Vacuum Pump

My wife and I have enjoyed using the vacuum device. You have to maintain a sense of humor. She says she loves "pumping me up."

— *Stan*

Help With Erections

Penile injections work great in providing me with reliable and sustained erections, and they aren't as scary as they seem. It's a really tiny needle, and the erection is worth it. I had a penis-ache side effect until I tapered to a lower dose.

— *Don*

Facing Changes in Erectile Functioning

In terms of my impotence, my surgeon uses the word "partial." It's not a problem all the time, or only to certain degrees. I waited about a year before I finally accepted the fact that things were not going to be like they used to be. Penile injections are a wonderful thing for me. My sex life's better than it ever was.

— *Ron*

sac. In the 3-piece implant, the reservoir is tucked behind the groin muscles and the pump is placed inside the loose skin of the scrotum sac.

Generally, the bigger the reservoir, the greater the amount of fluid available to produce an erection. As a result, compared to rigid or semi-rigid implants and the 2 other models of inflatable implants, the 3-piece implant shows the most promising results in terms of the length and thickness of the erection as well as the softness of the penis when not inflated. However, men generally observe that when the penis is not inflated, it remains soft but always a little fuller than a naturally flaccid penis.

Choosing the right implant for you. We encourage you to have thorough discussions not only with your health care team, but also with other professionals (such as a sex therapist, see below) about the pros and cons of each type of implant. You will want to include your partner in the decision-making process as well to ensure that you both understand the procedure and so you will both be able to discuss your fears and/or questions with your health care team. Sexual and/or couple counseling is often recommended and helps both partners to enjoy their sex life after penile implant surgery.

SEXUAL THERAPY

Sex therapy, also called sexual counseling, is a brief type of psychotherapy and usually consists of 10 to 20 sessions either for an individual or for both partners. A sex therapist is a licensed mental health professional (for example, a psychiatrist, social worker, or psychologist) with specialized training in treating sexual problems (see the *Resources* section of this book for more information).

The underlying principle of sex therapy is that sexuality is a lovemaking skill that is learned throughout your sexual life. Negative sexual and/or life experiences not only affect lovemaking skills, but can also create bad sexual habits or lead to sexual problems. These habits or problems may be corrected using sexual education methods and learning sexual techniques.

Sex therapy is based on a concrete, practical approach to learning sexual techniques and often relies on giving homework assignments of therapeutic exercises to practice in between sessions. Some exercises may be specific to a sexual problem or aim to improve the overall quality of sexual and partner relationships.

COPING WITH DECREASED SEXUAL DESIRE

One aspect of your sexuality that may have changed since your prostate cancer diagnosis is your level of sexual desire. Most men and their partners report a decrease in their desire for sexual activities during cancer treatment that may be directly related to the effects of treatments or to other consequences of cancer. Just as a man's erectile and orgasm responses fluctuate, sexual desire fluctuates over his sexual lifespan and is influenced by a combination of physical and psychological factors.

PHYSICAL FACTORS

Physical factors that may diminish sexual desire mainly relate to the side effects of lowered or absent testosterone and fatigue, low energy, or nausea. Hormone treatments such as LHRH analogs, antiandrogens, or orchiectomy have the goal of either stopping testosterone from being made or blocking it from entering cells in the prostate. These treatments are especially likely to affect your sexual desire (see worksheet on page 310).

Men treated for prostate cancer also frequently use prescription medications that can interfere with sexual desire, including opioid painkillers, antidepressants, or anti-anxiety drugs.

PSYCHOLOGICAL FACTORS

The way you and your partner react to your treatments—your communication, attitude, frame of mind, and emotions—can significantly affect sexual desire.

Your sexual desire has many sources of influence, and because most of them are under your control, you are able to positively affect your desire. Some men are able to maintain their sexual desire by remaining sexually active and communicating openly with their partners. They also learn from their health care team about available methods to effectively deal with these side effects.

COPING WITH ORGASM AND EJACULATION PROBLEMS

Orgasm refers to the moment of most intense pleasure during sex; ejaculation is the release of semen during orgasm. Changes in a man's ability to feel the pleasure of orgasm and ejaculate semen can occur after treatment for prostate cancer, and include difficulty reaching an orgasm, loss of the intensity of orgasmic pleasure, or having a dry orgasm. Premature ejaculation may be an indirect result of side effects from treatment.

DRY ORGASM

Radical prostatectomy involves removing the prostate and seminal vesicles, which produce most of the seminal fluid, and tying off the vas deferens (the tubes that bring sperm from the testicles to the urethra). Radiation therapy to the prostate also destroys much of the tissue in the prostate and seminal vesicles, reducing semen production radically. Hormonal therapy lessens semen because testosterone controls how much semen is made in the glands.

When the production of semen is stopped, the sensation of orgasm may be the same, but there is no ejaculation of semen. This is referred to as a dry orgasm.

WEAK ORGASM

When a man reaches orgasm after prostate cancer, the feeling may be less intense. It is unclear if this relates to having less semen, to weaker desire and arousal, or to having an orgasm without an erection. It is possible to improve the intensity of orgasm with time and practice.

PREMATURE EJACULATION

Although premature ejaculation is not directly related to cancer treatment, when men have erection problems, they may also have trouble controlling ejaculation after treatment. As a result, they may find themselves ejaculating too quickly and becoming frustrated if they are not able to detect the point at which they will orgasm or if their usual methods of delaying ejaculation do not seem to work. This premature ejaculation can be dealt with using simple, practical methods. Talk to your doctor about methods that may work for you.

Although you may feel unsettled about these changes, remember that you will always be able to feel the pleasurable sensations of orgasm. Cancer treatments do not affect pelvic contractions, and most treatments rarely interfere with your capacity to have orgasms.

MANAGING PAIN DURING INTIMACY

Being in pain is sometimes a side effect of cancer treatments and may interfere with your sexual response. A small number of men have pain during an erection, others feel pain at the moment of ejaculation, and some men simply feel sore or uncomfortable. Men who have undergone radical prostatectomy may experience aching in the testicles during sex. After radiation therapy, men may feel a sharp pain at ejaculation. (This pain usually stems from irritation in the urethra and should progressively decrease within a few weeks of your last session of radiation treatment.) Alert your health care team to any pain you have and discuss treatment options that may exist.

PERSONAL CHANGES

Coping with prostate cancer often means facing a series of changes in your personal lifestyle. Some of these changes are temporary. Others last longer and may affect the way you behave, the way you feel about yourself, or how you relate to your loved ones, including your partner.

CHANGES IN YOUR SELF-ESTEEM

Incontinence may impact self-image, and sexual problems may challenge feelings of masculinity. Living with diminished sexual potency, having little or no sexual energy, or losing part of the orgasmic experience may affect feelings of self-worth.

For the majority of partners, sexual satisfaction is not based on the rigidity or length of your penis but on the quality of your sexual exchanges and communication, as well as feelings of mutual closeness and caring. Try to remember that an orgasm can often be attained without penetration.

What Can I Do About Treatment-Related Changes in Intimacy?

CHANGES IN YOUR SEXUAL RELATIONSHIP

Periodic shifts from lovers to patient-caregiver roles will likely temporarily change the frequency and quality of your sexual relationship. Every person and couple reacts differently to the changes we've discussed, and people place varied levels of importance on treatment side effects. The worksheet in Figure 30.1 offers a simple method of evaluating your treatment outcomes that may help guide how you cope with side effects.

EVALUATING TREATMENT OUTCOMES

The worksheet on page 310 is meant to help you evaluate what has changed in your life and determine how important these changes are for you and your partner. Keep in mind that the most important thing to recognize may not be how an aspect has changed, but how bothered you and your partner are by it. As you think through these changes, consider the following questions:

- Why is that treatment change so important for me?
- What specifically bothers me about that treatment change?
- What other areas of my life have been affected by or are related to that change?

Set aside a time to discuss your results with your partner. Couples are often pleasantly surprised to find out how they each feel about changes or are relieved that many aspects of their relationships have remained or even improved since prostate cancer. Couples also often find this exercise useful because it serves to remind them of their strengths and gives them a better idea of the areas of their relationship they could work to strengthen.

EVALUATING TREATMENT OUTCOMES WORKSHEET

The purpose of this questionnaire is to help you identify the various aspects of your life that may have changed since your prostate cancer treatments (column I) and evaluate how important and/or bothersome these are for you (column II). Then you are asked to list the 3 aspects of your life that have changed the most and the 3 that are most important and/or bothersome.

Column I: based on the scale below, rate the various aspects of your life that that may have changed since your prostate cancer treatments:

Considerable or complete deterioration (1)

Slight or moderate deterioration (2)

No changes (3)

Slight or moderate improvement (4)

Considerable or complete improvement (5)

Not applicable (N/A)

Column II: based on the scale below, rate how important and/or bothersome these changes are for you:

Not at all (1)

Slightly (2)

Moderately (3)

Very (4)

Extremely (5)

Non-applicable (N/A)

SEXUAL RELATIONSHIPS	Column I (1 to 5 or N/A)	Column II (1 to 5 or N/A)
1. Your ability to get an erection		
2. Your ability to maintain your erection		
3. The rigidity of your erection to allow for penetration		
4. Your sexual desire		
5. Your sexual energy or stamina		
6. Your sexual thoughts, ideas or fantasies		
7. Your sexual pleasure		
8. The frequency of your sexual initiations		
9. The frequency of your sexual activities		
10. The quality of your sexual activities		
11. The degree to which you feel excited or aroused		
12. The frequency of your orgasms		
13. Your ability to control your ejaculation		

	Column I (1 to 5 or N/A)	Column II (1 to 5 or N/A)
14. The quality of your orgasms		
15. Your ability to sexually satisfy your partner		
16. Your overall sexual satisfaction		
COUPLE RELATIONSHIPS		
17. The degree of closeness between you and your partner		
18. Your overall couple communication		
19. Your sexual communication (e.g., desires, preferences)		
20. Your mutual display of affection or love		
21. Your satisfaction with the frequency of couple time		
22. Your satisfaction with the quality of couple time		
23. Your overall satisfaction with your couple relationship		
OTHER ASPECTS		
24. Your bladder control		
25. Your overall energy level		
26. Your self-esteem		
27. Your physical appearance (e.g., specific parts of your body or overall)		
28. Your body image (e.g., how attractive or satisfied you feel about your body)		

Based on your scores in **column I**, list the 3 aspects that have changed the most since your prostate cancer treatments.

1. _____

2. _____

3. _____

Based on your scores in **column II**, list the 3 aspects that are most important and/or bothersome to you.

1. _____

2. _____

3. _____

BEING PREPARED FOR DOCTOR'S APPOINTMENTS

Appointments with your doctor are often brief and focused on a specific aspect of your treatment. You may want to prepare a list of questions for your doctor, potentially including the following:

- What can I expect in terms of recovery time for my _____ issue (for example, desire, erectile dysfunction, incontinence, pain, depressed mood)?
- What are my chances at recovery?
- Can you tell me more about treatment methods that might help me deal with this?
- Are there any side effects from taking medications to deal with this issue?
- Will these methods interfere with any ongoing cancer treatments?
- Can you provide a referral to someone who can help me cope with this issue?

MANAGING EXPECTATIONS ABOUT SIDE EFFECTS

One of the challenges of dealing with the side effects of treatment is not knowing if they will be temporary and how long side effects will last.

LONG-TERM SIDE EFFECTS

Chronic side effects are sometimes called late side effects because they may take months or years to develop and are usually long-term. Even with procedures minimizing damage, such as nerve-sparing surgery, some men still permanently suffer from incontinence or erectile dysfunction. Erectile dysfunction problems usually develop long after radiation or hormonal therapy, sometimes up to 24 months afterward, due to irreversible vascular, nervous, or tissue damage.

TEMPORARY SIDE EFFECTS

Acute side effects, or early side effects, are temporary; they occur soon after treatment begins and end within a few weeks after treatment. Fortunately, most side effects from prostate cancer treatments are temporary and will go away with time. For example, incontinence problems from radical prostatectomy or radiation therapy are often short term, and normal bladder control usually returns within several weeks or months. Moreover, pain during an erection or during ejaculation, hot flashes, or diminished sexual desire due to low levels of or a lack of testosterone or to the stress of undergoing treatment will likely subside once treatment is finished. Erectile dysfunction problems may also be temporary.

It is difficult to predict the length and extent of your recovery. Give yourself several months or a year after your last treatment to develop a better idea of your long-term outcome. In the meantime, there are plenty of strategies you can try to evaluate your chances of recovery and restore your sexual life.

STRATEGIES TO IMPROVE INTIMATE AND SEXUAL RELATIONSHIPS

For couples with prostate cancer, managing illness-related issues may add stress and create strain on their relationships. The degree of closeness between you and your partner will be strongly influenced by how you both manage and communicate your emotions. It may also help to set goals of trying to provide each other with mutual support and listening or actively working together to solve problems.

MAKING INTIMATE TIME TOGETHER A PRIORITY

In the active phases of your treatments, your communication with your partner may have been mostly about care and other treatment issues. You and your partner may have spent less time together doing relaxing, fun activities.

Healthy sexuality starts with taking time to build intimacy together. Couple closeness can grow through planned occasions or time spent in relaxed, enjoyable activities that may or may not include sex. Here are some approaches to carving out time together:

- Identify a block of 3 to 4 hours during the week when you will least likely have problems scheduling or be physically indisposed and mark it in your weekly calendar.

- Select activities you both find relaxing and fun.

- Remember that your scheduled time together is not limited to having sex but is for doing any activities that bring you closer to each other.

- If you must discuss sensitive subjects, set a time limit and determine a future time to talk about these subjects

NON-DEMAND MUTUALLY PLEASURING EXERCISES

Resuming sexual activities after prostate cancer may pose a special challenge: how to cope with sexual anticipations or fears while learning to modify your sexual routine to account for your side effects of treatment or physical limitations. As a result, you may have postponed sexual activities until you felt better either physically or emotionally.

The most secure way to resume your sex life is to use a gradual, progressive approach and to make sure that you and your partner feel comfortable at every step. Sensual, non-demand mutually pleasuring exercises with no performance

Intimacy Beyond Sex

Sexual intercourse is only one way of showing affection toward your mate. You don't have to avoid showing any kind of affection or withdraw completely. A hug, a kiss, a touch—those 3 little things mean an awful lot and will in a lot of instances be satisfying. You can still have a feeling of closeness with each other.

— Dave R.

Becoming Closer Through Challenges

Having an erection or not being able to have an erection is not the bottom line for lovemaking. Intimacy is the bottom line, and I think we all want that. In talking with other patients and their families, I heard that many men and women were getting closer through the prostate cancer experience. The patients I've talked to have discovered this for themselves, and it's very heartening to see.

— Fred

goal (such as expecting to have an erection, to attempt penetration, or to have an orgasm) can allow you to regain intimacy with your partner in a relaxed, non-pressured context.

How non-demand mutually pleasuring exercises may help couples. These exercises involve focusing on sensual, pleasurable aspects of sexual encounters by mutually exploring each other's bodies. Exploration consists of touching, stroking, caressing, or massaging and gradually moves from sensual to erotic and sexual caresses. Partners also communicate their preferences and give each other feedback through hand guiding. Guiding is especially helpful in genital caressing because it may be difficult to verbally express the amount of pressure, location, and speed that feel most pleasurable.

- Exercises begin with mutual caresses of each other's entire bodies, avoiding the breast and genital areas.

- Partners then move on to explore the genitals and/or breasts without reaching the point of orgasm.

- At later sessions, partners have the option of asking each other to continue caressing to the point of orgasm through manual, oral, or other types of stimulation.

- The final exercises consist of exploring penetration. Initial exercises involve containment without movement and progress to gentle thrusting, including intermittent pauses to allow a focus on sensations. Partners are encouraged to explore with various types of penetration and different rotating angles and movements.

MAKING INTERCOURSE MORE COMFORTABLE

After a number of non-genital and genital exercises, you and your partner may feel ready to explore or attempt sexual intercourse. Penetration exercises are a good way to try new lovemaking positions without worrying about sexual performance. Because your favorite position may no longer be possible, may not feel as comfortable, or may be slightly-to-moderately painful, you may need to discover alternate lovemaking positions or make some adjustments.

Treatment side effects such as fatigue, shortness of breath, muscle ache, or weakness may limit your exploration of certain positions. For example, the "missionary position" (the man lying on top of the woman) may take too much effort because it requires sustained muscle strength and flexibility. You may want to try an alternate position, for example, one in which you are facing each other.

You may also experiment with various pelvic rotations or angles, allow yourself to rest on stable objects (such as a bed or table) for support, or introduce pillows to soften impact. Experimenting with different positions is a mutual learning experience and may involve multiple slight adjustments to make sure your encounters grow increasingly comfortable and enjoyable.

HEALTHY COMMUNICATION

Satisfying sexual relationships depend not only on the closeness of a couple, but also on the partners' abilities to communicate with and listen to each other. By communication, we mean the verbal and nonverbal expression of messages as well as listening with the body. Communication has the power to bring partners closer together.

Many factors influence our ability to communicate and/or to listen. These factors range from the nature of the topic being discussed to the way thoughts and emotions are managed. For couples with prostate cancer, resuming sexuality often includes the sensitive aspects of:

- making sexual advances
- how to decline a sexual advance
- telling the partner about changes in sexual preferences or desires
- sharing sexual fears or anxieties

Emotions such as sadness, guilt, or anger that may have been triggered by prostate cancer are often difficult to manage. Emotions may impair your ability to communicate by causing you to withdraw or to be defensive, critical, or accusatory.

Healthy communication is based on open expression and active listening. Communication skills may be learned through practicing a set of basic rules. These rules are often associated with effective speaking skills and are the basis of active listening versus passive listening. Some examples are provided below, and reading suggestions are provided in the *Resources* of this book. You may want to begin by reviewing these rules against your current skills and further discuss them with your partner:

- Try using the pronoun "I" to express your desires in a positive way. You might say "I would prefer this type of caress" as opposed to "Stop, that hurts!"
- When making a criticism, include positive feelings you have about your partner.
- Focus on understanding (not necessarily agreeing) by trying to put yourself in your partner's shoes or by looking at a situation from his or her perspective.
- Be specific. Avoid vague, generalized statements (such as those that use the words "always" or "never").
- Actively listen by asking questions and making head movements or sounds.

- Summarize or verify your partner's message to make sure you don't misinterpret actions or jump to faulty conclusions.

Communication and openness also refer to how flexible you and your partner can be at finding new, creative ways of bringing each other sexual pleasure, such as trying different types of sexual activities, body positions, or caresses. For example, if the first medical treatment you try is not successful, you may want to discuss more radical, but potentially more effective measures.

CONTINUE TO LEARN AND GROW

Knowledge is a very powerful way to restore your feelings of control and boost your self-esteem. Pose questions to your health care team about treatment outcomes and address any doubts or concerns you have, including your sexual concerns. Turn to reliable information sources such as those listed in the *Resources* section of this book, and ask your health care team for other sources of information. This will not only help you feel confident about your treatment decision but also provide you with ways for you and your partner to improve the quality of your relationship.

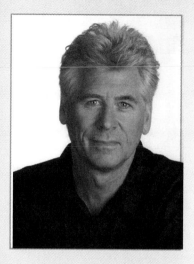

BARRY
BOSTWICK,
ACTOR

They say God doesn't give you anything you can't handle, but handling it can be a lot of hard work.

WHEN MY PROSTATE CANCER WAS DISCOVERED, I was playing the mayor of New York on the show "Spin City," and like my character, I didn't have a clue about how to face such a challenge. I was just another guy facing prostate cancer, and I dealt with it like any other "real" man, with confusion, fear, and some loud and copious weeping. And of course, a lot of leaning on my wise and patient wife, Sherri Ellen.

Before being diagnosed with prostate cancer, I'd never survived anything more serious than a bad opening night or a screwed-up relationship. I had always been relatively healthy, took care of myself with physical exercise and dance classes, had meditated for 20 years, and didn't eat red meat, smoke, take drugs, or drink too much. But I turned out to be the 1 out of 3 who would get prostate cancer in his lifetime. I never thought that "one" would be me! I always wanted to be somebody, but I guess I should have been more specific!

People say survivors often realize that a cancer experience opens their eyes to the possibilities of life and the love of family and friends. Well, I already appreciated the joys of life and the love of my family. But when I made it through prostate cancer, I did think it was time to examine my usefulness in the world. So one of my personal goals has been to help men examine their health habits and to encourage them to pursue all available screening procedures—in other words, to send men to their urologists begging for digital rectal exams and tests. Another goal is to raise public awareness about the need for more funding for prostate cancer.

My doctor feels my cancer was successfully treated with surgery. But when I'm forced to revisit the past by going for my bi-yearly PSA test, I once again feel vulnerability and sadness over the loss and diminishment of certain physical functioning…and when I face the statistics, charts, and odds of recurrence, it still scares me.

They say God doesn't give you anything you can't handle, but handling it can be a lot of hard work. I am a prostate cancer survivor and I intend to live a long, long time…so far so good.

RESEARCH IN
PROSTATE CANCER

THE FOLLOWING SECTION EXPLORES EXCITING RESEARCH
areas and specific studies that may pave the way for new developments in prostate cancer
prevention, screening, and care.

The role of genetics in cancer is explained, as well as the promising
power of molecular biology and how it may aid doctors in determining
which patients should pursue watchful waiting, which patients should
be treated, and which treatments might work best.

Clinical trials allow for the development of new treatments for
prostate cancer (and many other diseases). A chapter in this section is
dedicated to explaining specific clinical trials currently underway and
what researchers hope to learn in order to better address the needs of
men who are likely to develop prostate cancer or men who have been
diagnosed and are seeking treatment. If you are interested in partici-
pating, your health care team can advise you further about which trials may be suitable for you.

**Shaping the Future of
Cancer Care**

Clinical trials allow for the
development of new treatments
for prostate cancer and many
other diseases.

CHAPTER 31

MOLECULAR BIOLOGY

Jonathan C. Berger
Carrie W. Rinker-Schaeffer, PhD

ALMOST DAILY, TELEVISION AND NEWSPAPERS report a new discovery claiming that it may eventually result in a revolutionary new treatment for cancer. For a man with prostate cancer and his family, as well as for the public, these reports can be both exciting and confusing. In general, the media have neither the time nor the expertise to fully explain scientific discoveries or accurately assess their limitations or potential importance. In this chapter, we will give a brief overview of some exciting advances in the field of basic prostate cancer research and answer some of the common questions men with prostate cancer have about how these studies may impact their life and treatment.

What Is Molecular Biology?

Molecular biology is the study of life at a submicroscopic level. Molecules are arrangements of atoms that make up all matter. Molecular biologists study the molecules that are important to the functioning of living cells and try to determine how the behavior of these molecules affects a particular organism as a whole. In cancer research, molecular biologists study the molecules that determine how a cell grows, how it interacts with its environment, and what goes wrong with this machinery when cancer develops.

What Is a Gene?

A gene is a specific sequence of deoxyribonucleic acid (more commonly known as DNA) that stores information telling a cell how to grow and function properly. DNA is organized into structures called chromosomes. Each cell in our body has 46 chromosomes. When a human is conceived, 23 chromosomes in each of its cells are inherited from its mother and 23 are inherited from its father. These 46 chromosomes encode (specify the genetic code for) genes that are collectively referred to as the genome. The genome is copied and carried through every cell division.

With all of the excitement in recent years about the sequencing of the human genome, people often want to know exactly what genes do. Perhaps the best way to think of the genome is as a set of instructions, or a blueprint. This blueprint tells a cell how to behave: whether it should live, divide, or die, or whether it should become a muscle cell, a brain cell, a prostate cell, or any other type of cell.

To undertake a second analogy, a chromosome is simply a package for storing information, similar to a compact disc or a record. In this analogy, each gene on a chromosome represents a song on that record. Each of our cells has machinery that functions like a record player and is able to translate the information encoded in DNA. Instead of music, the songs contain instructions that tell the cell what job it needs to do.

How Are Genes Involved in Cancer?

Every time a cell divides, it must copy all of its genes. Most of the time, the copies that are made are flawless. However, occasionally a small mistake is made. These mistakes are called mutations. Mutations can occur randomly, but they can also be created when a cell is affected by certain stresses. Sun exposure, for instance, causes mutations in skin cells that may lead to skin cancer.

Mutations are very rare and usually do not cause problems, but when a mutation occurs in a gene that controls cell growth, it can start the cancer process. Usually several mutations in certain vital genes are necessary to convert a normal cell into a cancer cell. In this way, cancer is a genetic disease, so the study of genes is a very important and fundamental area of cancer research.

What Does Genetic Predisposition Mean?

As noted earlier, genes are passed down from parents to children. When people say, "You have your father's eyes," it is because eye color and shape are traits determined by your parents' genes. People come in all shapes and sizes because everyone's genes are a little different.

The term "genetic predisposition" means that small differences in the genes that a person inherits from his or her parents may increase or decrease his chances of developing cancer. That is why people might say that prostate cancer "runs in the family."

Genetic predisposition is an important determinant of whether an individual will develop cancer, but it is not the only factor. In fact, most cancers (including most prostate cancers) are not "inherited." (See chapter 2 for more information about risk factors.)

Individuals with a strong family history of some cancers can undergo genetic testing to determine whether they have inherited some of these genetic predispositions. At this time, however, such testing is not available for prostate cancer.

How Does Research in Molecular Biology Affect Cancer Care?

Basic research may change the way men with prostate cancer are cared for in several ways. Molecular research may affect how cancers are diagnosed, staged, and treated. For many patients, therapy such as surgery or radiation can successfully treat prostate cancer, while for patients with more advanced disease, it does not. Some men choose not to undergo active therapy at all, choosing instead "watchful waiting" because their disease is limited at the time of diagnosis and their age or other health problems suggest that therapy is not likely to lengthen or improve their lives.

Prostate cancers may grow at different rates and may need to be treated accordingly. Therefore a major challenge for doctors and men with prostate cancer is determining whether a patient should be treated and how. Basic researchers are currently exploring ways to answer these questions.

IMPROVED SCREENING

The prostate-specific antigen (PSA) blood test is a valuable screening tool for identifying men who may have prostate cancer. However, not all men with an elevated PSA have prostate cancer, and not all men with a low PSA are guaranteed to be cancer-free. Much of the basic science research in prostate cancer has been focused on developing new tests that may supplement PSA screening.

Through genomics, the study of how genes interact and function, researchers have discovered a gene associated with an inherited form of prostate cancer in some families. A man with the ribonuclease L (RNASEL) gene may be more likely to develop prostate cancer. RNASEL helps protect against infections and causes defective cells to die. If the gene is inactivated, prostate cancer may be allowed to develop.

A future blood test could determine whether a man with a family history of prostate cancer had inherited a mutation in RNASEL that may lead to prostate cancer. Such men might start screening at a younger age or undergo screening more often than men without genetic risk factors.

Researchers might also be able to target a cancer therapy at this inactivated gene and reverse prostate cancer. (See *Targeted Therapy* on page 326.)

A blood test could someday help determine whether a man with a high prostate-specific antigen (PSA) level has prostate cancer. Proteomics, a new science that studies the proteins produced by a cell, has led to the discovery of PCa-24, a protein that appears to be present only when prostate cancer exists in the body. If developed, a blood test for this protein could distinguish between prostate cancer and benign prostatic hyperplasia (BPH; which may also cause a man's PSA level to rise), avoiding unnecessary biopsies. Men with prostate cancer who do not show high PSA levels could also be diagnosed through a screening test for PCa-24.

MORE EFFECTIVE STAGING AND PROGNOSIS

Doctors currently use several tests to try to predict the course of prostate cancer in an individual. They may look at a man's PSA level, Gleason score, bone scans, MRIs, CT scans, and other studies. But these tests only provide indications, not accurate predictions. Some cancers with low Gleason scores may still spread, and some with high scores will stay confined to the prostate. Some men with low grade cancers may still develop metastatic disease.

Researchers are looking for ways to improve grading and staging so doctors can develop a clearer picture of how aggressive the cancer is in a particular person. These studies are already complete for patients with some types of leukemias.

THE P53 GENE

We can currently analyze some of the important genes in a prostate biopsy to determine whether they are mutated or not. Knowing which genes are not working correctly may help the doctor to tell how aggressive a cancer is. For example, researchers have looked at a gene called p53, which is commonly mutated in many cancers. Looking at p53 in radical prostatectomy samples shows that mutations are associated with higher grade, higher stage cancers and poorer prognosis. A test to discover whether a man with prostate cancer's p53 is mutated might guide doctors and patients to more or less aggressive therapy.

So why don't patients undergo a p53 test after diagnosis? At this time, p53 mutation is associated with poor prognosis in a patient only when it is found after the prostate is taken out. We don't yet know from looking at p53 in biopsy specimens how the cancer is likely to behave. This difference between biopsy samples and radical prostatectomy samples could be due to the fact that biopsy specimens allow doctors to look only at small regions of a tumor instead of the tumor as a whole. Although this seems to be a promising area of cancer research, p53 testing is not yet reliable for prostate biopsy samples.

PREDICTING EFFECTIVE TREATMENT

Because there are a variety of effective treatments for prostate cancer, doctors and patients are sometimes hard-pressed to decide how best to treat it. Choosing among surgery, radiation, hormonal therapy, or watchful waiting can be very difficult. Patients routinely consult several doctors, each of whom specializes in a different treatment, before they can make an informed decision. Researchers are currently trying to find ways to make treatment decisions less difficult.

ANDROGEN RECEPTORS

Researchers are looking at certain genes that may predict whether androgen deprivation will be an effective therapy. Androgens (male hormones) help prostate tissue grow by binding with a molecule called the androgen receptor. When testosterone or other androgens bind to the androgen receptor, a chain reaction of events occurs in prostate cells, causing them to grow. If this growth gets out of control, it results in prostate cancer.

Blocking androgen stimulation with drugs or surgery is a cornerstone of prostate cancer treatment (see chapter 22). However, some cancers do not respond to hormonal therapy, and there are several theories why. There may be a mutation in the androgen receptor that encourages or enables cancer cells to grow even without androgen. There may be other mutations in the cellular machinery associated with the androgen receptor that allow cells to grow. Prostate cancer cells may start making their own substances that stimulate other cancer cells. If any of these theories are true, looking for mutations in these genes may allow doctors and patients to more accurately choose the appropriate therapy. If the androgen receptor is found to be mutated, the patient and his medical team will know to rule out hormonal therapy because it is not likely to work. Knowing this could help the patient avoid side effects, wasted time, and unnecessary expenses.

Certain mutations may be similarly associated with whether a prostatectomy or radiation treatment is likely to be effective.

TARGETED THERAPY

Targeted therapies use a variety of methods to either attack and kill cancer cells based on the specific ways they differ from normal cells, or compensate for those differences to make the cells less dangerous. As researchers learn more about the ways mutations change the shape and function of the molecules that regulate growth and spread of cancer cells, they can better design drugs that specifically exploit or repair these changes.

Hormonal therapies for prostate cancer are an early example of targeted therapies, but many researchers believe that future targeted therapies will be even more effective and have milder side effects.

GENE THERAPY

Now that scientists know cancer is caused by mutations in genes that control cell growth and division, they are trying to find ways to change the genes in a cancer cell to help the patient. For example, if a gene that ordinarily helps ensure that a cell does not grow out of control is mutated in such a way that it can no longer function, an effective therapy might involve introducing a normal version of the gene back into the cancer cell. This normal gene would presumably give the cell instructions to stop growing and dividing. The effort to introduce new genes into a cell or to alter the genes that are already there in the attempt to treat a disease is called gene therapy.

The logic behind gene therapy is very straightforward: the genes that are mutated in a cancer cell should be fixed. However, there are many technical challenges that make gene therapy very difficult. Making a cell do what it does not want to do is difficult, even in a laboratory. In actual patients, it is even more difficult.

To begin with, researchers must physically get the good genes into the cells, a tricky process. One way to do this may be by using specially modified viruses. Viruses are tiny organisms that cause problems in the human body by putting their genes into our cells. Researchers are trying to take out viral genes that normally cause illness and replace them with the correct copies of genes that have been mutated in cancer cells, using the virus as a delivery system.

Other strategies for gene therapy involve more than simply replacing a broken gene. Some strategies involve making a cancer cell respond to certain drugs that it ordinarily ignores. Another idea is to make cells create some of the proteins that the human immune system can recognize and fight. This strategy is called immunomodulating gene therapy.

When Will Gene Therapy Be Available to Patients?

Though scientists and clinicians are very excited about gene therapy, there are technical challenges to making it work well. Some early studies have been completed in humans, but at this time, they have not been shown to improve outcomes in prostate cancer patients. Consequently, gene therapy will not be a generally available treatment for prostate cancer patients for at least the next several years. There are a number of ongoing studies involving gene therapy, and we encourage you to speak with your doctor if you are interested in participating in a clinical trial.

CHAPTER 32

OTHER PROSTATE CANCER RESEARCH

Samira Syed, MD
Ian M. Thompson, MD
Anthony W. Tolcher, MD

I N CHAPTER 26 WE EXPLORED WHAT CLINICAL TRIALS ARE, why men with prostate cancer may be interested in participating in them, and how to find out about clinical trials. In this chapter, we'll describe some important clinical trials that are currently underway, are still enrolling participants, or have recently been completed.

If you are interested in participating in a clinical trial, talk to your health care team about whether a clinical trial may be appropriate for you. You may want to research your options; the *Resources* section of this book provides information about organizations to contact to learn about clinical trials.

Prostate Cancer Research

The research studies in this chapter may be of interest to men at risk of prostate cancer as well as men already diagnosed with prostate cancer. The exciting ongoing research into prostate cancer prevention, screening, and treatment includes studies of diet, genetics, changes in current treatments, and cancer vaccines.

PROSTATE CANCER PREVENTION STUDIES

PROSTATE CANCER PREVENTION TRIAL (FINASTERIDE)

The Prostate Cancer Prevention Trial studied over 18,000 men without prostate cancer. Although the bulk of the study is complete, researchers are still collecting follow-up data and formulating recommendations based on their findings.

In this study, participants received either the medication finasteride (Proscar, which lowers the body's levels of the androgen DHT and is used to treat benign prostatic hyperplasia, BPH) or a placebo (an inactive substance whose effects are compared against the effects of a given treatment; a "sugar pill") for 7 years. At the end of the study, men who received finasteride showed a 25 percent lower risk of developing prostate cancer than the men who did not take the drug. However, those who did develop prostate cancer seemed to have higher grade cancers. Investigators are continuing to follow participants and test blood and tissue samples collected during the trial. This research is needed to clarify the results and establish recommendations for most men.

SELECT: THE SELENIUM AND VITAMIN E CANCER PREVENTION TRIAL

SELECT, the Selenium and Vitamin E Cancer Prevention Trial, has enrolled over 32,000 men in a study to determine if selenium or vitamin E, alone or in combination, can reduce the risk of prostate cancer. The National Cancer Institute-sponsored study is available at over 400 sites around the United States and Canada.

OTHER PREVENTION TRIALS

Two other large-scale phase III prostate cancer prevention trials are also ongoing at institutions throughout the United States. One of these studies is examining a cyclooxygenase-2 (COX-2) inhibitor, rofecoxib (Vioxx), a drug that is normally used to reduce arthritis-related pain. The other study is examining the effects of dutasteride (Avodart), a medication similar to finasteride (Proscar), which has been studied in the Prostate Cancer Prevention Trial (see page 329). The eligibility requirements for participating in these studies vary considerably.

PROSTATE CANCER SCREENING STUDIES
PROSTATE, LUNG, COLORECTAL, AND OVARIAN (PLCO) STUDY

Another important ongoing study is the Prostate, Lung, Colorectal, and Ovarian (PLCO) cancer screening study, sponsored by the Division of Cancer Prevention of the National Cancer Institute. The study is being conducted at a number of sites around the United States and is examining whether screening for prostate cancer through prostate-specific antigen (PSA) testing and digital rectal examinations (DREs) reduces the risk of death from cancer. The results of this study are likely to have a major impact. It will likely be several years before the results of this study are known.

OTHER SCREENING STUDIES

A number of new studies are being developed to examine how new screening methods could improve prostate cancer detection. One serious concern about detecting more cases of prostate cancer is the risk that some of the cancers detected would grow so slowly that the risk that they would spread and cause problems during a man's lifetime is very low. As screening methods become more sensitive, cancers that might not ever cause problems might be found and treated, resulting in unnecessary worry, unnecessary treatment, and troublesome side effects. But at present, no one can reliably predict which tumors will spread and which will not.

To address this issue, the Early Detection Network of the National Cancer Institute is mounting a major effort to determine if a new technique called proteomics, which uses technologically complex machines to measure the levels of PSA and the other 100,000 proteins that are in the blood. The broader analysis of proteins may help diagnose prostate cancer and distinguish which cancers are likely to be aggressive. This could allow for more balanced diagnosis and differentiation between prostate tumors that are likely to create serious health problems and those that aren't. (See page 324 of chapter 31 for information about the PCa-24 protein.)

EARLY-STAGE PROSTATE CANCER TREATMENT STUDIES

Traditionally, early-stage prostate cancer refers to tumors that are, in the doctor's best estimate, confined to the prostate and have not spread. The majority of men diagnosed in the United States, especially those men diagnosed by a periodic PSA or DRE, are diagnosed with early-stage disease. For these men, there are many treatment options.

A number of clinical trials currently underway are examining how best to treat this disease in its early stages. Some of these are phase II trials testing new treatments to determine if and how they affect the tumor. Examples of these might include studies of increasing radiation doses, new methods of implanting radioactive seeds, and combinations of chemotherapy and surgery.

While phase II trials are important steps in clinical testing, fundamental advances in the treatment of prostate cancer result from large-scale, phase III studies in which one treatment is compared with another.

Two ongoing studies are comparing the effectiveness of treatment and observation to determine if radical prostatectomy reduces a man's risk of death from prostate cancer.

PIVOT

In the ongoing Prostatectomy Intervention versus Observation Trial (PIVOT), 1,000 men with localized prostate cancer receive either observation or surgery. Researchers will compare outcomes and quality of life in the 2 groups of men.

RANDOMIZED TRIAL COMPARING RADICAL PROSTATECTOMY WITH WATCHFUL WAITING IN EARLY PROSTATE CANCER

The initial results of a study examining similar issues in Scandinavia have been published. Follow up of the 700 men lasted an average of 6 years. While the initial results suggest that there was no difference in survival in the 2 groups of men, the men who were managed with observation had a significantly greater risk of having cancer spread to their bones, which typically results in eventual death from prostate cancer.

The majority of these men were diagnosed through biopsies and had tumors that could be felt through a DRE. Only 10 percent were diagnosed through PSA testing, which typically identifies cancer years before symptoms develop.

SPIRIT

A very important phase III study in the United States is enrolling men to help answer another compelling question. The SPIRIT study, administered by the American College of Surgeons Oncology Group, is designed to determine whether radioactive seed implantation (brachytherapy) or radical prostatectomy better treats cancer that has not spread from the prostate. SPIRIT is available at a number of institutions around the United States. Eligible men are randomly assigned to receive either brachytherapy or surgery as a treatment for prostate cancer. An important component of the study beyond the assessment of the control of the cancer also is the examination of other quality of life issues such as sexual and urinary function.

SOUTHWEST ONCOLOGY GROUP STUDY

For some men with localized prostate cancer, the information obtained from an initial prostate biopsy indicates the risk of recurrence after treatment. Three pieces of information contribute to this assessment: PSA, Gleason score, and clinical stage; the higher each of these values, the higher the risk that the disease will recur after treatment. For men who undergo radical prostatectomy, an even more precise estimate of disease control can be provided by the examination of the entire prostate after it is removed.

Southwest Oncology Group Study 9921 is currently enrolling men whose risk of cancer recurrence after radical prostatectomy is 40 percent or more. In this study, participants who undergo radical prostatectomy are randomly assigned to receive either 2 years of only hormonal therapy or a combination of chemotherapy medication called mitoxantrone (Novantrone) and hormones.

This study is structured similarly to breast cancer studies 20 or more years ago in which it was discovered that the addition of chemotherapy after breast surgery saved lives for women at a higher risk of relapse. This question remains to be answered for prostate cancer; this study will help answer the question.

LOCALLY ADVANCED PROSTATE CANCER TREATMENT STUDIES

Two recent clinical trials have helped determine the most appropriate therapy for a man whose prostate cancer has spread beyond the prostate. This assessment of cancer spread is generally made by either physical examination (in which the physician can feel the tumor outside the prostate) or by a CT scan or other similar test. One of the most common treatments for these men is external beam radiation.

These 2 studies demonstrated that adding hormone treatment to radiation increases the chances of living longer cancer-free. Because of the side effects of hormones, however, the additional hormone may not be appropriate for all men, but the results showing longer, cancer-free lives demonstrate the powerful impact of clinical trials on helping to control prostate cancer.

METASTATIC PROSTATE CANCER TREATMENT STUDIES

A man with prostate cancer whose disease never spreads will almost never die of his cancer. Conversely, a man whose disease spreads has a high risk of dying from it. Therefore a tremendous amount of research has focused on metastatic prostate cancer.

INTERMITTENT HORMONAL THERAPY STUDIES

Hormonal therapy has been the mainstay of treatment for metastatic prostate cancer for the past 50 years, but while treatment often leads to a dramatic initial response, ultimately the tumor grows even in the absence of androgens, the cancer progresses, and death occurs. In some animal studies, it has been shown that if hormones are given intermittently, the tumor can be controlled for a longer period of time by preventing the creation of hormone-resistant cancer cells.

Intermittent therapy is currently being tested in a large-scale National Cancer Institute clinical trial in which men with metastatic prostate cancer are randomly assigned to receive continuous hormonal therapy or intermittent hormonal therapy. The goal of the study is to examine the differences in survival of the 2 treatments and to compare these differences with the side effects and quality of life in the 2 groups.

CHEMOTHERAPY STUDIES

Hormonal therapy won't cure most men with advanced prostate cancer. The majority of men with advanced prostate cancer eventually become resistant to hormone therapy. Typically, chemotherapy is considered at this point because certain chemotherapy combinations have been shown to decrease tumor burden and improve symptoms caused by the cancer. Chemotherapy has also prolonged survival in men with advanced metastatic cancer.

Therefore a number of clinical trials are examining if additional therapy given at the time of diagnosis can improve survival. Traditionally, chemotherapy given after hormonal therapy does not control prostate cancer because the cancer is often advanced and may be too extensive to respond to treatment.

Fortunately, abundant evidence now shows that several classes of chemotherapy will kill prostate cancer cells and have a reasonable chance of reducing PSA, decreasing cancer-related side effects such as pain, or shrinking tumors that have metastasized to other areas in the body. Several key studies are currently enrolling men with advanced prostate cancer who are being randomly assigned to receive either hormonal therapy alone ("standard" treatment) or hormonal therapy with chemotherapy. The results of these studies are expected to be available in the very near future. The results are hoped to change the way metastatic cancer is treated and reduce the number of men who die from the disease.

STUDIES OF NEWER TYPES OF TREATMENT

Given the modest benefits of available chemotherapy, a number of clinical trials are in progress that are evaluating both new chemotherapy combinations and novel agents that may improve the outcome of men with metastatic disease. Many of these newer agents target specific parts of prostate cancer cells, which may allow them to be more effective than chemotherapy while causing fewer side effects. The new generation of agents being investigated for prostate cancer that does not respond to hormonal therapy includes but is not limited to the areas below.

New chemotherapy agents and combinations. Researchers are studying new chemotherapeutic agents that show promising activity against prostate cancer in pre-clinical studies, as well as combinations of biological/targeted agents and chemotherapy. For example, calcitriol, a form of vitamin D, has recently shown promising results when combined with the chemotherapy drug docetaxel (Taxotere).

Drugs to cut cancer cells' nourishment. Like other cancers, prostate cancer depends on angiogenesis, the growth of new blood vessels, to nourish the cancer cells and allow a tumor to grow. Analysis of angiogenesis in prostate cancer specimens may help predict prognosis. Cancers that stimulate many new vessels to grow result in a poorer patient prognosis. New drugs are being studied that may be useful in stopping prostate cancer growth by keeping new blood vessels from forming. Some antiangiogenic drugs, such as thalidomide (Thalomid), are already being tested in clinical trials.

Drugs to control cell life and death. Researchers are looking at developing drugs to target signal transduction pathways. These are networks of proteins that send signals from the cell surface to genes within the cell that control the production of proteins that help regulate the cell cycle and cell death. A few of these drugs, called signal transduction inhibitors, are already being used successfully against other types of cancer.

Antibodies. Monoclonal antibodies are manmade versions of immune system proteins that target and attach to a specific part of prostate cancer cells. These antibodies may direct the body's immune system to kill the cancer cells on their own, or they may be used to guide other forms of therapy (chemotherapy drugs or radioactive materials) to the cancer cells. One example now being studied is a monoclonal antibody targeting prostate-specific membrane antigen (PSMA), found on the surface of prostate cells.

Vaccines. Anticancer vaccines are, in some ways, similar to vaccines used to prevent diseases caused by viruses, such as polio, measles, and mumps. These antiviral vaccines usually contain weakened viruses or parts of a virus that cannot cause the disease. The vaccine stimulates the body's immune system to destroy the more harmful type of virus.

Several types of vaccines for boosting the body's immune response to prostate cancer cells are being tested in clinical trials. One technique removes dendritic cells (a part of the immune system) from the patient's blood and exposes them to PSMA. These cells are then put back into the body, where they induce other immune system cells to attack the patient's prostate cancer. Other prostate cancer vaccines use genetically modified viruses that contain PSA. The patient is then injected with the virus. His immune system responds to the virus and also becomes sensitized to cancer cells containing PSA and destroys these cells. At this time, prostate cancer vaccines are available only in clinical trials.

Drugs to encourage cancer cells to self-destruct. Agents that promote apoptosis (programmed cell death) of cancer cells may also hold promise.

The hope is that cancer will respond to these new drugs and that the treatments will improve survival in men with prostate cancer that does not respond to hormonal therapy.

About the Resources

Listings in this section represent organizations that operate on a national level and provide some type of service or resource to consumers related to cancer, cancer research, or public health. This list is designed to offer a starting point for seeking information, support, and needed resources. Most of the organizations listed here can be contacted via phone, fax, or e-mail, and some through their Web site. Many of the Web sites provide much of the same information that is available by postal mail. Some organizations are solely Web-based and will require Internet access. Keep in mind that new Web sites appear daily while old ones expand, move, or disappear entirely. Some of the Web sites or content outlined below may change. Often, a simple Internet search will point to the new Web site for a given organization. The American Cancer Society Web site provides links to outside sources of cancer information as well (http://www.cancer.org; click on Cancer Resource Center).

There is a vast amount of information on the Internet. This information can be very valuable to the general public in making decisions about their health. However, since any group or individual can publish on the Internet, it is important to consider the credentials and reputation of the organization providing information. Internet information should not be a substitute for medical advice.

The American Cancer Society does not necessarily endorse the agencies, organizations, corporations, and publications represented in this resource guide. This guide is provided for assistance in obtaining information only.

AMERICAN CANCER SOCIETY RESOURCES

American Cancer Society
Toll-Free: 800-ACS-2345
Web site: http://www.cancer.org

The American Cancer Society is the nationwide community-based volunteer health organization dedicated to eliminating cancer as a major health problem by preventing cancer, saving lives and diminishing suffering from cancer, through research, education, advocacy, and service.

For more information about prostate cancer, educational materials (Spanish materials are available), patient programs, and services within your community, call 800-ACS-2345 or visit http://www.cancer.org to locate your division office for your state or region. The publications listed in the front of this book are available for sale through the Society's toll-free number and Web site and include information about caregiving, couples facing cancer, pain control, and making informed decisions.

Additional materials related to prostate cancer available from the Society include:

· *After Diagnosis: Prostate Cancer: Understanding Your Treatment Options*

· *Caring for the Patient with Cancer at Home: A Guide for Patients and Families*

· *Facts on Prostate Cancer and Prostate Cancer Testing*

· *Guidelines for the Early Detection of Prostate Cancer*

· *Managing Incontinence After Treatment for Prostate Cancer*

· *Prostate Cancer: Treatment Guidelines for Patients*

· *Sexuality and Cancer: For the Man Who Has Cancer and His Partner*

Let's Talk About It (LTAI)
Phone: 800-ACS-2345
Web site: http://www.cancer.org

Let's Talk About It is a free community-based program developed by the American Cancer Society and 100 Black Men of America to increase awareness and knowledge of prostate cancer among African-American men. The program provides to communities easy, step-by-step ways to organize prostate cancer awareness events to empower African-American men and their loved ones to reduce their risk of prostate cancer and make informed decisions about detecting and treating the disease.

National Prostate Cancer Coalition (NPCC)
1154 15th Street
Washington, DC 20005
Phone: 202-463-9455
Toll-Free: 888-245-9455
Fax: 202-463-9456
Web site: http://www.pcacoalition.org

The National Prostate Cancer Coalition (NPCC) is a nonprofit, grassroots advocacy organization that is dedicated to eliminating prostate cancer as a serious health concern for men and their families. The organization reaches state coalition and other national constituencies seeking to end the problem of prostate cancer. NPCC publishes a free email-based newsletter, AWARE. The Web site provides information about NPCC, prostate cancer, and early detection.

Paget Foundation
120 Wall Street, Suite 1602
New York, NY 10005-4001
Phone: 212-509-5335
Toll-Free: 800-23-PAGET (800-237-2438)
Fax: 212-509-8492
E-mail: pagetfdn@aol.com
Web site: http://www.paget.org

The Paget Foundation is a national, nonprofit, voluntary health agency which provides patient information on prostate cancer metastatic to bone, Paget's disease of bone, and other conditions. The Paget Foundation Web site offers the information above online.

Prostate Cancer Education Council (PCEC)
5299 DTC Boulevard, Suite 345
Greenwood Village, CO 80111
Phone: 303-316-4685
Toll-Free: 866-477-6788
Fax: 303-320-3835
E-mail: pcec@pcaw.com
Web site: http://www.pcaw.com

PCEC offers free or low-cost prostate cancer screenings across the country and educates men and the women in their lives, as well as the medical community, about the prevalence of prostate cancer, the importance of early detection, and available treatment options. The national Prostate Cancer Awareness Week program is one of the oldest and largest organized screening efforts in the United States and offers free screenings for prostate cancer.

Prostate Cancer Foundation
1250 4th Street, Suite 360
Santa Monica, CA 90401
Phone: 310-570-4700
Toll-Free: 800-757-CURE (800-757-2873)
Fax: 310-570-4701
Web site: http://www.prostatecancerfoundation.org

Formerly known as CaP Cure (The Association for the Cure of Cancer of the Prostate), Prostate Cancer Foundation is a nonprofit public charity dedicated to finding cures and controls for prostate cancer. Prostate Cancer Foundation does not provide medical advice or treatment information other than clinical trial information. Limited treatment information can be found on their Web site. Prostate Cancer Foundation provides: general information on prostate cancer, clinical trial information, survivor stories, and nutritional data.

Us TOO! International, Inc.
5003 Fairview Avenue
Downers Grove, IL 60515
Phone: 630-795-1002
Toll-Free: 800-80US-TOO (800-808-7866; metro
Chicago callers should use the local number)
Fax: 630-795-1602
Web site: http://www.ustoo.org

Us TOO is a nonprofit organization providing
information, counseling, and educational meetings
to assist men with prostate cancer (and their families) in making decisions about their treatment
with confidence and support. Us TOO offers a
hotline which answers caller inquiries, provides
literature, and makes referrals to its network of
support groups. (They do not provide doctor or
hospital referrals.) The Us TOO Web site includes:
information about prostate cancer, a listing of
local support groups, a clinical trials listing,
an online literature order form, and newsletter
articles. *Some Spanish materials are available.*

PROSTATE CANCER TREATMENT AND SIDE EFFECT INFORMATION

**American Association of Sex Educators,
Counselors, and Therapists (AASECT)**
P.O. Box 5488
Richmond, VA 23220-0488
Fax: 804-644-3290
E-mail: aasect@aasect.org
Web site: http://www.aasect.org

AASECT is a nonprofit, interdisciplinary
professional organization. Members include sex
educators, sex counselors, sex therapists, physicians,
nurses, social workers, psychologists, allied health
professionals, clergy members, lawyers, sociologists,
marriage and family planning specialists and
researchers, as well as students in relevant professional disciplines. Members share an interest in
promoting understanding of human sexuality and
healthy sexual behavior. AASECT can provide a list
of AASECT-certified counselors and/or therapists.
To obtain a list, send a stamped, self-addressed
business-size envelope to the above address.

American Brachytherapy Society (ABS)
12100 Sunset Hills Road, Suite 130
Reston, VA 20190-3221
Phone: 703-234-4078
Fax: 703-435-4390
Web site: http://www.americanbrachytherapy.org

The ABS is a nonprofit organization that seeks
to benefit patients by providing information,
promoting high standards of practice of brachytherapy, benefit health care professionals by
encouraging improved and continuing education
for health care professionals involved in the treatment of cancer, and promote research. The Web
site includes information for patients considering
brachytherapy.

**American College of Surgeons (ACoS)
Commission on Cancer**
633 North Saint Clair Street
Chicago, IL 60611-3211
Phone: 312-202-5000;
312-202-5085 Cancer Programs
Fax: 312-202-5009 or 312-202-5011
E-mail: postmaster@facs.org
Web site: http://www.facs.org

The ACoS' Commission on Cancer accredits
cancer programs of health care organizations in
the United States. This voluntary approval program
includes a site visit to evaluate the program's
compliance with specific standards in 10 major
areas—from prevention to end-of-life care. This
organization also provides tips and information on
selecting a surgeon and some of the fees involved.
A link to a searchable database of certified
physicians is also available.

American Society for Therapeutic Radiology and Oncology (ASTRO)
12500 Fair Lakes Circle, Suite 375
Fairfax, VA 22033-3882
Phone: 703-502-1550
Toll-free: 800-962-7876
Fax: 703-502-7852
Web site: http://www.astro.org

ASTRO is the largest radiation oncology society in the world. ASTRO provides a booklet, *Treating Cancer with Radiation Therapy*, about radiation therapy for cancer treatment, as well as a video on prostate cancer. The ASTRO Web site includes an overview of radiation therapy, a searchable database of radiation oncologists, answers to frequently asked questions, and other links to health Web sites.

American Foundation for Urologic Disease
1000 Corporate Boulevard, Suite 410
Linthicum, MD 21090
Phone: 410-689-3990
Toll-Free: 800-828-7866
Fax: 410-689-3998
Web site: http://www.afud.org

The American Foundation for Urologic Disease supports national urologic research, education, awareness, and advocacy programs. Services include: information and literature on urologic diseases and disorders, a national directory of prostate cancer support and self-help groups, and a prostate cancer resource guide. Their Web site includes information on urologic conditions including prostate cancer, BPH, prostatitis, urinary incontinence, and erectile dysfunction. *Spanish materials are available.*

American Urological Association (AUA)
1000 Corporate Boulevard
Linthicum, MD 21090
Toll-Free (US only): 866-746-4282
(866-RING-AUA)
Phone: 410-689-3700
Fax: 410-689-3800
Web site: http://www.urologyhealth.org

The American Urological Association is an educational nonprofit urological association. AUA online patient information addresses urological conditions including BPH and prostatitis as well as prostate cancer, screening, and treatment options. The Web site also provides an online directory service of urologists and a glossary.

Chemotherapy Foundation
183 Madison Avenue, Suite 403
New York, NY 10016-4501
Phone: 212-213-9292 (call for free literature)
Fax: 212-213-3831

The Chemotherapy Foundation is a nonprofit organization dedicated to the control, cure, and prevention of cancer through innovative medical therapies. It conducts professional education symposia to enable oncologists to incorporate treatment advances into the care of patients and provides free literature for patients on chemotherapy and prostate cancer.

National Association for Continence
P.O. Box 1019
Charleston, SC 29240
Toll-Free: 800-252-3337 (800-BLADDER)
E-mail: memberservices@nafc.org
Web site: http://www.nafc.org

National Association for Continence is a national, private, nonprofit organization dedicated to improving the quality of life for people with incontinence by educating the public about the causes, prevention, diagnosis, treatments, and management alternatives for incontinence. Publications and services include a quarterly newsletter, database of health care professionals, index of incontinence products and services, support group development information, brochures, audio/visuals, and books.

Radiation Therapy Oncology Group (RTOG)
1101 Market Street, 14th Floor
Philadelphia, PA 19107
Phone: 215-574-3205
Fax: 215-923-1737
Web site: http://www.rtog.org

RTOG is a national cancer study research organization and a National Cancer Institute Cooperative Group Program. The Web site provides extensive clinical trial information.

Society for Sex Therapy and Research (SSTAR)
409 12th St. SW
P.O. Box 96920
Washington, DC 20090-6920
Phone: 202-863-1648
Web site: http://www.sstarnet.org

The Society for Sex Therapy and Research (SSTAR) is a community of professionals who have clinical and/or research interests in human sexual concerns. Its goals are to facilitate communication among clinicians who treat problems of sexual identity, sexual function, and reproductive life and to provide a forum for exchange of ideas between those interested in research in human sexuality and those whose primary activities are patient care. The Web site offers books for consumers and clinicians.

GENERAL CANCER INFORMATION

American Society of Clinical Oncology (ASCO)
1900 Duke Street, Suite 200
Alexandria, VA 22314
Toll-Free: 888-651-3038
Phone: 703-299-0150
Fax: 703-299-1044
Web site: http://www.plwc.org

The ASCO is an international medical society representing about 10,000 cancer specialists involved in clinical research and patient care. The ASCO *People Living with Cancer* Web site is a resource for cancer patients, doctors, and researchers and includes patient guides, a glossary of cancer terms, an ASCO member oncologist locator, news and information about different cancers and drug treatments, information about cancer legislation, summaries of government reports, and links to related sites.

Association of Community Cancer Centers (ACCC)
11600 Nebel Street, Suite 201
Rockville, MD 20852-2557
Phone: 301-984-9496
Fax: 301-770-1949
Web site: http://www.accc-cancer.org

This national organization includes over 600 medical centers, hospitals, and cancer programs. This Web site contains a searchable database of cancer centers listed by state as well as information about oncology drugs (registration is required), and specific cancers.

Cancer Research Institute (CRI)
681 Fifth Avenue
New York, NY 10022
Toll-Free: 800-99-CANCER (800-992-2623)
Phone: 212-688-7515
Fax: 212-832-9376
Web site: http://www.cancerresearch.org

An institute funding cancer research and providing public information on cancer immunology and cancer treatment, the CRI helps patients locate immunotherapy clinical trials, and offers a cancer reference guide and other informational booklets, including *What to Do If Prostate Cancer Strikes*.

Intercultural Cancer Council (ICC)
6655 Travis, Suite 322
Houston, TX 77030-1312
Tel: 713-798-4617
Fax: 713-798-6222
E-mail: info@iccnetwork.org
Web site: http://iccnetwork.org/

The Intercultural Cancer Council is a nonprofit organization that promotes policies, programs, partnerships, and research to eliminate the unequal burden of cancer among racial and ethnic minorities and medically underserved populations in the United States and its associated territories. The Web site provides: cancer fact sheets on different medically underserved populations (such as African Americans, Asian Americans, and Hispanics and Latinos), as well as cancer news updates.

National Cancer Institute (NCI)
NCI Public Inquiries Office
Building 31, Room 10A03
31 Center Drive, MSC 2580
Bethesda, MD 20892-2580
Toll-Free: 800-4-CANCER (800-422-6237)
Web site: http://www.cancer.gov

This government agency provides cancer information through several services (see list below). The Physicians' Data Query (PDQ) database contains a directory of 10,000 doctors whose practices center on cancer treatment. *Spanish-speaking staff and Spanish materials are available.*

CANCERLIT (Bibliographic Database)
Web site: http://www.cancer.gov/cancerinfo/literature

This searchable site is maintained by the NCI and contains cancer articles published in medical and scientific journals, books, government reports, and articles that were presented at national meetings. A link to the Physicians' Data Query (PDQ) search engine is provided which allows you to search for clinical trials by state, city, and type of cancer.

CancerTrials
Web site: http://www.cancer.gov/clinicaltrials

Maintained by the NCI, this site offers information about ongoing cancer clinical trials and explanations of what a trial is and what is involved. A link to the PDQ search engine allows you to search for clinical trials by state, city, and type of cancer.

Cancer Topics
Web site: http://cancer.gov/cancerinformation
Web site (Spanish version):
http://www.cancer.gov/espanol
Web site (online ordering):
https://cissecure.nci.nih.gov/ncipubs/

This comprehensive Web site contains information on diagnosis, treatment, support, resources, literature, clinical trials, prevention and risk factors, and testing. The PDQ section provides a treatment option overview for patients and addresses treatment options for cancer by stages (800-4-CANCER or http://www.cancer.gov/cancerinfo/pdq/treatment/prostate/patient). Up to 20 publications can be ordered online. The publications list is searchable. *Some publications are available in Spanish.*

Cancer Information Service (CIS)
Toll-Free: 800-4-CANCER (800-422-6237)
Web site: http://cis.nci.nih.gov

The CIS provides information to consumers and health care professionals. The Web site contains a wealth of information including pamphlets and brochures on cancer diagnosis, treatment, research, and prevention. *Spanish-speaking staff members are available.*

Center to Reduce Cancer Health Disparities
6116 Executive Boulevard
Suite 602 MSC 8341
Rockville, MD 20852
Phone: 301-496-8589
Fax: 301-435-9225
E-mail: crchd@mail.nih.nci.gov
Web site: http://crchd.nci.nih.gov/

The Center to Reduce Cancer Health Disparities is the keystone of NCI's efforts to reduce the unequal burden of cancer in our society. As the organizational locus for these efforts, the center directs the implementation of and supports initiatives that advance understanding of the causes of health disparities and develop and integrate effective interventions to reduce or eliminate these disparities. The Web site includes patient, family, and caregiver information, news and updates, and other information.

National Center for Complementary and Alternative Medicine (NCCAM)
Web site: http://altmed.od.nih.gov
Toll-Free: 888-644-6226

The NCCAM, part of the National Institutes of Health (NIH), facilitates research and evaluation of unconventional medical practices and distributes this information to the public. Their Web site provides information on some complementary and alternative methods promoted as treatments for different diseases.

National Comprehensive Cancer Network (NCCN)
500 Old York Road
Jenkintown, PA 19046
Toll-Free: 800-909-NCCN
Phone: 215-690-2300
Fax: 215-690-0280
Web site: http://www.nccn.org

The NCCN is a nonprofit organization that is an alliance of 19 cancer centers. The American Cancer Society has partnered with NCCN to translate the NCCN Clinical Practice Guidelines into a patient-friendly resource with easy-to-understand information for patients and family members. An overview of treatment guidelines for patients with prostate cancer are found on page 160. Call the American Cancer Society for the latest guidelines or view them online at either http://www.cancer.org or http://www.nccn.org.

National Library of Medicine (includes Medline)
Web site: http://www.nlm.nih.gov

This National Institutes of Health Web site provides a search engine for health, medical, and scientific literature and research as well as links to other government resources. Medline (http://medlineplus.gov/) is a searchable site with health information from the National Library of Medicine about conditions including cancer. It includes lists of hospitals and physicians, a medical encyclopedia and a medical dictionary, information on prescription and nonprescription drugs, health information from the media, and links to thousands of clinical trials. *Spanish materials are available.*

PubMed
Web site: http://www.ncbi.nlm.nih.gov/PubMed

As part of the National Library of Medicine (NLM), this Web site provides access to literature references in Medline and other databases, with links to online journals. The site is searchable by key word.

OncoLink
OncoLink Editorial Board
University of Pennsylvania Cancer Center
3400 Spruce Street-2 Donner
Philadelphia, PA 19104-4283
Web site: http://www.oncolink.com

This Web site provides information on cancer including educational materials about prostate cancer, support groups, financial questions, and other resources for people with cancer.

PATIENT AND FAMILY SERVICES

AARP (formerly the American Association of Retired Persons)
Pharmacy Services
Dept. # 258390
P.O. Box 40011
Roanoke, VA 24022
Toll-Free: 800-456-2277
Web site: http://www.aarp.org
Web site (for Pharmacy Service):
http://www.aarppharmacy.com

The AARP is a nonprofit membership organization with a commitment to older adults. It provides a variety of services to its members including information on managed care, Medicare, Medicaid, long-term care, and other issues of interest. Membership is open to anyone 50 years old or older. The Web site includes information on a member pharmacy service that offers discounts on drugs used for cancer treatment and pain relief.

American Cancer Society Hope Lodges
Toll-free: 800-ACS-2345

The Hope Lodge is a temporary residential facility providing sleeping rooms and related facilities for people with cancer who are undergoing outpatient treatment and their family members. Approval from a physician or referring agency is necessary.

Americans with Disabilities Act (ADA)
United States Department of Justice
950 Pennsylvania Avenue, NW
Civil Rights Division
Disability Rights Section-NYAV
Washington, D.C. 20530
Phone: 800-514-0301
Fax: 202-307-1198
Web site: http://www.ada.gov

Specialists at the ADA information line answer
questions about titles II and III of the ADA. The
ADA Web site includes a text version of the ADA
and available publications. Many publications
can be ordered through the automated fax
system; call the information line for directions.
*Spanish-speaking staff and Spanish materials are
available.*

Angel Flight America
Toll-free: 800-446-1231
Web site: http://www.angelflightamerica.org

Angel Flight provides access to free air transportation to specialized health care facilities or distant
destinations due to family, community, or national
crisis. The Web site has a search by zip code
function that enables a patient to find the regional
office nearest to the departure location as well as a
map showing the regions served by Angel Flight
America.

Cancer Care, Inc.
275 Seventh Avenue
New York, NY 10001
Toll-Free (Counseling): 800-813-HOPE
(800-813-4637)
Phone: 212-712-8080
Fax: 212-712-8495
Web site: http://www.cancercare.org
Web site (Spanish version):
http://www.cancercare.org/EnEspanol/
EnEspanolmain.cfm

A nonprofit social service agency, Cancer Care,
Inc. provides counseling and guidance to help
people with cancer, their families, and friends
cope with the impact of cancer. The Web site
includes detailed information on specific cancers
and cancer treatment, cancer pain, clinical trials,

a searchable database of regional and national
resources, and links to other sites. The organization also provides videos, free support groups
(online, telephone, and face-to-face), workshops,
seminars and clinics, a newsletter, and other
publications to interested consumers. *Spanish-
speaking staff members are available.*

Cancer Survivors Network
American Cancer Society
1599 Clifton Road, NE
Atlanta, GA 30329-4251
Toll-Free: 800-ACS-2345
Web site: http://www.acscsn.org

This network provides an online community that
welcomes cancer survivors, friends, and families to
share and communicate with others with similar
interests and experiences. The program offers a
vibrant community of real people supporting one
another and sharing personal experiences with
cancer. The Web site enables registered members
to have live, private chats, to create personal Web
pages to share experiences, thoughts, and wisdom,
to help people create personal support communities
of people who share common concerns and
interests, and offers information about resources.

Health Insurance Association of America
555 13th Street, NW, Suite 600 East
Washington, DC 20004
Toll-Free: 800-879-4422
Phone: 202-824-1600
Fax: 202-824-1722
Web site: http://www.hiaa.org

This association represents most United States
health insurance companies. The Web site
contains insurance guides and general insurance
information, and an annual directory and survey
of hospitals, along with other information.

I Can Cope
American Cancer Society
Toll-Free: 800-ACS-2345
Web site: http://www.cancer.org

This educational program is provided in a
supportive environment for adults with cancer
and their loved ones. The program offers several
courses designed to help participants cope with

their cancer experience by increasing their knowledge, positive attitude, and skills. The program is conducted by trained health care professionals in communities throughout the U.S., often with hospital co-sponsorship, as well as in other countries. It offers straightforward cancer information and answers to questions about human anatomy, cancer development, diagnosis, treatment, side effects, new research, communication, emotions, sexuality, self-esteem, and community resources. The program also provides information, encouragement, and practical hints through presentations and class discussions. All classes are free.

Look Good…Feel Better (LGFB) for Men
American Cancer Society
Toll-Free: 800-395-LOOK
Web site: http://www.cancer.org

LGFB provides a brochure for men undergoing chemotherapy or radiation treatment. The brochure also features a tear-out sheet containing steps to help men with skin care and other information.

Make Today Count
Mid-American Cancer Center
1235 East Cherokee
Springfield, MO 65804-2263
Toll-Free: 800-432-2273
Phone: 417-885-2273
Fax: 417-888-8761

This is a support organization for people affected by cancer or other life-threatening illness.

Man to Man
American Cancer Society
Toll-Free: 800-ACS-2345
Web site: http://www.cancer.org

The Man to Man program helps men cope with prostate cancer by offering community-based education and support for patients and their family members. In addition, Man to Man plays an important role in community education about prostate cancer and screening. A core component of the program is the self-help and/or support group. Volunteers organize these free monthly meetings where speakers and participants learn about and

discuss information about prostate cancer, treatment, side effects, and how to cope with prostate cancer and its treatment. Man to Man programs, services, and activities vary. Your local program may also include other services and activities such as: one-on-one visits with a prostate cancer survivor, community education (speaker's bureau), the Man to Man newsletter, outreach to high-risk groups, such as African-American men, and outreach and collaboration with health care providers. Some Man to Man groups may invite wives and partners to attend meetings. In other locations, wives and partners may meet separately in a group setting called Side by Side.

Medicare Hotline
Department of Health and Human Services
Toll-Free: 800-MEDICAR
Web site: http://www.medicare.gov

The official U.S. Government site for Medicare provides information on eligibility, enrollment, premiums, coverage, payment and billing, insurance, prescription drugs, and frequently asked questions. Call the toll-free number to receive information about local services.

National Coalition for Cancer Survivorship (NCCS)
1010 Wayne Avenue, Suite 770
Silver Spring, MD 20910
Toll-Free: 877-NCCS-YES (877-622-7937; general information and publications)
Phone: 301-650-9127
Fax: 301-565-9670
Web site: http://www.canceradvocacy.org

The NCCS is a survivor-led advocacy organization working in the area of cancer survivorship and support. NCCS seeks to empower survivors by educating all those affected by cancer and speaking out on issues related to quality cancer care. The Web site offers links to online cancer resources, support groups, survivorship programs, a newsletter, and an audio program that teaches skills to help people with cancer meet the challenges of their illness.

National Family Caregivers Association (NFCA)
10400 Connecticut Avenue, Suite 500
Kensington, MD 20895-3944
Toll-Free: 800-896-3650
Phone: 301-942-6430
Fax: 301-942-2302
Web site: http://www.nfcacares.org

This organization is a national, nonprofit, membership association whose mission is to promote caregiving through education and advocacy. NFCA publishes *Take Care!* a newsletter (free for family caregivers) that includes can-do advice, helpful resources, and stories about family caregivers. The NFCA provides referrals to national resources for caregivers and offers a bereavement kit for caregivers. The NFCA Web site provides a report on the status of family caregivers and ten tips for family caregivers.

National Self-Help Clearinghouse
Graduate School and University Center of the City University of New York
365 Fifth Avenue, Suite 3300
New York, NY 10016
Phone: 212-817-1822
Fax: 212-817-2990
Web site: http://www.selfhelpweb.org

This nonprofit organization provides access to regional self-help services.

Partnership for Caring: America's Voices for the Dying
1620 Eye Street NW, Suite 202
Washington, DC 20006
Phone: 202-296-8071
Fax: 202-296-8352
Toll-Free: 800-989-9455 (Hotline)
E-mail: pfc@partnershipforcaring.org
Web site: http://www.partnershipforcaring.org

Partnership for Caring: America's Voices for the Dying is a national, nonprofit organization that partners individuals and organizations with the goal of improving how society cares for dying people and their loved ones. Services include: counseling via their 24-hour hotline; publications and videos; information about speaking with family and friends about end-of-life issues; advance directives (living wills and/or medical powers of attorney forms) tailored to each state's legal requirements; and information about state laws on issues such as refusing medical treatment, withdrawing life supports, honoring advance directives, and managing pain.

Pharmaceutical Research and Manufacturers Association of America (PHRMA)
1100 15th Street, NW, Suite 900
Washington, DC 20005
Phone: 202-835-3400
Fax: 202-835-3414
Web site: http://www.phrma.org

PHRMA provides information about member pharmaceutical companies and drugs that are currently available, in use in clinical trials, or under development. The Web site includes a directory of patient assistance programs for prescription drugs and a database of new medications for cancer and other diseases.

Social Security Administration
Department of Health and Human Services
Toll-Free: 800-772-1213
Web site: http://www.ssa.gov

Call the toll-free number to receive information about local services or visit the Web site to learn more about benefits, disability, and other frequently asked-about topics.

TRICARE (formerly CHAMPUS)
Web site: http://www.tricare.osd.mil

TRICARE is part of the military health care system. The Web site offers a link to TRICARE regional offices and a list of phone numbers.

Wellness Community
919 18th Street NW, Suite 54
Washington, DC 20006
Toll-Free: 888-793-WELL
Phone: 202-659-9709
Fax: 202-659-9301
E-mail: help@thewellnesscommunity.org
Web site: http://www.thewellnesscommunity.org

The Wellness Community is a nonprofit organization whose mission is to help people with cancer and their families enhance their health and well-being by providing a professional program of emotional support, education, and hope. Support groups are facilitated by licensed psychotherapists. Bereavement support groups are also available. Referrals are provided to their 25 facilities across the nation. The Web site has information about relaxation, talking with children when a parent has cancer, a study sponsored by the Wellness Community investigating the benefits of a professionally facilitated, online support group for women with breast cancer.

OTHER ORGANIZATIONS PROVIDING HEALTH INFORMATION AND SUPPORT

Agency for Healthcare Research and Quality (AHRQ)
Publications Clearinghouse
P.O. Box 8547
Silver Springs, MD 20907-8547
Toll-Free: 800-358-9295
Web site: http://www.ahrq.gov

The AHRQ, an office within the U.S. Department of Health and Human Services' Public Health Service, is responsible for supporting research designed to improve the quality of health care, reduce its cost, and broaden access to essential services. One of AHRQ's highest priorities is providing consumers with science-based, easily understandable information that will help them make informed decisions about their own personal health care, including selection of the highest quality health plans and most appropriate health care services.

The American Geriatrics Society Foundation for Health in Aging (FHA)
Toll-Free: 800-563-4916
Web site: http://www.healthinaging.org/
public_education/

The FHA's patient education resources were developed in collaboration with the American Geriatrics Society (AGS) and are based on the new major AGS clinical practice guideline for health care providers entitled *The Management of Persistent Pain in Older Persons.* The FHA Web site provides practical and easy-to-use tools to help older adults and their caregivers better manage persistent pain in consultation with their physicians and other health care providers, including: a pain diary and a medication and supplement diary; guides to pain medications, how to assess pain in those with dementia, and information about eldercare at home. Materials may be downloaded and printed from the Web site. Call to obtain hard copies or to place bulk orders.

American Psychological Association (APA)
750 First Street, NE
Washington, DC 20002-4242
Toll-Free: 800-374-2721
Phone: 202-336-5500
Web site: http://www.apa.org

This organization has a Division on Health Psychology that addresses a range of health issues including cancer. The APA provides a hotline patients can use to obtain literature and discuss psychological conditions, and referrals to state psychological associations to locate a psychologist in a specific area. The APA Web site provides a help center with information about psychological issues. *Spanish-speaking staff members are available.*

Joint Commission on Accreditation of Healthcare Organizations (JCAHO)
One Renaissance Boulevard
Oakbrook Terrace, IL 60181
Toll-Free (for filing complaints about a health care organization): 800-994-6610
Phone: 630-792-5000
Fax: 630-792-5005
Web site: http://www.jcaho.org

This is an independent nonprofit organization that evaluates and accredits more than 19,500 health care organizations in the United States, including hospitals, health care networks, and health care organizations that provide home care, long-term care, behavioral health care, and laboratory and ambulatory care services. JCAHO provides information to the public about accreditation status and selecting quality care. Performance reports of accredited organizations and guidelines for choosing a health care facility are available to the public and can be obtained by calling JCAHO or visiting their Web site.

Memorial Sloan-Kettering Cancer Center (MSKCC)
AboutHerbs
Web site: http://www.mskcc.org/mskcc/html/11570.cfm

Memorial Sloan-Kettering Cancer Center's *AboutHerbs* Web site provides information for consumers about herbs, botanicals, and alternative or unproven cancer therapies, including details about adverse effects, interactions, and potential benefits or problems.

National Association of Social Workers
750 First Street NE, Suite 700
Washington, DC 20002-4241
Toll-Free: 800-638-8799
Phone: 202-408-8600
Fax: 202-336-8340
Web site: http://www.naswdc.org

This organization is concerned with advocacy, work practice standards and ethics, and professional standards for agencies employing social workers. The Web site provides a national register of clinical social workers for local referrals. *Spanish-speaking staff members are available.*

Oncology Nursing Society (ONS)
501 Holiday Drive
Pittsburgh, PA 15220-2749
Toll-Free: 866-257-4ONS
Fax: 877-369-5497
Web site: http://www.ons.org

This organization is a national membership organization of registered nurses involved in oncology care whose mission is to promote professional standards for oncology nursing, research, and education. Nonmembers can access the ONS Web site to find information about cancer treatment, survivorship, and end-of life issues.

Quackwatch
Web site: http://www.quackwatch.com

This Web site provides a guide to fraudulent claims about alternative medicines and questionable health products. The site is searchable by keyword.

World Health Organization (WHO)
WHO Publications Center USA
49 Sheridan Avenue
Albany, NY 12210
Phone: 202-974-3000
Fax: 202-974-3663
Web site: http://www.who.org

The WHO is an agency of the United Nations which promotes technical cooperation for health among nations, carries out programs to control and eradicate disease, and strives to improve the quality of human life. The WHO Web site includes data on cancer, a list of publications, and links to related Web sites. *Spanish materials are available.*

3DCRT: see three-dimensional conformal radiation therapy.

5-alpha reductase: an enzyme that converts testosterone to a more active hormone called dihydrotestosterone (DHT).

5-alpha reductase inhibitors: Drugs such as finasteride (Proscar or Propecia) that prevent the conversion of testosterone to a more active hormone called dihydrotestosterone (DHT). They may help reduce the risk of prostate cancer.

A

ablative therapy: treatment that removes or destroys the function of an organ, for example, removing the ovaries or testicles or having some types of treatment that cause these organs to stop working.

adenocarcinoma: cancer that starts in the glandular tissue, such as the prostate.

adrenal glands: glands located on top of each kidney. Their main function is to produce hormones that control metabolism, fluid balance, and blood pressure. In addition, they produce small amounts of "male" hormones (androgens) and "female" hormones (estrogens and progesterone).

adjuvant therapy: treatment used in addition to the main treatment. It usually refers to hormonal therapy, chemotherapy, or radiation added after primary treatment to increase the chances of curing the disease or keeping it in check.

advanced cancer: general term describing stages of cancer in which the disease has spread from the primary site to other parts of the body. When the cancer has spread only to the surrounding areas, it is called locally advanced. If it has spread to distant parts of the body, it is called metastatic.

agonist: a manmade version of a naturally occurring substance. Also called an analog. See also LHRH agonist.

alpha blocker: a drug that relaxes smooth muscle tissue. Alpha blockers are sometimes used to help men who have difficulty urinating due to benign prostatic hyperplasia (BPH) or other causes.

alternative therapy: use of an unproven therapy instead of standard (proven) therapy. Some alternative therapies may have dangerous or even life-threatening side effects. For others, the main danger is that a patient may lose the opportunity to benefit from standard therapy. The American Cancer Society recommends that patients considering use of any alternative or complementary therapy discuss this with their health care team. See also complementary therapy.

androgen: any male sex hormone. The major androgen is testosterone.

androgen ablation: see combination hormonal therapy.

androgen blockade: use of drugs to disrupt the actions of male hormones.

androgen-dependent: term used to describe prostate cells, benign or malignant, that are stimulated to grow and multiply by male hormones and suppressed by drugs that disrupt the action of male hormones.

androgen deprivation therapy (ADT): see hormonal therapy

androgen receptors: when androgens bind with these molecules, they help prostate tissue grow.

anemia: low red blood cells.

anesthesia: the loss of feeling or sensation as a result of drugs or gases. General anesthesia causes loss of consciousness (makes you go into a deep sleep). Local or regional anesthesia numbs only a certain area of the body.

angiogenesis: the formation of new blood vessels. Some cancer treatments work by blocking angiogenesis, thus preventing blood from reaching the tumor.

antiandrogens: drugs that block the body's ability to use androgens. They are taken as pills, once or 3 times a day. Antiandrogens are usually used in combination with orchiectomy or LHRH agonists. Several drugs of this type are currently available: flutamide (Eulexin), bicalutamide (Casodex), and nilutamide (Nilandron).

antibody: a protein produced by the body's immune system cells and released into the blood. Antibodies defend the body against foreign agents, such as bacteria. These agents contain certain substances called antigens. Each antibody works against a specific antigen. See also antigen.

anticonvulsants or antidepressants: adjuvant medications not only used for convulsions or to treat depression, but also used along with a primary cancer pain medicine to control burning and tingling pain, such as pain caused by nerve damage or spinal compression.

antiemetic: a drug that prevents or relieves nausea and vomiting, which are common side effects of chemotherapy.

antigen: a substance that causes the body's immune system to react, often resulting in the production of antibodies. For example, the immune system's response to antigens that are part of bacteria and viruses helps people resist infections. Cancer cells have certain antigens that can be found by laboratory tests. They are important in cancer diagnosis and in gauging response to treatment. Other cancer cell antigens play a role in immune reactions that may help the body's resistance against cancer.

antioxidants: molecules such as some vitamins that block the actions of activated oxygen molecules, known as free radicals, that can damage cells.

artificial sphincter: an inflatable cuff implanted around the upper urethra to squeeze the urethra shut and provide urinary control.

aspiration: the process of drawing out by suction.

atypical: not usual; abnormal. Often refers to the appearance of cancerous or precancerous cells. See also, hyperplasia.

B

BPH: see benign prostatic hyperplasia.

benign: not cancerous; not malignant.

benign prostatic hyperplasia: non-cancerous enlargement of the prostate that may cause problems with urination such as trouble starting and stopping the flow. Also referred to as BPH.

biopsy: the removal of a sample of tissue to see if cancer cells are present. There are several kinds of biopsies. In a fine needle aspiration biopsy (sometimes used to check pelvic lymph nodes), a very thin needle is used to draw out fluid and cells. In a core biopsy, a larger needle is used to remove a thin cylinder of tissue. For a sextant biopsy, 6 core biopsy samples are taken, 1 each from the top, middle and bottom of each side of the prostate. Saturation biopsies, which involve taking more than 40 cores, are done only in cases in which there is a high suspicion of prostate cancer and multiple negative biopsies or when a thorough mapping of the prostate is desired.

bisphosphonates: drugs that slow down the action of bone-eating cells called osteoclasts, thereby slowing the spread of cancer in the bones. Bisphosphonates are used in breast cancer and multiple myeloma (a type of bone cancer) and are now being studied for possible use in men with prostate cancer that has spread to the bones.

bladder: a hollow organ with flexible, muscular walls that stores urine.

bladder neck contracture: scar formed at the site of reconstruction of the urethra and bladder after prostatectomy, which may impede the flow of urine.

bone scan: an imaging test that gives important information about the bones, including the location of cancer that may have spread to the bones. It can be done on an outpatient basis and is painless, except for the needle stick when a low-dose radioactive substance is injected into a vein. Pictures are taken to see where the radioactivity collects, pointing to an abnormality.

bowel irritability: a rare and temporary irregular pattern of bowel activity and increased frequency of bowel movements due to radiation.

bowel preparation: the use of enemas and strong oral laxatives; for example, before radical prostatectomy.

brachytherapy: internal radiation treatment given by placing radioactive material directly into the tumor or close to it. Also called interstitial radiation therapy or seed implantation.

C

CAB: combined androgen blockade. See combination hormonal therapy.

CAT scan: see computed tomography

CT scan: see computed tomography

cancer: cancer is not just one disease but rather a group of diseases. All forms of cancer cause cells in the body to change and grow out of control. Most types of cancer cells form a lump or mass called a tumor. The tumor can invade and destroy healthy tissue. Cells from the tumor can break away and travel to other parts of the body, where they can continue to grow. This spreading process is called metastasis. When cancer spreads, it is still named after the part of the body where it started. For example, if prostate cancer spreads to the bones, it is still prostate cancer, not bone cancer.

Some cancers, such as blood cancers, do not form a tumor. Not all tumors are cancer. A tumor that is not cancer is called benign. Benign tumors do not grow and spread the way cancer does. They are usually not a threat to life. Another word for cancerous is malignant.

cancer care team: the group of health care professionals who work together to find, treat, and care for people with cancer. The cancer care team may include any or all of the following and others: primary care physician, pathologist, oncology specialists (medical oncologist, radiation oncologist), surgeons (including surgical specialists such as urologists, gynecologists, neurosurgeons, etc.), nurses, oncology nurse specialists, and oncology social workers. Whether the team is linked formally or informally, there is usually one person who takes the job of coordinating the team.

cancer cell: a cell that divides and reproduces abnormally and can spread throughout the body. See also metastasis.

cancer-related checkup: a routine health examination for cancer in persons without obvious signs or symptoms of cancer. The goal of the cancer-related checkup is to find the disease, if it exists, at an early stage, when chances for cure are greatest. Depending on the person's sex and age, this checkup may include a digital rectal examination, clinical breast examinations, Pap smears, PSA blood test, and skin examinations. See also detection.

capsule: the outer surface of the prostate.

carcinogen: any substance that causes cancer or helps cancer grow. For example, tobacco smoke contains many carcinogens that greatly increase the risk of lung cancer.

carcinoma: a malignant tumor that begins in the lining layer (epithelial cells) of organs. At least 80 percent of all cancers are carcinomas. Almost all prostate cancers are carcinomas, specifically adenocarcinomas.

castration: surgery to remove the testicles; the medical term is orchiectomy.

catheter (urinary): a thin, flexible tube through which fluids enter or leave the body; for example, a tube to drain urine (known as a "Foley catheter").

cavernous nerves: nerves that control erections.

cell: the basic unit of which all living things are made. Cells replace themselves by splitting and forming new cells (mitosis). The processes that control the formation of new cells and the death of old cells are disrupted in cancer.

"chemical castration": the use of hormonal therapy to achieve very low levels of testosterone without surgical removal of the testicles.

chemotherapy: treatment with drugs to destroy cancer cells. Chemotherapy is often used with surgery or radiation to treat cancer when the cancer has spread, when it has come back (recurred), or when there is a strong chance that it could recur.

clinical trials: research studies to test new drugs or other treatments to compare current, standard treatments with others that may be better. Before a new treatment is used on people, it is studied in the laboratory. If lab studies suggest the treatment will work, the next step is to test its value for patients. These human studies are called clinical trials.

combination hormonal therapy: complete blockage of androgen production that may include castration (orchiectomy) or LHRH agonists, plus the use of antiandrogens; also called combined androgen blockade (CAB), total hormonal ablation, total androgen blockade, or total androgen ablation.

combined androgen blockade (CAB): see combination hormonal therapy.

complementary therapy: therapy used in addition to standard therapy. Some complementary therapies may help relieve certain symptoms of cancer, relieve side effects of standard cancer therapy, or improve a patient's sense of well-being. The American Cancer Society recommends that patients considering use of any alternative or complementary therapy discuss this with their health care team. See also alternative therapy.

complete blood count: a complete blood count (CBC) is a test that provides information about bone marrow function and if it is safe to perform other studies, such as biopsies of the prostate. Patients who will undergo a prostate needle biopsy or have symptoms which could be related to low blood counts may have this test performed.

computed tomography (CT): an imaging test in which many x-ray images are taken from different angles of a part of the body. These images are combined by a computer to produce cross-sectional pictures of internal organs. Except for the injection of a dye (needed in some but not all cases), this is a painless procedure that can be done in an outpatient clinic. It is often referred to as a "CT" or "CAT" scan.

conformal proton beam radiation therapy: a technique that uses proton beams instead of conventional radiation. Protons are parts of atoms that cause little damage to tissues they pass through but are very effective in killing cells at the end of their path. This means that proton beam radiation may be able to deliver more radiation to the cancer while reducing side effects of nearby normal tissues.

contrast material: a substance such as a dye given into a vein or by mouth to make a radiology image clearer. Because various body tissues absorb this material differently, the image produced shows greater contrast between types of tissues, allowing abnormalities such as tumors to be seen more clearly.

core biopsy: see biopsy.

"cure": in prostate cancer, this usually refers to a PSA level so low that it can't be detected by the PSA lab test (usually after 5 or 10 years).

cryosurgery: use of extreme cold to freeze the prostate and destroy cancer cells. Also called cryoablation.

curative treatment: treatment aimed at producing a cure. Compare with palliative treatment.

cystoscope: a slender tube with a lens and a light. It is placed into the bladder through the urethra and the doctor can then view the inside of these organs.

cystoscopy: examination of the bladder with an instrument called a cystoscope.

cytology: the branch of science that deals with the structure and function of cells. Also refers to tests to diagnose cancer and other diseases by examination of cells under the microscope.

D

DHT: see dihydrotestosterone.

DNA: see deoxyribonucleic acid.

DRE: see digital rectal examination.

dehydroepiandrosterone (DHEA): a steroid hormone some researchers believe may increase prostate cancer risk and promote the growth of prostate cancer.

deoxyribonucleic acid (DNA): holds genetic information on cell growth, division, and function.

detection: finding disease. Early detection means that the disease is found at an early stage, before it has grown large or spread to other sites. Note: many forms of cancer can reach an advanced stage without causing symptoms. Mammography can help to find breast cancer early, and the PSA blood test can help find early prostate cancer.

diagnosis: identification of a disease by its signs or symptoms and through the use of imaging procedures and laboratory findings. For some types of cancer, the earlier a diagnosis is made, the better the chance for long-term survival.

differentiation: the normal process through which cells mature so they can carry out the jobs they were meant to do. Cancer cells are less differentiated than normal cells. Grading is done to evaluate and report the degree of a cancer's differentiation. Well-differentiated cancer closely resembles normal prostate cells and glands and tends to be the slowest-growing and least dangerous cancer. Poorly differentiated cancer is often very aggressive and fast-growing.

digital rectal examination (DRE): an exam during which the doctor inserts a lubricated, gloved finger into the rectum to feel for anything not normal. Some tumors of the rectum and prostate gland can be felt during a DRE.

dihydrotestosterone (DHT): powerful form of male hormone produced by the action of a prostate enzyme on testosterone.

disease-free survival rate: the percentage of people with a certain cancer who still have no evidence of disease (cancer) a certain period of time (usually 5 years) after treatment. This rate does not measure actual "survival," which is expressed by the 5-year survival rate.

doubling time: for cancer in general, the time it takes for a cell to divide and double itself. Cancers vary in doubling time from 8 to 600 days, averaging 100 to 120 days. Thus, a cancer may be present for many years before it can be felt. Compare to PSA doubling time.

drain: a small tube inserted into the space behind the pubic bone that comes out through the skin near the incision and carries any fluid collecting in this space out of the body.

E

EBRT: see external beam radiation therapy.

ED: see erectile dysfunction.

ejaculate: to release semen during orgasm; as a noun, semen.

epidemiology: the study of diseases in populations by collecting and analyzing statistical data. In the field of cancer, epidemiologists look at how many people have cancer; who gets specific types of cancer; and what factors (such as job hazards, family patterns, personal habits such as smoking and diet, and environment) play a part in the development of cancer.

epididymis: a system of tiny tubes within the scrotum but outside the testicles through which sperm travel after forming and where they are stored until they mature; they lead into the vas deferens.

epidural anesthesia: injection of anesthetic drugs into the space around the spinal cord. Used to numb the lower part of the body while allowing the patient to remain awake.

epithelial cells: the lining layer of organs.

erectile dysfunction (ED): not being able to have or keep an erection of the penis; impotence.

estrogen: a female sex hormone produced primarily by the ovaries, and in smaller amounts by the adrenal cortex. It is sometimes given to men with advanced prostate cancer to counteract the action of testosterone.

external beam radiation therapy (EBRT): radiation that is focused from a source outside the body on the area affected by the cancer. It is much like getting a diagnostic x-ray, but for a longer time and at a higher dose.

expectant management: see watchful waiting.

extraprostatic extension: cancer that penetrates through the prostatic capsule.

F

FNA: see fine needle aspiration biopsy.

false negative: test result implying a condition does not exist when in fact it does.

353

false positive: test result implying a condition exists when in fact it does not.

fecal incontinence: the inadvertent loss of stool; a potential side effect of radical prostatectomy.

finasteride: a drug that prevents the prostate from being affected by certain androgens. The trade name is Proscar.

fine needle aspiration (FNA) biopsy: a procedure in which a thin needle is used to draw up (aspirate) samples for examination under a microscope. See also biopsy.

five-year survival rate: the percentage of people with a given cancer who are expected to survive 5 years or longer with the disease. Five-year survival rates have some drawbacks. Although the rates are based on the most recent information available, they may include data from patients treated several years earlier. Advances in cancer treatment often occur quickly. Five-year survival rates, while statistically valid, may not reflect these advances. They should not be seen as a predictor in an individual case.

Foley catheter: a rubber tube inserted through the tip of the penis and into the bladder during surgery to drain urine directly from the bladder out of the body during recovery.

free-PSA ratio: a test that indicates how much PSA circulates unbound (alone) in the blood compared to the total amount of PSA. For total PSA results in the borderline range (4 to 10 ng/mL), a low percent free-PSA (25 percent or less) means that a prostate cancer is more likely to be present and suggests the need for a biopsy. See also prostate-specific antigen.

free radicals: molecules that can damage cells.

frequency: the need to urinate often.

frozen section: a very thin slice of tissue that has been quick-frozen and then examined under a microscope. This method is sometimes used during an operation because it gives a quick diagnosis, and can tell a surgeon whether or not to continue with a procedure. The diagnosis is confirmed in a few days by a more detailed study called a permanent section. See also permanent section.

G

gene: a segment of DNA that contains information on hereditary characteristics such as hair color, eye color, and height, as well as susceptibility to certain diseases.

gene therapy: the effort to introduce new genes into a cell or to alter the genes that are already there in the attempt to treat a disease such as prostate cancer.

genetic predisposition: small differences in the genes a person inherits from his or her parents that may increase or decrease his chances of developing cancer.

genomics: the study of how genes interact and function.

gland: a cell or group of cells that produce and release substances used nearby or in another part of the body. The prostate is an example of a gland.

glans: the head of the penis.

Gleason grade: the most often used prostate cancer grading system is called the Gleason s ystem. A pathologist assigns a Gleason grade ranging from 1 through 5 based on how much cancer cells look like normal prostate cells. Those that look a lot like normal cells are graded as 1, while those that look the least like normal cells are graded as 5. See also Gleason score; grade.

Gleason score: a method of classifying prostate cancer cells. Because prostate cancers often have areas with different grades, a grade is assigned to the 2 areas that make up most of the cancer. These 2 grades are added together to give a Gleason score between 2 and 10. The higher the Gleason score, the faster the cancer is likely to grow and the more likely it is to spread beyond the prostate. See also Gleason grade.

grade: the grade of a cancer reflects how abnormal it looks under the microscope. There are several grading systems for different types of cancers, such as the Gleason grades for prostate cancer. Each grading system divides cancer into those with the greatest abnormality, the least abnormality, and those in between.

Grading is done by a pathologist, who examines tissue from the biopsy. Cancers with more abnormal-appearing cells tend to grow and spread more quickly and have a worse prognosis (outlook).

H

HDR brachytherapy: see high dose rate brachytherapy.

HIFU: see high-intensity focused ultrasound.

HPC1: inherited DNA changes in a gene called HPC1 may make prostate cancer more likely to develop in some men. These changes appear to be responsible for about 10 percent of prostate cancers. Research on this gene is still preliminary and a genetic test is not yet available.

half life: the time it takes for 50 percent of the radiation in a substance to be released.

hernia: a defect in the muscles of the abdominal wall that may cause a bulge as well as pain and pressure.

hesitancy: inability to start the stream of urine promptly.

high dose rate (HDR) brachytherapy: a form of treatment involving insertion of small plastic catheters into the prostate gland, guided by transrectal ultrasound (TRUS). A radioactive source (iridium-192) is then placed in the catheters and is removed a short time later. It is usually given once a week for 2 or 3 weeks and is often used in combination with external beam radiation. Unlike standard brachytherapy (which uses lower doses of radiation over a longer period of time), the radioactive seeds are not left in the body.

high-intensity focused ultrasound: an investigational procedure in which high-intensity sound energy is channeled through a small probe that can be inserted into the rectum to destroy cancerous tissue.

hormonal therapy: also called androgen deprivation therapy (ADT), this is treatment with hormones, using drugs that interfere with hormone production or hormone action, or the surgical removal of hormone-producing glands. Hormonal therapy may kill cancer cells or slow their growth. It is a common form of treatment for advanced prostate cancer.

hormone: a chemical substance released into the body by the endocrine glands such as the thyroid, adrenal, or ovaries. The substance travels through the bloodstream and sets in motion various body functions. Testosterone and estrogen are examples of male and female hormones.

hormone naïve: also called hormone sensitive, this describes cancer that has not been treated with hormonal therapy.

hormone refractory: term for prostate cancer cells that no longer respond to hormonal therapy; also known as androgen independent or hormone independent.

hot flash: sudden rush of body heat causing reddening and sweating; a common side effect of some types of hormonal therapy. Also called a hot flush.

hyperplasia: too much growth of cells or tissue in a specific area, such as the lining of the prostate. Hyperplasia is not cancer, however. See also, benign prostatic hyperplasia.

hyperthermia: also called heat therapy; the application of heat in treating diseases, including cancer.

hypothalamus: a small area of the brain that senses when testosterone levels are too high or too low and stimulates production when necessary.

I

IGF-1: see insulin-like growth factor-1.

IM: see intramuscular.

IMRT: see intensity modulated radiation therapy.

IV: see intravenous.

IVP: see intravenous pyelogram.

imaging studies: methods used to produce a picture of internal body structures. Some imaging methods used to help diagnose or stage cancer are x-rays, bone scans, CT scans, magnetic resonance imaging (MRI), and ultrasound.

immune system: the complex system by which the body resists infection by germs such as bacteria or viruses and rejects transplanted tissues or organs. The immune system may also help the body fight some cancers.

impotence: not being able to have or maintain an erection of the penis.

incidence: the number of new cases of a disease that occur in a population each year. Compare to prevalence.

incision: cut made during surgery.

incontinence, urinary: partial or complete loss of urinary control. See also stress incontinence, urge incontinence, overflow incontinence.

indolent: posing a minimal threat; defined as a total tumor volume of less than 0.5 cubic centimeters cancer confined to the prostate, and not Gleason pattern 4 or 5.

insulin-like growth factor-1 (IGF-1): researchers have recently noted that men with high blood levels of this hormone-like substance may be more likely to develop prostate cancer.

intensity modulated radiation therapy (IMRT): an advanced method of conformal radiation therapy in which the beams are aimed from several directions and the intensity (strength) of the beams is controlled by computers. This allows more radiation to reach the treatment area while reducing the radiation to healthy tissues. See also 3-dimensional conformal radiation therapy.

intermittent hormonal therapy: a type of prostate cancer treatment in which hormonal drugs are stopped after a man's blood PSA level drops to a very low level and remains stable for a while. If the PSA level begins to rise, the drugs are started again.

internal radiation: treatment involving implantation of a radioactive substance; see also brachytherapy.

interstitial radiation therapy: a type of internal radiation or brachytherapy treatment in which a radioactive implant is placed directly into the tissue (not in a body cavity).

intramuscular (IM): injected into a muscle.

intravenous (IV): A method of supplying fluids and medications using a needle inserted in a vein.

intravenous pyelogram (IVP): a special kind of x-ray procedure. A dye injected into the blood-stream travels to the kidneys, ureters and bladder and helps to clearly outline these organs on x-rays.

invasive cancer: cancer that has spread beyond the layer of cells where it first developed to involve adjacent tissues.

investigational: under study; often used to describe drugs used in clinical trials that are not yet available to the general public.

K

Kegel exercises: exercises to strengthen bladder muscles. These exercises may help men and women with certain forms of incontinence.

L

LDR: see low dose rate (LDR) brachytherapy

LH: see luteinizing hormone.

LHRH: see luteinizing hormone-releasing hormone.

LHRH agonists: see luteinizing hormone-releasing hormone agonists.

LHRH analogs: see luteinizing hormone-releasing hormone agonists.

LHRH antagonists: see luteinizing hormone-releasing hormone (LHRH) antagonists

Laetrile: a compound produced from the pits of fruits; several cases of cyanide poisoning have been linked to its use. Laetrile use is illegal in the US.

laparoscope: a long, slender tube inserted into the abdomen through a very small incision. The laparoscope allows the surgeon to view lymph nodes near the prostate and remove these pelvic lymph nodes using special surgical instruments operated through the laparoscope.

laparoscopic lymphadenectomy: removal of lymph nodes with a laparoscope.

laparoscopic radical prostatectomy: surgery to remove the prostate in which several small incisions are made in the abdomen. Specially designed instruments are inserted to view and remove the prostate.

libido: sex drive.

local anesthesia: see anesthesia.

local recurrence: see recurrence.

localized prostate cancer: cancer that is confined to the prostate gland.

low dose rate (LDR) brachytherapy: also called a permanent seed implant, this is a form of radiation therapy in which radioactive materials in the form of "seeds," each about the size and shape of a grain of rice, are deposited in the prostate and left in place indefinitely.

luteinizing hormone (LH): pituitary hormone that stimulates the testicles to produce testosterone.

luteinizing hormone-releasing hormone (LHRH): a hormone produced by the hypothalamus, a tiny gland in the brain, that affects levels of LH in the body and therefore affects testosterone levels.

luteinizing hormone-releasing hormone (LHRH) agonists: manmade hormones, chemically similar to LHRH. They block the production of the male hormone testosterone and are sometimes used as a treatment for prostate cancer. LHRH agonists approved for use in the US include leuprolide (Lupron) and goserelin (Zoladex). See also luteinizing hormone-releasing hormone.

luteinizing hormone-releasing hormone (LHRH) antagonists: medicine that lowers testosterone levels in the blood; thought to work in a similar way to LHRH agonists.

lycopenes: vitamin-like antioxidants that help prevent damage to DNA and may help lower prostate cancer risk. These substances are found in tomatoes, grapefruit, and watermelon.

lymphadenectomy: surgical removal of lymph nodes. After removal, the lymph nodes are examined by microscope to see if cancer has spread; also called lymph node dissection. See also lymphatic system.

lymphatic system: also called the lymph system. The tissues and organs (including lymph nodes, spleen, thymus, and bone marrow) that produce and store lymphocytes (cells that fight infection) and the channels that carry the lymph fluid. The entire lymphatic system is an important part of the body's immune system. Invasive cancers such as prostate cancer sometimes penetrate the lymphatic vessels (channels) and spread (metastasize) to lymph nodes.

lymph: clear fluid that flows through the lymphatic vessels and contains cells known as lymphocytes. These cells are important in fighting infections and may also have a role in fighting cancer.

lymph nodes: small bean-shaped collections of immune system tissue, such as lymphocytes, found along lymphatic vessels. They remove cell waste and fluids from lymph. They help fight infections and also have a role in fighting cancer, although cancers sometimes spread through them. Also called lymph glands.

lymphocyte: a type of white blood cell that helps the body fight infection.

M

MRI: see magnetic resonance imaging.

magnetic resonance imaging (MRI): a method of taking pictures of the inside of the body. Instead of using x-rays, MRI uses a powerful magnet to send radio waves through the body; the images appear on a computer screen as well as on film. Like x-rays, the procedure is physically painless, but some people may feel confined inside the MRI machine.

malignant tumor: a mass of cancer cells that may invade surrounding tissues or spread (metastasize) to distant areas of the body.

Man to Man: American Cancer Society program of education and support for men with prostate cancer. Call 800-ACS-2345 to ask about program locations.

margin: edge of the tissue removed during surgery. A negative surgical margin is a sign that no cancer was left behind. A positive surgical margin indicates that cancer cells are found at the outer edge of the tissue removed and is usually a sign that some cancer remains in the body.

medical oncologist: a doctor who is specially trained to diagnose cancer and treat cancer with chemotherapy and other drugs.

metastasis: the spread of cancer cells to distant areas of the body by way of the lymph system or bloodstream.

mini-laparotomy prostatectomy: surgical removal of the prostate gland through smaller or "mini" incisions.

molecular biology: the study of life at a sub-microscopic level. In cancer research, molecular biologists study the molecules that determine how a cell grows, how it interacts with its environment, and what goes wrong with this machinery when cancer develops.

N

negative margin: see margin.

neoadjuvant therapy: treatment given before radiation or surgery. For example, neoadjuvant hormonal therapy is sometimes used to shrink the prostate tumor prior to brachytherapy to make it more effective.

neoplasm: an abnormal growth (tumor) that starts from a single altered cell; a neoplasm may be benign or malignant. Cancer is a malignant neoplasm.

nerve graft: replacing nerves that control erections with small nerves taken from the side of the foot in an attempt to retain erectile functioning.

"nerve-sparing" prostatectomy: radical prostatectomy in which the surgeon attempts to maintain potency by leaving in the neurovascular bundles that control erection.

neurovascular bundle: one of 2 groups of nerves and blood vessels that run alongside the prostate and help the penis become erect. Removal or injury of these bundles during surgery, or damage from radiation therapy, can lead to impotence.

node: lymph node; see lymphatic system.

nomogram: computer-based tools that offer simplified estimates of prognoses and may help a doctor and patient better understand if the patient's cancer is likely to pose health risks.

nurse practitioner: a registered nurse with a master's or doctoral degree. Licensed nurse practitioners diagnose and manage illness and disease, usually working closely with a doctor. In many states, they may prescribe medications.

O

oncogenes: genes that promote cell growth and multiplication. These genes are normally present in all cells. But oncogenes may undergo changes that activate them, causing cells to grow too quickly and form tumors.

oncologist: a doctor with special training in the diagnosis and treatment of cancer.

oncology: the branch of medicine concerned with the diagnosis and treatment of cancer.

oncology clinical nurse specialist: a registered nurse with a master's degree in oncology who specializes in the care of cancer patients. Oncology nurse specialists may prepare and administer treatments, monitor patients, pre-scribe and provide supportive care, and teach and counsel patients and their families.

oncology social worker: a person with a master's degree in social work who is an expert in coordinating and providing non-medical care to patients. The oncology social worker provides counseling and assistance to people with cancer and their families, especially in dealing with the non-medical issues that can result from cancer, such as financial problems, housing (when treat-ments must be administered at a facility away from home), and child care.

opioids: the strongest pain relievers available, available by prescription only; morphine is one example.

orchiectomy: surgery to remove the testicles; castration.

overflow incontinence: needing to get up often during the night to urinate, taking a long time to urinate, and have a dribbling stream with little force. Overflow incontinence is usually due to blockage or narrowing of the bladder outlet, by either cancer or scar tissue.

P

p53: one of the tumor suppressor genes. Changes of this and similar genes may also be responsible for making some prostate cancers more likely to grow and spread more rapidly than others.

PAP: see prostatic acid phosphatase.

PC-SPES: a form of complementary/alternative therapy consisting of a mixture of 8 herbs (including saw palmetto) containing a range of plant chemicals and trace minerals. PC-SPES was removed from the US market in February 2002 because some PC-SPES capsules were found to be contaminated with compounds identical to or similar to other prescription drugs that could cause serious health problems.

PCa-24: a protein that appears to be present only when prostate cancer exists in the body. If developed, a blood test for this protein could distinguish between prostate cancer and BPH, avoiding unnecessary biopsies.

PIN: see prostatic intraepithelial neoplasia.

PSA: see prostate-specific antigen.

PSA density (PSAD): PSAD is determined by dividing the PSA level by the prostate volume (its size as measured by transrectal ultrasound). A higher PSAD indicates greater likelihood of cancer. See also prostate-specific antigen.

PSA doubling time (PSADT): the amount of time it takes for the PSA level to double. This is sometimes useful in helping to determine if cancer is present or has recurred. See also prostate-specific antigen.

PSA velocity (PSAV): a measurement of how quickly the PSA level rises over a period of time. This has been suggested as a way to improve the accuracy of PSA testing. A higher PSAV indicates greater likelihood of cancer being present. See also prostate-specific antigen.

palliative treatment: therapy that relieves symptoms, such as pain or blockage of urine flow, but is not expected to cure the cancer. Its main purpose is to improve the patient's quality of life.

palpation: using the hands to examine. A palpable mass is one that can be felt.

pathologist: a doctor who specializes in diagnosis and classification of diseases by lab tests such as examining tissue and cells under a microscope. The pathologist determines whether a tumor is benign or cancerous, and, if cancerous, the exact cell type and grade.

pathology report: a report outlining the cell type and extent of your cancer.

pelvic lymph node dissection: removal of the lymph nodes in the pelvis.

pelvic nodes: pelvic lymph nodes; the lymph nodes, located within the pelvis, to which prostate cancer is most likely to spread. These nodes are often removed and examined for cancer (pelvic lymph node dissection) prior to radical prostatectomy.

pelvis: the part of the skeleton that forms a ring of bones in the lower trunk and that supports the spine and legs. Cancer may spread (metastasize) to these bones. Pelvis is also used to refer to the general region of the lower trunk surrounded by these bones.

penile implant or prosthesis: artificial device placed in the penis during surgery to restore erections.

penile injection: involves placing a needle into a specific part of the penis and injecting medication that produces an erection.

penile suppository: a small pellet of medication that is placed into the tip of the penis to produce an erection.

penis: the male organ of copulation.

perineal biopsy: the doctor places a finger in the patient's rectum to feel the prostate and then inserts the biopsy needle through a small incision in the skin of the perineum. This method has been abandoned by many urologists in favor of a transrectal ultrasound–guided biopsy.

perineal prostatectomy: an operation in which the prostate is removed through an incision in the skin between the scrotum and anus.

perineum: the area between the anus and the scrotum.

perineural invasion: invasion of cancer cells into areas around nerves in the prostate gland. This is sometimes reported by pathologists looking at prostatectomy specimens, but it is not thought to affect a man's prognosis.

peripheral zone: the largest part of the prostate, near the outer edges of the gland. It is where most prostate cancers occur.

permanent section: a method of preparation of tissue for microscopic examination. The tissue is soaked in formaldehyde, processed in various chemicals, surrounded by a block of wax, sliced very thin, attached to a microscope slide and stained. This usually takes 1 to 2 days. It provides a clear view of the sample so that the presence or absence of cancer can be determined.

phase I clinical trial: intensive and closely-monitored studies conducted at a limited number of institutions in the US. The primary purpose is to determine if a new treatment is safe and to establish the highest dose that can be given safely.

phase II clinical trial: all participants receive a standard dose of treatment (determined from a phase I study) and are repeatedly examined to determine if they respond.

phase III clinical trial: often randomized trials, these are studies in which eligible patients are randomly assigned to one treatment or another. Generally, hundreds of patients and several institutions are involved in phase III clinical trials, which have the potential to change the standard of care for treatment and prevention.

phosphodiesterase inhibitors: drugs, such as sildenafil (Viagra), that can help men achieve an erection. Not all forms of impotence respond to these drugs, however.

placebo: a substance or other kind of treatment that seems therapeutic, but is actually inactive.

placebo effect: the real effect of placebos in some patients.

platelet: a part of the blood that plugs up holes in blood vessels after an injury. Chemotherapy can cause a drop in the platelet count, a condition called thrombocytopenia that carries risk of excessive bleeding.

positive margin: see margin.

prevalence: a measure of the proportion of persons in the population with a particular disease at a given time. Compare with incidence.

primary site: the place where cancer begins. Primary cancer is usually named after the organ in which it starts. For example, cancer that starts in the prostate is always prostate cancer even if it spreads (metastasizes) to other organs such as bones or lymph nodes.

primary treatment: the first, and usually the most important, treatment.

prognosis: a prediction of the course of disease; the outlook for the chances of survival.

prognostic factors: everything that could affect that person's disease and outcomes.

ProstaScint scan: like the bone scan, the ProstaScint scan uses low level radioactive material to find cancer that has spread beyond the prostate. But the radioactive material for the ProstaScint scan is attached to an antibody made in a lab to recognize and stick to a particular substance. In this case, the antibody sticks to prostate-specific membrane antigen (PSMA), a substance found only in normal and cancerous prostate cells. This test detects spread of prostate cancer to bone as well as lymph nodes and other organs, and that it can clearly distinguish prostate cancer from other cancers and benign disorders. It is most commonly used to look for cancer if the PSA level is elevated after treatment.

prostate: a gland found in men just below the bladder and in front of the rectum. The prostate makes a fluid that is part of semen. The tube that carries urine (the urethra) runs through the prostate.

prostate-specific antigen (PSA): a gland protein made by the prostate. Levels of PSA in the blood often go up in men with prostate cancer. The PSA test is used to help find prostate cancer as well as to monitor the results of treatment.

prostatectomy: surgical removal of all or part of the prostate gland.

prostatic acid phosphatase (PAP): a blood test, like the PSA test, that may be done when looking for evidence of prostate cancer. Unlike the PSA test, the PAP test is not useful for prostate cancer screening.

prostatic intraepithelial neoplasia (PIN): a condition in which there are changes in the microscopic appearance of prostate epithelial cells. The condition is not cancer, but it may lead to the development of cancer.

prostatic urethra: the part of the urethra that runs through the prostate.

prostatitis: inflammation of the prostate. Prostatitis is not cancer.

proteomics: a new technique that uses technologically complex machines to measure the levels of PSA and the other 100,000 proteins in the blood. Analysis of these proteins may help diagnose prostate cancer and distinguish which cancers are likely to be aggressive.

protocol: a formal outline or plan, such as a description of what treatments a patient will receive and exactly when each should be given. See also regimen.

proton: a radioactive particle used in some forms of radiation therapy. See also conformal proton beam radiation therapy.

R

RT-PCR test: a very sensitive test for finding small numbers of prostate cancer cells in blood samples. It is still uncertain if or how the test should be used in considering treatment options.

rad: stands for "radiation absorbed dose," a measurement of the amount of radiation absorbed by tissues. The term rad is being replaced by cGy (centigray).

radiation oncologist: a doctor who specializes in using radiation to treat cancer.

radiation therapy: treatment with high-energy rays (such as x-rays) to kill or shrink cancer cells. The radiation may come from outside of the body (external beam radiation) or from radioactive materials placed directly in the tumor (brachytherapy or internal radiation).

Radiation therapy may be used to reduce the size of a cancer before surgery, to destroy any remaining cancer cells after surgery, or, in some cases, as the main treatment.

radical prostatectomy: surgery to remove the entire prostate gland, the seminal vesicles, and nearby tissue.

radical perineal prostatectomy: surgical removal of the prostate through an incision in the area between the scrotum and anus.

radical retropubic prostatectomy: surgery to remove the prostate through an incision in the lower abdomen.

radiologist: a doctor with special training in diagnosis of diseases by interpreting x-rays and other types of diagnostic imaging studies, for example, CT and MRI scans.

radiopharmaceuticals: a group of drugs that include radioactive elements, such as strontium-89 or samarium-153, and that are given intravenously (IV) to treat bone pain related to metastatic prostate cancer. See also strontium-89.

rectum: the lower part of the large intestine leading to the anus.

recurrence: "residual" cancer that was not destroyed during treatment. Local recurrence means that the cancer is present in the same place as the original cancer. Regional recurrence means that the cancer is present in the lymph nodes near the primary site. Distant recurrence is when cancer metastasizes after treatment to distant organs or tissues (such as the lungs, liver, bone marrow, or brain).

red blood cells: blood cells that contain hemoglobin, the substance that carries oxygen to other tissues of the body.

refractory: no longer responsive to a certain therapy.

regimen: a strict, regulated plan (such as diet, exercise, or other activity) designed to reach certain goals. In cancer treatment, a plan to treat cancer. See also protocol.

regional involvement: the spread of cancer from its original site to nearby areas such as lymph nodes, but not to distant sites.

regression: reduction of the size of the tumor or the extent of the cancer.

rehabilitation: activities to help a person adjust, heal, and return to as full and productive a life as possible after injury or illness. This may involve physical restoration (such as the use of prostheses, exercises, and physical therapy), counseling, and emotional support.

relapse: reappearance of cancer after a disease-free period. See also recurrence.

relative 5-year survival rate: the percentage of people with a certain cancer who have not died from it within 5 years. This number is different from the 5-year survival rate in that it does not include people who have died from unrelated causes. Relative survival rates are important for prostate cancer because many men with it are older and may die from other health problems.

remission: complete or partial disappearance of the signs and symptoms of cancer in response to treatment; the period during which a disease is under control. A remission may not be a cure.

resectoscope: instrument used in transurethral resection of the prostate (TURP), allowing the surgeon direct inspection of the prostatic urethra and adjacent prostatic tissue.

response: outcome derived from treatment or reaction to a drug or any other therapy.

retention: see urinary retention.

retrograde ejaculation: a condition, often occurring after radiation, radical, prostatectomy, or TURP, in which orgasm causes semen to enter the bladder, as opposed to exiting the body through the penis. Also known as a dry orgasm.

retropubic: behind the pubic bone.

retropubic prostatectomy: see radical retropubic prostatectomy.

ribonuclease L (RNASEL): a gene that helps protect against infections and causes defective cells to die. If the gene is inactivated, prostate cancer may be allowed to develop. A man with RNASEL may be more likely to develop prostate cancer.

risk factor: anything that increases a person's chance of getting a disease such as cancer. Different cancers have different risk factors. Some risk factors, like a person's age or race, can't be changed. Others are linked to cancer-causing factors in the environment or to personal choices such as diet and exercise.

S

saw palmetto: an herbal extract from the berries of the saw palmetto tree that is sometimes used for BPH. It is not a proven treatment for prostate cancer.

screening: the search for disease, such as cancer, in people without symptoms. For example, screening measures for prostate cancer include digital rectal examination and the PSA blood test. Screening may refer to coordinated programs in large populations.

scrotum: pouch of skin that holds the testicles.

selenium: a few clinical trials indicate that this antioxidant may reduce the risk of prostate cancer. Studies into its potential benefits are underway.

semen: fluid released during orgasm, containing sperm and seminal fluid.

seminal vesicles: glands at the base of the bladder and next to the prostate that release fluid into the semen during orgasm. Cancer that spreads beyond the prostate gland may invade the seminal vesicles.

serum: blood serum is the liquid portion of the blood; the portion of blood that is not solid— that is, not red blood cells, white blood cells, and platelets.

sextant biopsy: see biopsy.

side effects: unwanted effects of treatment, such as hair loss caused by chemotherapy and fatigue caused by radiation therapy.

sign: an observable physical change caused by an illness. Compare to symptom.

simulation: a process involving special x-ray pictures that are used to plan radiation treatment so that the area to be treated is precisely located and marked for treatment.

sphincter, urethral: muscle that squeezes the urethra shut and provides urinary control.

spinal cord compression: any process that results in pressure on the spinal cord, the spinal nerve trunks, or both; can occur when prostate cancer spreads to the spine.

St. John's wort: an herb that may be used to treat mild or moderate depression. It has been shown to diminish the effects of chemotherapy and some other drugs.

staging: the process of finding out whether cancer has spread and if so, how far. There is more than 1 system for staging.

The TNM system, which is used most often, gives 3 key pieces of information:

T refers to the size of the tumor

N describes how far the cancer has spread to nearby nodes

M shows whether the cancer has spread (metastasized) to other organs of the body

Letters or numbers after the T, N, and M give more details about each of these factors. To make this information somewhat clearer, the TNM descriptions can be grouped together into a simpler set of stages, labeled with Roman numerals. In general, the lower the number, the less the cancer has spread. A higher number means a more serious cancer.

The 2 types of staging are:

clinical staging: an estimate of the extent of cancer based on physical examination and diagnostic imaging tests.

pathologic staging: an estimate of the extent of cancer by direct study of tissue removed during surgery.

standard therapy: the most commonly used and most widely accepted form of treatment; see therapy.

stereotactic body radiation therapy: investigational external beam radiation therapy technique in which a large, precise radiation dose is directed at a small tumor area and allows the course of treatment to be reduced.

stress incontinence: passing a small amount of urine when coughing, laughing, sneezing, or exercising.

stricture, urethral: a narrowing of the urethra due to scar tissue which blocks flow of urine and can result in overflow incontinence. This can be treated by surgically removing the scar tissue stretching the urethra.

strontium-89: a radioactive substance that is used for treatment of bone pain due to metastatic prostate cancer. It is injected into a vein and is attracted to areas of bone containing metastatic cancer. The radiation given off by the strontium 89 kills the cancer cells, and relieves the pain caused by bone metastases.

subcapsular orchiectomy: the surgical removal of the inside glandular tissue of the testicles, leaving the outer shells of the testicles in place to avoid an empty scrotum.

suprapubic catheter: a tube that drains urine from the bladder outside of the body through a hole in the skin of the lower abdomen.

survival rate: see 5-year survival rate.

symptom: a change in the body caused by an illness, as described by the person experiencing it. Compare to sign.

T

TNM: see staging.

TRUS: see transrectal ultrasound.

TURP: see transurethral resection of the prostate.

targeted therapies: these use a variety of methods to either attack and kill cancer cells based on the specific ways they differ from normal cells, or compensate for those differences to make the cells less dangerous.

temporary brachytherapy: see high dose rate brachytherapy.

testicles: the male reproductive glands found in the scrotum. The testicles (or testes) produce sperm and the male hormone testosterone.

testosterone: the main male hormone, made primarily in the testes. It stimulates blood flow, growth in certain tissues, and the secondary sexual characteristics. In men with prostate cancer, it can also encourage growth of the tumor.

therapy: any of the measures taken to treat a disease. See also standard therapy, alternative therapy, complementary therapy, and unproven therapy.

thermocouples: devices used in cryotherapy that measure the temperature within the prostate to ensure that a temperature of –40 degrees Celsius is reached for tumor cells and to prevent freezing in areas of normal tissue that should not get cold.

"thermoseeds": non-radioactive metallic pellets inserted directly into the prostate that generate heat when placed into a magnetic field, providing hyperthermia inside a prostate tumor.

three-dimensional conformal radiation therapy (3DCRT): this treatment uses sophisticated computers to very precisely map the location of the cancer within the prostate. The patient is fitted with a plastic mold resembling a body cast to keep him still so that the radiation can be more accurately aimed. Radiation beams are then aimed from several directions. This reduces the effects on normal tissues and may allow higher doses of radiation to be used.

tissue: a group of cells, united to perform a particular function in the body.

total androgen blockade: see combination hormonal therapy.

transition zone: innermost area of the prostate, surrounding the urethra. This is where benign prostatic hyperplasia (BPH) develops.

transrectal biopsy: the most common biopsy technique, involving inserting the biopsy needle through the rectum to withdraw sample tissue.

transrectal ultrasound (TRUS): an imaging test in which a probe, inserted into the rectum, gives off sound waves to create a picture of the prostate on a screen to help detect or find the location of tumors.

transrectal ultrasound–guided biopsy: a small biopsy needle is placed into a guide attached to a transrectal ultrasound device and inserted through the rectum.

transurethral resection of the prostate (TURP): an operation that involves removing a part of the prostate gland that surrounds the urethra (the tube through which urine exits the bladder). The procedure is used for some men with prostate cancer who cannot have a radical prostatectomy because of advanced age or other serious illnesses. This operation can be used to relieve symptoms caused by a tumor, but it is not expected to cure this disease or remove all of the cancer. TURP is used more often to relieve symptoms of benign prostatic hyperplasia (BPH).

tumor: an abnormal lump or mass of tissue. Tumors can be benign (not cancerous) or malignant (cancerous).

tumor flare: an increase or surge in testosterone levels as a result of increased testosterone production by the adrenal glands. May cause bone pain or, rarely, more serious complications.

tumor marker: a substance produced by cancer cells—and sometimes by normal cells as well. Tumor markers can be found in large amounts in the blood or urine of some patients with cancer.

tumor suppressor genes: genes that slow down cell division or cause cells to die at the appropriate time. Alterations that inactivate these genes can lead to too much cell growth and development of cancer.

tumor volume: measure of the amount of cancer present.

U

unproven therapy: any therapy that has not been scientifically tested and approved.

ureters: tubes carrying urine from each kidney to the bladder.

urethra: the tube that carries urine from the bladder to the outside. In women, this tube is fairly short; in men it is longer, passing through the penis, and it also carries the semen.

urge incontinence: a sudden and uncontrollable urge pass urine. This problem occurs when the bladder becomes too sensitive to stretching by urine accumulation.

urgency: feeling that you need to urinate right away.

urinary retention: inability to empty the bladder; inability to urinate.

urethral warming device: a device inserted through the penis into the bladder that decreases potential complications associated with freezing the urethra during cryotherapy.

urologist: a doctor who specializes in treating problems of the urinary tract in men and women, and of the genital area in men.

V

vacuum pump: a device that creates an erection by drawing blood into the penis; a ring placed at the base of the penis traps the blood and sustains the erection.

vas deferens: one of 2 muscular tubes that carry sperm from the testicles to the urethra.

Viagra (sildenafil citrate): a drug used to treat impotence caused by medical (rather than psychological) problems. Viagra can cause side effects such as headache, hot flashes, indigestion, sensitivity to light, and other visual problems and should not be used with nitrates, a type of heart medication. Viagra can cause heart attacks in men who already have certain heart conditions.

vasectomy: surgery in which a segment of each vas deferens is removed to prevent release of sperm and thus provide contraception.

vitamin E: an antioxidant vitamin that may help prevent prostate cancer.

W

watchful waiting: a form of management of prostate cancer in which it is closely monitored (usually with PSA blood tests and DREs) instead of active treatment such as surgery or radiation therapy. This may be a reasonable choice for older men with small tumors that might grow very slowly. If the situation changes, active treatment can be started. Also known as expectant management.

white blood cells: one of several types of blood cells that help defend the body against infections. Certain cancer treatments such as chemotherapy can reduce the number of these cells and make a person more likely to get infections.

X

x-ray: a form of radiation that can be used at low levels to produce an image of the body on film or at high levels to destroy cancer cells.

REFERENCES

CHAPTER 1

American Cancer Society. Detailed guide: prostate cancer. Available at http://www.cancer.org/docroot/CRI/CRI_2_3x.asp?dt=36. Accessed March 5, 2004.

Gjengsto P, Halvorsen OJ, Akslen LA, Frugard J, Hoisaeter PA. Benign growth of different prostate zones in aging men with slightly elevated PSA in whom prostate cancer has been excluded: a prospective study of 510 patients. *Urology.* September 2003;62(3):447-50.

MacNeal JE. Pathology of benign prostatic hyperplasia. Insight into etiology. *Urol Clin North Am.* 1992;17:477-486.

Partin AW, Coffey DS. The molecular biology, endocrinology, and physiology of the prostate and seminal vesicles. In: Walsh PC, Retik AB, Vaughan ED Jr, et al, eds. *Campbell's Urology.* 8th ed. Philadelphia: Saunders; 2002:1237-1296.

U.S. Library of Medicine and the National Institutes of Health. Medline Plus Medical Encyclopedia. Prostate cancer. Available at: http://www.nlm.nih.gov/medlineplus/ency/imagepages/18038.htm. Accessed: March, 2004.

U.S. Library of Medicine and the National Institutes of Health. Medline Plus Medical Encyclopedia. Prostatectomy-series: Normal. Available at: http://www.nlm.nih.gov/medlineplus/ency/presentations/100046_5.htm. Accessed: March, 2004.

Zaviacic M. The adult human female prostatic homologue and male prostate gland: a comparative enzyme-histochemical study. *Acta Histochem.* 1985;77:19-31.

CHAPTER 2

American Cancer Society. *Cancer Facts and Figures 2003.* Available at: http://www.cancer.org/docroot/STT/stt_0.asp. Accessed October 30, 2003.

American Cancer Society. *Cancer Facts and Figures 2004.* Available for download at: http://www.cancer.org/docroot/STT/stt_0.asp. Accessed January, 2004.

American Cancer Society. Detailed guide: prostate cancer. Available at http://www.cancer.org/docroot/CRI/CRI_2_3x.asp?dt=36. Accessed January 1, 2004.

American Cancer Society. DHEA. Available at: http://www.cancer.org/docroot/ETO/content/ETO_5_3X_Dhea.asp?sitearea=ETO. Accessed May 13, 2004.

Basler JW, Piazza GA. Nonsteroidal anti-inflammatory drugs and cyclooxygenase-2 selective inhibitors for prostate cancer chemoprevention. *J Urol.* February 2004;171(2 Pt 2):S59-62;discussion S62-3.

Bostwick DG. Prostate-specific antigen. Current role in diagnostic pathology of prostate cancer. *Am J Clin Pathol.* October 1994;102(4 Suppl 1):S31-7.

Bostwick DG, Burke HB, Djakiew D, et al. Human Prostate Cancer Risk Factors. *Cancer.* Submitted 2003.

Boyle P. Screening for prostate cancer: have you had your cholesterol measured? *BJU International.* 2003;92: 191-199.

Bruner DW, Moore D, Parlanti A, Dorgan J, Engstrom P. Relative risk of prostate cancer for men with affected relatives: Systematic review and meta-analysis. *Int. J. Cancer.* 2003;107:797-803.

Calle EE, Rodriguez C, Walker-Thurmond K, Thun MJ. Overweight, Obesity, and Mortality from Cancer in a Prospectively Studied Cohort of U.S. Adults. *N Engl J Med.* 2003;348:1625-1638. April 24, 2003.

Cerhan JR, Torner JC, Lynch CF, et al. Association of smoking, body mass, and physical activity with risk of prostate cancer in the Iowa 65+ Rural Health Study (United States). *Cancer Causes Control.* March 1997;8(2):229-38.

Clark LC, Dalkin B, Krongrad A, et al. Decreased incidence of prostate cancer with selenium supplementation: results of a double-blind cancer prevention trial. *Br J Urol.* 1998;81:730-4.

Coffey DS. Similarities of prostate and breast cancer: Evolution, diet, and estrogens. *Urology.* April 2001;57(4 Suppl 1):31-8.

Crawford ED. Epidemiology of prostate cancer. *Urology.* December 22, 2003;62(6 Suppl 1):3-12.

Deutsch E, Maggiorella L, Eschwege P, Bourhis J, Soria JC, Abdulkarim B. Environmental, genetic, and molecular features of prostate cancer. *Lancet Oncol.* May 2004;5(5):303-13.

Gann PH. Risk Factors for Prostate Cancer. *Rev. Urol.* 2002;4:Suppl. 5, S3-S10.

Heinonen OP, Albanes D, Virtamo J, et al. Prostate cancer and supplementation with alpha-tocopherol and beta-carotene: incidence and mortality in a controlled trial. *J Natl Cancer Inst.* 1998;90:440-6.

Hsing AW, Tsao L, Devesa SS. International trends and patterns of prostate cancer incidence and mortality. *Int. J. Cancer.* 2000;85:60-67.

Klein EA, Thompson IM, Lippman SM, et al. SELECT: the next prostate cancer prevention trial. Selenum and Vitamin E Cancer Prevention Trial. *J Urol.* 2001;166:1311-5.

Kushi L, Giovannucci E. Dietary fat and cancer. *Am J Med.* 2002 Dec 30;113 Suppl 9B:63S-70S.

Memorial Sloan Kettering Cancer Center. Dehydroepiandrosterone. About Herbs. Available at: http://www.mskcc.org/mskcc/html/11571.cfm?RecordID=625. Accessed May 13, 2004.

Messina MJ. Emerging evidence on the role of soy in reducing prostate cancer risk. *Nutr Rev.* 2003 Apr;61(4):117-31. Review.

Michaud DS, Augustsson K, Rimm EB, Stampfer MJ, Willet WC, Giovannucci E. A prospective study on intake of animal products and risk of prostate cancer. *Cancer Causes Control.* 2001 Aug;12(6):557-67.

National Cancer Institute. Statistical Research and Applications Branch. DEVCAN: Probability of Developing or Dying of Cancer Software, Version 5.1. 2003. Available at: http://srab.cancer.gov/devcan. Accessed: October, 2003.

National Cancer Institute. Cancer rates and risks. Surveillance, Epidemiology and End Results. Available at: http://seer.cancer.gov/publications/. Accessed October 30, 2003.

National Safety Council. What are the odds of dying? Available at: http://www.nsc.org/lrs/statinfo/odds.htm. Accessed October 30, 2003

Parkin DM, Whelan SL, Ferlay J, Raymond L, Young J, eds. 1997. *Cancer Incidence in Five Continents,* Vol. VII. IARC Scientific Publications No. 143. Lyon, IARC.

Platz EA, Leitzmann MF, Michaud DS, Willett WC, Giovannucci E. Interrelation of energy intake, body size, and physical activity with prostate cancer in a large prospective cohort study. *Cancer Res.* December 1, 2003;63(23):8542-8.

Ries LAG, Eisner MP, Kosary CL, et al, eds. Adapted from *SEER Cancer Statistics Review, 1975-2000,* National Cancer Institute, Bethesda, Maryland. Available at: http://seer.cancer.gov/csr/1975_2002,2003.

Sabichi AL, Lippman SM. COX-2 inhibitors and other NSAIDs in bladder and prostate cancer. *Prog Exp Tumor Res.* 2003;37:163-78.

Shames DA. Risks of testosterone replacement. *N Engl J Med.* May 6, 2004;350(19):2004-6.

Thompson IM, Goodman PJ, Tangen CM, et al. The influence of finasteride on the development of prostate cancer. *N Engl J Med.* 2003;349:215-24.

U.S. Department of Health and Human Services. *The Health Consequences of Smoking: A Report of the Surgeon General.* Executive summary. May 27, 2004. Available at: http://www.cdc.gov/tobacco/sgr/sgr_2004/pdf/executivesummary.pdf.

CHAPTER 3

American Cancer Society. *Cancer Prevention and Early Detection Facts and Figures 2003.* Available at: http://www.cancer.org/docroot/STT/stt_0.asp. Accessed December 2003.

Barry M, Fowler F, O'Leary M, et al. The American Urological Association symptom index for benign prostatic hyperplasia. *J Urol* 1992;148:1549-57.

Brawn PN, Johnson EH, Speights VO, et al. Incidence, racial differences and prognostic significance of prostate carcinomas diagnosed with obstructive symptoms. *Cancer.* 1994;74(5):1607-1611.

Brown CT, O'Flynn E, Van Der Muelen J, Newman S, Mundy AR, and Emberton M. The fear of prostate cancer in men with lower tract symptoms: should symptomatic men be screened? *BJU Int.* 2003;91(1):30-32.

Dodds PR, Caride VJ, Lytton BL. The role of vertebral veins in the dissemination of prostatic carcinoma. *J Urol.* 1981;126:753-755.

Kim ED, Grayhack T. Clinical symptoms and signs of prostate cancer. In: Vogelzang, NJ, Scardino PT, Shipley WU, and Coffey DS, eds. *Comprehensive Textbook of Genitourinary Oncology.* Baltimore, MD: Lippincott Williams and Wilkins; 2000:525-532.

Lawton CA, Cantrell JE, Derus SW, Murray KJ, Byhard RW, Wilson JF. Prostate cancer: are racial differences in clinical stage and survival explained by differences in symptoms. *Radiology.* 1994;192:37-40.

Marshall VF, Fuller NF. Hematospermia. *J Urol.* 1983;129:377-378.

Masters JG, Rice ML. Improvement in urinary symptoms after radical prostatectomy: a prospective evaluation of flow rates and symptom scores. *BJU Int.* 2003;91(9):795-797.

National Kidney and Urologic Diseases Information Clearinghouse. Medical tests for prostate problems. National Institute of Diabetes and Digestive and Kidney Diseases, National Institutes of Health. Available at: http://kidney.niddk.nih.gov/ kudiseases/pubs/medtestprostate/index.htm. Accessed March, 2004.

Paquette EL, Sun L, Paquette LR, Connelly R, Mcleod DG, Moul JW. Improved prostate cancer-specific survival and other disease parameters: impact of prostate specific antigen testing. *Urology.* 2002;60(5):756-759.

Powell IJ. Prostate cancer and African-American men. *Oncology.* 1997;11:599-605.

Rosenthal MA, Rosen D, Raghavan D, et al. Spinal cord compression in prostate cancer: a 10 year experience. *Br J Urol.* 1992;69:530-533.

Schmidt JD, Mettlin CJ, Natarajan N, et al. Trends in patterns of care for prostate cancer, 1974-1983: results of surveys by the American College of Surgeons. *J Urol.* 1986;136(2):416-421.

Stamey TA, Donaldson AN, Yemoto CE, McNeal JE, Sozan S, Gill H. Histological and clinical findings in 896 consecutive prostates treated only with radical retropubic prostatectomy: Epidemiologic significance of annual changes. *J Urol.* 1998;160:2412-2417.

Stormont TJ, Farrow GM, Meyers RP, et al. Clinical stage Bo or T1c prostate cancer: nonpalpable disease identified by elevated prostate-specific antigen concentration. *Urology.* 1993;41(1):3-8.

Surya BV, Provet JA. Manifestations of advanced prostate cancer: prognosis and treatment. *J Urol.* 1989;142:921-927.

Venable DD, Hastings D, Misra RP. Unusual metastatic patterns of prostate adenocarcinoma. *J Urol.* 1983;130:980-985.

CHAPTER 4

American Cancer Society. ACS cancer detection guidelines: cancer-related checkup. Available at: http://www.cancer.org/docroot/PED/content/ PED_2_3X_ACS_Cancer_Detection_Guidelines_ 36.asp?sitearea=PED. Accessed March, 2004.

American Cancer Society. Detailed guide: prostate cancer. Available at: http://www.cancer.org/docroot/ CRI/CRI_2_3x.asp?dt=36. Accessed January, 2004.

Catalona WJ, Smith DS, Ratliff TL, et al. Detection of organ confined prostate cancer is increased through prostate-specific antigen-based screening. *JAMA.* 1993;270:948-54.

de Konig HJ, Auvinen A, Berenguer Sanchez A, et al. Large-scale randomized prostate cancer screening trials: program performances in the European Randomized Screening for Prostate Cancer trial and the Prostate, Lung, Colorectal and Ovary Cancer Trial. *Int J Cancer.* 2002;97(2): 237-44.

National Cancer Institute. Surveillance: prostate-specific antigen (PSA) testing. Surveillance, Epidemiology and End Results Program (SEER). Available at: http://seer.cancer.gov/studies/ surveillance/study6.html. Accessed May 24, 2004.

Schroeder FH, Roobol-Bouts M, Vis AN, et al. PSA based early detection of prostate cancer-validation of screening without rectal examination. *Urology.* 2001;57:83-90.

Stephenson RA. Population-based prostate cancer trends in the PSA era: data from Surveillance, Epidemiology and End Results Program (SEER). Monogr. *Urol.* 1998;19:3-19.

U.S. Preventive Services Task Force. Recommendations and rationale: screening for prostate cancer. December 2002. Available at: http://www.ahrq.gov/ clinic/3rduspstf/prostatescr/prostaterr.htm. Accessed March 2004.

CHAPTER 5

Catalona WJ, Smith DS, et al. Measurement of prostate-specific antigen in serum as a screening test for prostate cancer. *N Engl J Med.* 1991;324:1156-1161.

Chodak GW, Keller P, et al. Assessment of screening for prostate cancer using the digital rectal examination. *J Urol.* 1989;141:1136-1138.

Haas GP, Sakr WA. Epidemiology of prostate cancer. *CA Cancer J Clin.* 1997;47:273-87.

Jacobsen SJ, Bergstralh EJ, Katusic SK, et al. Screening digital rectal examination and prostate cancer mortality: a population-based case-control study. *Urology.* 1998;52:173-9.

Schroder FH, van der Maas P, et al. Evaluation of the digital rectal examination as a screening test for prostate cancer. Rotterdam section of the European Randomized Study of Screening for Prostate Cancer. *J Natl Cancer Inst.* 1998;90, 1817-1823.

CHAPTER 6

American Cancer Society. Detailed guide: prostate cancer. Available at: http://www.cancer.org/ docroot/CRI/CRI_2_3x.asp?rnav=cridg&dt=36. Accessed January, 2004.

American Cancer Society. Tumor markers. Available at: http://www.cancer.org/docroot/PED/content/PED_2_3X_Tumor_Markers.asp?sitearea=PED. Accessed November 11, 2003.

Bazinet M, Meshref AW, Trudel C, et al. Prospective evaluation of prostate-specific antigen density and systematic biopsies for early detection of prostatic carcinoma. Urology. 1994;43:44-51.

Benson MC, Whang IS, Olsson CA, McMahon DJ, Cooner WH. The use of PSA density to enhance the predictive value of intermediate levels of serum PSA. J Urol. 1992;147:817-821.

Benson MC, Whang IS, Pantuck A, et al. Prostate-specific antigen density: A means of distinguishing benign prostatic hypertrophy and prostate cancer. J Urol. 1992;147:815-816.

Brawer M, Cheli C, Neaman I, et al. Complexed prostate-specific antigen provides significant enhancement of specificity compared with total prostate specific antigen for detecting prostate cancer. J Urol. 2000;163:1476-1480.

Brawer MK, Aramburu EAG, Chen GL, Preston SD, Ellis WJ. The inability of PSA index to enhance the predictive value of PSA in the diagnosis of prostatic carcinoma. J Urol. 1993;150:369-373.

Brawer MK, Meyer GE, Letran JL, et al. Measurement of complexed PSA improves specificity for early detection of prostate cancer. Urology. 1998;52:372-378.

Carter H, Morrell CH, Pearson JD, et al. Estimation of prostatic growth using serial PSA measurements in men with and without prostate disease. Cancer Research. 1992;52:3323-3328.

Catalona WJ, Partin AW, Slawin KM, et al. Use of the percentage of free prostate-specific antigen to enhance differentiation of prostate cancer from benign prostatic disease: A prospective multicenter clinical trial. JAMA. 1998;279:1542-1547.

Chen Y, Luderer AA, Thiel RP, Carlson G, Cuny CL, Soriano TF. Using proportions of free to total prostate-specific antigen, age, and total prostate-specific antigen to predict the probability of prostate cancer. Urology. 1996;47:518-524.

Christensson A, Bjork T, Nilsson O, et al. Serum prostate-specific antigen complexed to alpha 1-antichymotrypsin as an indicator of prostate cancer. J Urol. 1993;150:100-105.

Christensson A, Laurell CB, Lilja H. Enzymatic activity of prostate-specific antigen and its reaction with extracellular serine proteinase inhibitors. Eur J Biochem. 1990;194:755.

Christensson A, Lilja H. Complex formation between protein C inhibitor and prostate-specific antigen in vitro and in human semen. Eur J Biochem. 1994;220:45-53.

Dalkin BL, Ahmann FR, Kopp JB. PSA levels in men older than 50 years without clinical evidence of prostatic carcinoma. J Urol. 1993;150:1837-1839.

Etzioni R, Shen Y, Petteway JC, Brawer MK. Age-specific PSA: A reassessment. Prostate. 1996;7:70-77.

Higashihara E, Nutahara K, Kojima M, et al. Significance of serum free prostate-specific antigen in the screening of prostate cancer. J Urol. 1996;156:1964-68.

Luderer AA, Chen Y, Thiel R, et al. Measurement of the proportion of free to total PSA improves diagnostic performance of PSA in the diagnostic gray zone of total PSA. Urology. 1995;46:187-94.

Mettlin C, Littrup PJ, Kane RA, et al. Relative sensitivity and specificity of serum PSA level compared with age-referenced PSA, PSA density and PSA change. Cancer. 1994;74:1615-1620.

National Cancer Institute. Questions and answers about the prostate-specific antigen (PSA) test. Available at: http://cis.nci.nih.gov/fact/5_29.htm. Accessed March 12, 2004.

Nixon RG, Gold MH, Blase AB, Meyer GE, Brawer MK. Comparison of three investigative assays for the free form of prostate-specific antigen. J Urol. 1998;160:420-425.

Nixon RG, Wener MH, Brawer MK, Parson RE, Blase AB, Strobel SA. Biological variation of free prostate-specific antigen. J Urol. ed. 157. 1997;4:109A.

Oesterling JE, Jacobsen SJ, Chute CG, et al. Serum PSA in a community-based population of healthy men: Establishment of age-specific reference ranges. JAMA. 1993;270:860-864.

Piironen T, Pettersson K, Suonpaa M, et al. In vitro stability of free prostate-specific antigen (PSA) and prostate-specific antigen (PSA) complexed to alpha-1-antichymotrypsin in blood samples. Urology. 1996;48:81-87.

Porter JR, Hayward R, Brawer MK. The significance of short-term PSA change in men undergoing ultrasound guided prostate biopsy. J Urol (Suppl). Vol. 264, 1994:293A.

Rommel FM, Augusta VE, Breslin JA, et al. The use of PSA and PSAD in the diagnosis of prostate cancer in a community based urology practice. J Urol. 1994;151:88-93.

Roth HJ, Christensen-Stewart S, Brawer MK. A comparison of three free and total PSA assays. PCPD. 1998;1:326-331.

Stenman U, Leinonen J, Alfthan H, Rannikko S, Tuhkanen K, Althan O. A complex between PSA and alpha-1-antichymotrypsin is the major form of PSA in serum of patients with prostatic cancer: Assay of the complex improves clinical sensitivity for cancer. Cancer Research. 1991;51:222.

Tchetgen MB, Song JT, Strawderman M, Jacobsen SJ, Oesterling JE. Ejaculation increases the serum prostate-specific antigen concentration. *Urology.* 1996;47:511-516.

Woodrum DL, Brawer MK, Partin AW, Catalona WJ, Southwick PC. Interpretation of free prostate-specific antigen: clinical research studies for the detection of prostate cancer. *J Urol.* 1998;159:5-12.

Zhang WM, Finne P, Leinonen J, et al. Characterization and immunological determination of the complex between prostate-specific antigen and alpha-2-macroglobulin. *Clin Chem.* 1998;44:2471-9.

CHAPTER 7

American Cancer Society. Detailed guide: prostate cancer: can prostate cancer be found early? Available at: http://www.cancer.org/docroot/CRI/content/CRI_2_4_3X_Can_prostate_cancer_be_found_early_36.asp?sitearea=. Accessed December 3, 2003.

American Cancer Society. Detailed guide: prostate cancer: how is prostate cancer diagnosed? Available at: http://www.cancer.org/docroot/CRI/content/CRI_2_4_3X_How_is_prostate_cancer_diagnosed_36.asp?sitearea=. Accessed May 23, 2004.

Fleshner N, Klotz L. Role of "saturation biopsy" in the detection of prostate cancer among difficult diagnostic cases. *Urology.* July 2002;60(1):93-7.

Mallick S, Humbert M. Local anesthesia before transrectal ultrasound guided prostate biopsy: comparison of 2 methods in a prospective, randomized clinical trial. *J Urol.* February 2004;171(2 Pt 1):730-3.

Matlaga BR, Eskew LA, McCullough DL Prostate biopsy: indications and technique. *J Urol.* January 2003;169(1):12-9. Review.

Stewart CS, Leibovich BC, Weaver AL. Prostate cancer diagnosis using a saturation needle biopsy technique after previous negative sextant biopsies. *J Urol.* July 2001;166(1):86-91;discussion 91-2.

CHAPTER 8

American Cancer Society. Detailed guide: prostate cancer: can prostate cancer be found early? Available at: http://www.cancer.org/docroot/CRI/content/CRI_2_4_3X_Can_prostate_cancer_be_found_early_36.asp?sitearea=. Accessed January, 2004.

American Cancer Society. Imaging (radiology) tests. Available at: http://www.cancer.org/docroot/PED/content/PED_2_3X_Imaging_Radiology_Tests.asp?sitearea=PED. Accessed January 26, 2004.

National Kidney and Urologic Diseases Information Clearinghouse. National Institutes of Health. Medical Tests for Prostate Problems: Transrectal Ultrasound and Prostate Biopsy. Available at: kidney.niddk.nih.gov/kudiseases/ pubs/prostate/. Accessed February, 2004.

Schulam PG, Kawashima A, Sandler C, Barron BJ, Lamki LM, Goldman SM. Urinary tract imaging: Basic Principles. In: Walsh PC, Retik AB, Vaughan ED, Wein AJ, eds. *Campbell's Urology.* 8th ed. Philadelphia, PA: W.B. Saunders; 2002.

Terris MK. Ultrasonography and biopsy of the prostate. In: Walsh PC, Retik AB, Vaughan ED, Wein AJ, eds. *Campbell's Urology.* 8th ed. Philadelphia, PA: W.B. Saunders;2002.

CHAPTER 9

Allsbrook Jr. WC, Mangold KA, Johnson MH, et al. Interobserver reproducibility of Gleason grading of prostatic carcinoma: urologic pathologists. *Hum Pathol.* 2001;32: 74.

American Cancer Society. Testing biopsy and cytology specimens for cancer. Available at: http://www.cancer.org/docroot/PED/content/PED_2_3X_Testing_Biopsy_and_Cytology_Specimens_for_Cancer.asp?sitearea=PED. Accessed April, 2004.

Blute ML, Bostwick DG, Seay TM, et al. Pathologic classification of prostate carcinoma: the impact of margin status. *Cancer.* 1998;82: 902.

Bostwick DG. Gleason grading of prostatic needle biopsies. Correlation with grade in 316 matched prostatectomies. *Am J Surg Pathol.* 1994;18: 796.

Bostwick DG. Staging prostate cancer—1997: current methods and limitations. *Eur Urol.* 1997;32 Suppl 3: 2

Bostwick DG, Foster CS. Predictive factors in prostate cancer: current concepts from the 1999 College of American Pathologists Conference on Solid Tumor Prognostic Factors and the 1999 World Health Organization Second International Consultation on Prostate Cancer. *Semin Urol Oncol.* 1999;17: 222.

Bostwick DG, Grignon DJ, Hammond ME, et al. Prognostic factors in prostate cancer. *College of American Pathologists Consensus Statement 1999. Arch Pathol Lab Med.* 2000;124: 995.

Bostwick DG, Qian J, Schlesinger C. Contemporary pathology of prostate cancer. *Urol Clin North Am.* 2003;30: 181.

Cheng L, Darson MF, Bergstralh EJ, et al. Correlation of margin status and extraprostatic extension with progression of prostate carcinoma. *Cancer.* 1999;86: 1775.

Cheng L, Zincke H, Blute ML, et al. Risk of prostate carcinoma death in patients with lymph node metastasis. Cancer. 2001;91: 66.

Dundore PA, Cheville JC, Nascimento AG, et al. Carcinosarcoma of the prostate. Report of 21 cases. Cancer. 1995;76: 1035.

Egan AJ, Bostwick DG. Prediction of extraprostatic extension of prostate cancer based on needle biopsy findings: perineural invasion lacks significance on multivariate analysis. *Am J Surg Pathol.* 1997;21: 1496.

Epstein, JI. Diagnosis and reporting of limited adenocarcinoma of the prostate on needle biopsy. *Mod Pathol.* 2004

Greene DR, Taylor SR, Wheeler TM, et al. DNA ploidy by image analysis of individual foci of prostate cancer: a preliminary report. *Cancer Res.* 1991;51: 4084.

Grignon DJ, Bostwick DG, Civantos F, et al. Pathologic handling and reporting of prostate tissue specimens in patients receiving neoadjuvant hormonal therapy: report of the pathology committee. *Mol Urol.* 1999;3: 193.

Iczkowski KA, Cheng L, Qian J, et al. ASAP is a valid diagnosis. Atypical small acinar proliferation. *Hum Pathol.* 1999;30: 1403.

Jenkins RB, Qian J, Lieber MM, et al. Detection of c-myc oncogene amplification and chromosomal anomalies in metastatic prostatic carcinoma by fluorescence in situ hybridization. *Cancer Res.* 1997;57: 524.

Lau WK, Blute ML, Bostwick DG, et al. Prognostic factors for survival of patients with pathological Gleason score 7 prostate cancer: differences in outcome between primary Gleason grades 3 and 4. *J Urol.* 2001;166: 1692.

Leibovich BC, Cheng L, Weaver AL, et al. Outcome prediction with p53 immunostaining after radical prostatectomy in patients with locally advanced prostate cancer. *J Urol.* 2000;163: 1756.

Partin AW, Steinberg GD, Pitcock RV, et al. Use of nuclear morphometry, Gleason histologic scoring, clinical stage, and age to predict disease-free survival among patients with prostate cancer. *Cancer.* 1992;70: 161.

Powell IJ, Dey J, Dudley A, et al. Disease-free survival difference between African Americans and whites after radical prostatectomy for local prostate cancer: a multivariable analysis. *Urology.* 2002;59: 907.

Qian J, Hirasawa K, Bostwick DG, et al. Loss of p53 and c-myc overrepresentation in stage T(2-3) N(1-3) M(0) prostate cancer are potential markers for cancer progression. *Mod Pathol.* 2002;15: 35.

Qian J, Jenkins RB, Bostwick DG. Detection of chromosomal anomalies and c-myc gene amplification in the cribriform pattern of prostatic intraepithelial neoplasia and carcinoma by fluorescence in situ hybridization. *Mod Pathol.* 1997;10: 1113.

Qian J, Jenkins RB, Bostwick DG. Genetic and chromosomal alterations in prostatic intraepithelial neoplasia and carcinoma detected by fluorescence in situ hybridization. *Eur Urol.* 1999;35: 479.

Rasiah KK, Stricker PD, Haynes AM, et al. Prognostic significance of Gleason pattern in patients with Gleason score 7 prostate carcinoma. *Cancer.* 2003;98: 2560.

Saito S, Iwaki H. Mucin-producing carcinoma of the prostate: review of 88 cases. *Urology.* 1999;54: 141.

Sciarra A, Voria G, Monti S, et al. Clinical understaging in patients with prostate adenocarcinoma submitted to radical prostatectomy: predictive value of serum chromogranin A. *Prostate.* 2004;58: 421.

Srigley JR, Amin MB, Bostwick DG, et al. Updated protocol for the examination of specimens from patients with carcinomas of the prostate gland: a basis for checklists. Cancer Committee. *Arch Pathol Lab Med.* 2000;124: 1034.

Zhou M, Epstein JI. The reporting of prostate cancer on needle biopsy: prognostic and therapeutic implications and the utility of diagnostic markers. *Pathology.* 2003;35: 472.

CHAPTER 10

American Cancer Society. Detailed guide: prostate cancer: can prostate cancer be found early? Available at: http://www.cancer.org/docroot/CRI/content/CRI_2_4_3X_Can_prostate_cancer_be_found_early_36.asp?sitearea=. Accessed February 1, 2004.

Bostwick DG, Qian J, Frankel K. The incidence of high grade prostatic intraepithelial neoplasia in needle biopsies. *J Urol.* 1995 Nov;154(5):1791-4.

Cheville JC, Reznicek MJ, Bostwick DG. The focus of "atypical glands, suspicious for malignancy" in prostatic needle biopsy specimens: incidence, histologic features, and clinical follow-up of cases diagnosed in a community practice. *Am J Clin Pathol.* 1997;108:633-40.

Epstein JI. Atypical small acinar proliferation of the prostate gland. *Am J Surg Pathol.* November 1998;22(11):1430-1431.

Goldstein NS, Begin LR, Grody WW, Novak JM, Qian J, Bostwick DG. Minimal or no cancer in radical prostatectomy specimens. Report of 13 cases of the "vanishing cancer phenomenon". *Am J Surg Pathol.* September 1995;19(9):1002-9.

Iczkowski KA, Bassler TJ, Schwob VS, et al. Diagnosis of "suspicious for malignancy" in prostate biopsies: predictive value for cancer. *Urology*. May 1998;51(5):749-757;discussion 757-748.

Iczkowski KA, MacLennan GT, Bostwick DG. Atypical small acinar proliferation suspicious for malignancy in prostate needle biopsies: clinical significance in 33 cases. *Am J Surg Pathol*. 1997;21:1489-95.

Park S, Shinohara K, Grossfeld GD, et al. Prostate cancer detection in men with prior high grade prostatic intraepithelial neoplasia or atypical prostate biopsy. *J Urol*. 2001;165:1409-14.

CHAPTER 11

American Cancer Society. Depression. Available at: http://www.cancer.org/docroot/MBC/content/MBC _2_3X_Depression.asp?sitearea=MBC. Accessed May 2004.

Eton DT, Lepore SJ. Prostate cancer and health-related quality of life: A review of the literature. *Psycho-oncology*. 2002;11: 307-326.

Gray RE, Fitch M, Phillips C, Labrecque M, Fergus, K. To tell or not to tell: Patterns of disclosure among men with prostate cancer. *Psycho-oncology*. 2000;9: 273-282.

Klotz L. PSAdynia and PSA-related syndromes: A new epidemic. A case history and taxonomy. *Urology*. 1997;50: 831-832.

Kneier A, Rosenbaum E. "Coping: Ten steps toward emotional well-being when dealing with cancer." *Supportive Cancer Care*. Sourcebooks Trade. Naperville, IL: 2001.

Kornblith AB, Herr HW, Ofman US, Scher HI, Holland JC. Quality of life of patients with prostate cancer and their spouses: the value of a database in clinical care. *Cancer*. 1994;73:2791-2802.

Litwin MS, Flanders SC, Pasta DJ, Stoddard ML, Lubeck DP, Henning JM. Sexual function and bother after radical prostatectomy or radiation for prostate cancer: Multivariate quality-of-life analysis from CaPSURE. Cancer of the Prostate Strategic Urologic Research Endeavor. *Urology*. 1999;54, 503-508.

Roth AJ. The psychology of prostate cancer: In-depth report. Johns Hopkins White Paper Bulletins: Prostate Bulletin. Winter. 2004. 16-23.

Roth AJ, Kornblith AB, Batel-Copel L, Peabody E, Scher HI, Holland JC. Rapid screening for psychologic distress in men with prostate cancer. A pilot study. *Cancer*. 1998;82, 1904-1908.

Roth AJ, Passik S. Anxiety in men with prostate cancer may interfere with effective management of the disease. *Primary Care and Cancer*. 1996;16, 30.

Roth AJ, Rosenfeld B, Kornblith AB, et al. The Memorial Anxiety Scale for Prostate Cancer. Validation of a new scale to measure anxiety in men with prostate cancer. *Cancer*. 2003;97, 2910-2918.

Roth AJ, Scher H. Brief report: Sertraline relieves hot flashes secondary to medical castration as a treatment of advanced prostate cancer. *Psycho-oncology*. 1998;7, 129-132.

CHAPTER 12

American Cancer Society. *A Breast Cancer Journey: Your Personal Guidebook*. 2nd ed. Atlanta, GA: American Cancer Society; 2004.

American Hospital Association. *Patient Care Partnership: Understanding Expectations, Rights and Responsibilities*. Available at: http://www.hospitalconnect.com/aha/ ptcommunication/partnership/index.html. Accessed May 25, 2004.

CHAPTER 13

American Cancer Society. *A Breast Cancer Journey: Your Personal Guidebook*. 2nd ed. Atlanta, GA: American Cancer Society; 2004.

Laken V, Laken K. *Making Love Again*. East Sandwich, MA: Ant Hill Press; 2002.

Talcott JA. Quality of life in early prostate cancer. Do we know enough to treat? *Hematol Oncol Clin North Am*. 1996;10:691-701.

Talcott JA, Manola J, Clark JA, Kaplan I, Beard CJ, Mitchell SP, et al. Time course and predictors of symptoms after primary prostate cancer therapy. *J Clin Oncol*. 2003;21:3979-86.

CHAPTER 14

American Cancer Society. *A Breast Cancer Journey: Your Personal Guidebook*. 2nd ed. Atlanta, GA: American Cancer Society; 2004.

Centers for Medicare and Medicaid. Medicaid: A brief summary. Available at: http://cms.hhs.gov/ pf/printpage.asp?ref=http://63.241.27.78/ publications/overview-medicare-medicaid/ default4.asp? Accessed November 19, 2003.

Centers for Medicare and Medicaid. Medicare eligibility tool. Available at: http://www.medicare.gov/ home.asp?dest=NAV%7Chome%7CgeneralEnroll ment&version=defautlt&browser=IE%7C5%2E01 %7Cwin2000&language=Englis. Accessed November 19, 2003.

COBRA Insurance.com. What is COBRA insurance? Available at: http://www.cobrainsurance.com/ COBRA_Law.htm. Accessed November 19, 2003.

Cost Containment Research Institute. Free and low cost medical care. Available at: http://www.institutedc.org/medical.htm. November 19, 2003.

My Lawyer.com. Minding the gap in Medicare coverage. Available at: http://www.lawsguide.com/mylawyer/guideview.asp?layer=3&article=285. Accessed November 19, 2003.

US Department of Justice. American with Disabilities Act: questions and answers. Available at: http://www.usdoj.gov/crt/ada/q%26aeng02.htm. Accessed April 5, 2004.

US Department of Veterans. Enrollment in VA's health care system. Available at: http://www.appc1.va.gov/elig/page.cfm. Accessed November 19, 2003.

CHAPTER 15

American Cancer Society. Detailed guide: prostate cancer: how is prostate cancer staged? Available at: http://www.cancer.org/docroot/CRI/content/CRI_2_4_3X_How_is_prostate_cancer_staged_36.asp?sitearea=. Accessed January 8, 2004.

Flanigan RC, McKay TC, Olson M, Shankey TV, Pyle J, Waters WB. Limited efficacy of preoperative computed tomographic scanning for the evaluation of lymph node metastasis in patients before radical prostatectomy. *Urology*. September 1996;48(3):428-32.

Goossen TE, de la Rosette JJ, Hulsbergen-van de Kaa CA, van Leenders GJ, Wijkstra H. The value of dynamic contrast enhanced power Doppler ultrasound imaging in the localization of prostate cancer. *Eur Urol*. February 2003;43(2):124-31.

Greene FL, Page DL, Fleming ID, et al, eds. *AJCC Cancer Staging Manual*. 6th ed. New York, NY: Springer Verlag; 2002:340-341.

Grossfeld GD, Latini DM, Lubeck DP, et al. Predicting disease recurrence in intermediate and high-risk patients undergoing radical prostatectomy using percent positive biopsies: results from CaPSURE. *Urology*. April 2002;59(4):560-5.

Ismail M, Gomella LG. Ultrasound for prostate imaging and biopsy. *Curr Opin Urol*. September 2001;11(5):471-7.

Kane CJ, Amling CL, Johnstone PA, et al. Limited value of bone scintigraphy and computed tomography in assessing biochemical failure after radical prostatectomy. *Urology*. March 2003;61(3):607-11.

Sodee DB, Malguria N, Faulhaber P, Resnick MI, Albert J, Bakale G. Multicenter ProstaScint imaging findings in 2154 patients with prostate cancer. The ProstaScint Imaging Centers. *Urology*. December 20, 2000;56(6):988-93.

Wefer A, Hricak H. The prostate: Imaging and staging of prostate cancer. In: Kantoff PW, Carroll P, D'Amico A, eds. *Prostate Cancer*. Philadelphia, PA: Lippincott Williams & Wilkins; 2001 (296-).

CHAPTER 16

Cagiannos I, Karakiewicz P, Eastham JA, et al. A preoperative nomogram identifying decreased risk of positive pelvic lymph nodes in patients with prostate cancer. *J Urol*. November 2003;170(5):1798-1803.

Meng MV, Carroll PR. When is pelvic lymph node dissection necessary before radical prostatectomy? A decision analysis. *J Urol*. October 2000;164(4):1235-40.

Wolf JS Jr, Cher M, Dall'era M, Presti JC Jr, Hricak H, Carroll PR. The use and accuracy of cross-sectional imaging and fine needle aspiration cytology for detection of pelvic lymph node metastases before radical prostatectomy. *J Urol*. March 1995;153(3 Pt 2):993-9.

CHAPTER 17

American Cancer Society. Detailed guide: prostate cancer. Available at: http://www.cancer.org/docroot/CRI/CRI_2_3x.asp?rnav=cridg&dt=36. Accessed February, 2004.

Bostwick DG, Burke HB, Wheeler TM, et al. The most promising surrogate endpoint biomarkers for screening candidate chemopreventive compounds for prostatic adenocarcinoma in short-term phase II clinical trials. *J Cell Biochem*. 1994;19S:283-89.

Bostwick DG, Burke HB. Prediction of individual patient outcome in cancer: Comparison of artificial neural networks and Kaplan-Meier methods. *Cancer*. 2001;91:1643-46.

Bosze P, Bast RC, Berchuck A, et al. Consensus statements on prognostic factors in epithelial ovarian carcinoma. *Eur J Gynaec Oncol*. 2000;21:513-526.

Burke HB. Applying artificial neural networks to clinical medicine. *J Clin Ligand*. 1998;21:200-201.

Burke HB. Discovering clinically significant patterns in microarray generated data. *Mol Diagnosis*. 2000;5:349-357.

Burke HB. Increasing the power of surrogate endpoint biomarkers: the aggregation of predictive factors. *J Cell Biochem*. 1994;19S:278-82.

Burke HB. Integrating multiple clinical tests to increase predictive accuracy. In: Hanausek M, Walaszek Z, eds. *Methods in Molecular Biology*. Vol 20: Tumor Marker Protocols. Totowa, NJ: Humana Press Inc. 1998: 3-10.

Burke HB. Proteomics: Analysis of spectral data. *Applied Proteomics*. 2004. In press.

Burke HB, Goodman PH, Rosen DB, et al. Artificial neural networks improve the accuracy of cancer survival prediction. Cancer. 1997;79:857-62.

Burke HB, Henson DE. Evaluating prognostic factors. *CME J Gyn Onc*. 1999;4:244-252.

Burke HB, Henson DE. Specimen banks for prognostic factor research. *Arch Pathol Lab Med*. 1998;122:871-874.

Burke HB, Hoang A, Iglehart JD, Marks JR. Predicting response to adjuvant and radiation therapy in early stage breast cancer. *Cancer*. 1998;82:874-7.

Burke HB, Henson DE. Histologic grade as a prognostic factor in breast carcinoma. *Cancer*. 1997;80:1703-1705.

Lundin M, Lundin J, Burke HB, Toikkanen S, Pylkkanen L, Joensuu H. Artificial neural networks applied to survival prediction in breast cancer. *Oncology*. 1999;57:281-286.

CHAPTER 18

American Cancer Society and National Comprehensive Cancer Network. *Prostate Cancer Treatment Guidelines for Patients, Version IV/August 2004*. Atlanta, GA: 2004.

CHAPTER 19

American Cancer Society. *A Breast Cancer Journey: Your Personal Guidebook*. 2nd ed. Atlanta, GA: American Cancer Society; 2004.

American Cancer Society. *American Cancer Society's Guide to Pain Control: Understanding and Managing Cancer Pain*. Rev ed.. Atlanta, GA: American Cancer Society; 2004.

American Urological Association. *A Patient's Guide: The Management of Localized Prostate Cancer*. Prostate Cancer Clinical Guidelines Panel. 1995. Available at: http://www.auanet.org/timssnet/products/guidelines/patient_guides/ProstCaptguide.pdf.

Marks, Sheldon. *Prostate and Cancer: A Family Guide to Diagnosis, Treatment and Survival*. Boulder, CO: Perseus Publishing; 2003.

Walsh PC, Worthington JF. *Dr. Patrick Walsh's Guide to Surviving Prostate Cancer*. New York, NY: Warner Books; 2001.

CHAPTER 20

American Cancer Society. Detailed Guide: prostate cancer. Risks and Side Effects of Treatments. Available at: http://www.cancer.org/docroot/CRI/content/CRI_2_4_4X_Risks_and_Side_Effects_36.asp?sitearea=. Accessed May 24, 2004.

American Cancer Society. Experiencing incontinence? Available at: http://www.cancer.org/docroot/M2M/content/M2M_2_7_1x_Experiencing_Incontinence_15.asp?sitearea=. Accessed May 18, 2004.

American Cancer Society. Nerve grafting restores erectile function after prostatectomy. ACS News Center. March 22, 2001. Available at: http://www.cancer.org/docroot/NWS/content/NWS_1_1x_Nerve_Grafting_Restores_Erectile_Function_After_Prostatectomy.asp.

Bishoff JT, Motley G, Optenberg SA, et al. Incidence of fecal and urinary incontinence following radical perineal and retropubic prostatectomy in a national population. *J Urol*. 1998;160(2):454-8.

Boccon-Gibod L, Ravery V, Vordos D, Toublanc M, Delmas V, Boccon-Gibod L. Radical prostatectomy for prostate cancer: the perineal approach increases the risk of surgically induced positive margins and capsular incisions. *J Urol*. 1998;160(4):1383-5.

Boxer RT, Kaufman JJ, Goodwin WE. Radical prostatectomy for carcinoma of the prostate: 1971-1976: A review of 329 patients. *J Urol*. 1977;117:208-213.

Brady Urological Institute. Patient information: laparoscopic prostatectomy. Johns Hopkins Medical Institutions. Accessed June 9, 2004. Available at: http://urology.jhu.edu/MIS/LRP.html#button7.

Dahm P, Silverstein AD, Weizer AZ, et al. A longitudinal assessment of bowel related symptoms and fecal incontinence following radical perineal prostatectomy. *J Urol*. June 2003;169(6):2220-4.

Frazier HA, Roberston JE, Paulsen DF. Radical prostatectomy: The pros and cons of the perineal versus the retropubic approach. *J Urol*. 1992;147:888-890.

Guillonneau B, Krongrad A, Vallancien G. Laparoscopic radical prostatectomy: a technical manual. Private publication. 2000. Available at: http://www.krongrad-urology.com.

Haab F, Boccon-Gibbod L, Delmas V, Boccon-Gibod L, Toublanc M. Perineal versus retropubic radical prostatectomy for T1, T2 prostate cancer. *Br J Urol* .1994;74(5):626-9.

Holzbeierlein J, Hanson G, Mayo M, et al. Bowel dysfunction in patients undergoing radical prostatectomy: Results from the CaPSURE database. Unpublished data presented in part at the South Central Section of the American Urological Association, Boston MA 2003.

Hu JC, Elkin EP, Pasta DJ, Lubeck DP, Kattan MW, Carroll PR. Predicting quality of life after radical prostatectomy: Results from CAPSURE. *J Urol.* February 2004;171(2 pt 1):703-7.

Krongrad A. Laparoscopic radical prostatectomy. *Curr Urol Rep.* 2003;1:37-41.

Lance RS, Freidrichs PA, Kane C, et al. A comparison of radical retropubic with perineal prostatectomy for localized prostate cancer within the Uniformed Services Urology Research Group. *BJU Int.* 2001; 87(1):61-5.

Lepor H, Nieder AM, Ferrandino MN. Intraoperative and postoperative complications of radical retropubic prostatectomy in a consecutive series of 1,000 cases. *J Urol.* November 2001;166(5):1729-33.

Partin AW, Kattan MW, Subong EN, et al. Combination of prostate-specific antigen, clinical stage, and Gleason score to predict pathological stage of localized prostate cancer. A multi-institutional update. *JAMA* May 1997;277(18):1445-51.

Paulsen DF: Impact of radical prostatectomy in the management of clinically localized disease. *J Urol.* 1994;152:1826-1830.

Pound CR, Partin AW, Eisenberger MA, Chan DW, Pearson JD, Walsh PC. Natural history of progression after PSA elevation following radical prostatectomy. *JAMA* May 1999;281(17):1591-7.

Walsh PC, Lepor H, Eggleston JD. Radical prostatectomy with preservation of sexual function: Anatomical and pathological considerations. *Prostate.* 1983;4:473.

Weldon VE, Tavel FR. Potency sparing radical perineal prostatectomy: Anatomy, surgical technique, and initial results. *J Urol.* 1988;140:559-562.

Weyrauch HM. *Surgery of the Prostate.* Philadelphia: WB Saunders Co.; 1959, pp 172-230.

CHAPTER 21

American Cancer Society. Detailed guide: prostate cancer. Available at: http://www.cancer.org/docroot/CRI/CRI_2_3x.asp?rnav=cridg&dt=36. Accessed February 12, 2004.

Blander DS, Sanchez-Ortiz RF, Broderick GA. Sex Inventories: can questionnaires replace erectile dysfunction testing? *Urology.* 1999;54:719-723.

Curie M. *Radioactive Substances.* A translation from the French of the classical thesis presented to the Faculty of Sciences in Paris. New York: Philosophical Library; 1961.

Dearnaley DP, Khoo VS, Norman AR, et al. Comparison of radiation side-effects of conformal and conventional radiotherapy in prostate cancer: A randomised trial. *Lancet.* 1999;353:267-272.

Dosoretz AM, Stock RG, Cesaretti JA, Stone NN. Role of external beam radiation and hormonal therapy in low, intermediate and high risk patients treated with permanent radioactive seed implantation. *Int J Radiat Oncol Biol Phys.* 2003;54:20.

Gleason DF, Mellinger GT. Prediction of prognosis for prostatic adenocarcinoma by combined histological grading and clinical staging. *J Urol.* 1974;111:58.

Grimm PD, Blasko JC, Sylvester JE, Meier RM, Cavanagh W. 10-year biochemical (prostate-specific antigen) control of prostate cancer with 125I brachytherapy. *Int J Radiat Oncol Biol Phys.* 2001;51: 31-40.

Hanks GE, Hanlon AL, Schultheiss TE, et al. Dose escalation with 3D conformal treatment: five year outcomes, treatment optimization, and future directions. *Int J Radiat Oncol Biol Phys.* 1998;41:501-510.

Holm, HH, Juul N, Pederson JF, et al. Transperineal I-125 seed implantation in prostatic cancer guided by transrectal ultrasonography. *J Urol.* 1983;130:283-286.

Hu K, Wallner KE. Urinary incontinence in patients who have a TURP/TUIP following prostate brachytherapy. *Int J Radiat Oncol Biol Phys.* 1998;4:783-786.

Incrocci L, Slob AK, Levendag, PC. Sexual (dys)function after radiotherapy for prostate cancer: a review. *Int J Radiat Oncol Biol Phys.* 2002;52:681-693.

Janeway HH, Barringer BS, Failla G. *Radium Therapy in Cancer at the Memorial Hospital.* New York: Paul Hoeber; 1917.

Koper PC, Stroom JC, van Putten WL, et al. Acute morbidity reduction using 3DCRT for prostate carcinoma: A randomized study. *Int J Radiat Oncol Biol Phys.* 1999;43:727-734.

Kupelian PA, Potters L, Khuntia D, et al. Radical prostatectomy, external beam radiotherapy < 72 Gy, external beam radiotherapy > 72 Gy, permanent seed implantation, or combined seeds/external beam radiotherapy for stage T1-T2 prostate cancer. *Int J Radiat Oncol Biol Phys.* 2004;58(1):25-33.

Lattanzi J, McNeeley S, Pinover W, et al. A comparison of daily CT localization to a daily ultrasound-based system in prostate cancer. *Int J Radiat Oncol Biol Phys.* 1999;43:719-725.

Lawton CA, Won M, Pilepich MV, et al. Long-term treatment sequelae following external beam irradiation for adenocarcinoma of the prostate: analysis of RTOG studies 7506 and 7706. *Int J Radiat Oncol Biol Phys.* 1991;21:935-939.

Litwin MS, Hays RD, Fink A, et al. Quality-of-life outcomes in men treated for localized prostate cancer. *JAMA*. 1995;273:129-135.

Madalinska JB, Essink-Bot ML, de Koning HJ, et al. Health-related quality-of-life effects of radical prostatectomy and primary radiotherapy for screen-detected or clinically diagnosed localized prostate cancer. *J Clin Oncol*. March 15, 2001;19(6):1619-28.

Mate T, Kovacs G, Martinez A. High-rate brachytherapy of the prostate. In: Nag S, ed. *High Dose Rate Brachytherapy: A Textbook*. Armont: Futura; 1994: 55-371.

Merrick GS, Butler WM, Dorsey AT, Galbreath RW, Blatt H, Lief JH. Rectal function following prostate brachytherapy. *Int J Radiat Oncol Biol Phys*. 2000;48:667-674.

Merrick GS, Butler WM, Lief JH, Dorsey AT. Temporal resolution of urinary morbidity following prostate brachytherapy. *Int J Radiat Oncol Biol Phys*. 2000;47:121-128.

Merrick GS, Butler WM, Lief JH, et al. Efficacy of sildenafil citrate in prostate brachytherapy patients with erectile dysfunction. *Urology*. 1999;53:1112-1116.

Merrick GS, Butler WM, Wallner KE, et al. Prostate specific antigen spikes after permanent prostate brachytherapy. *Int J Radiat Oncol Biol Phys*. 2002;54:450-456.

Merrick GS, Wallner KE, Butler WM. Management of sexual dysfunction after prostate brachytherapy. *Oncology* (Huntingt). 2003;17:52-62.

Michalski, J, Mutic S, Eichling J, Ahmed, N. Radiation exposure to family and household members prostate brachytherapy. *Int J Radiat Oncol Biol Phys*. 2003;56:764-768.

Michalski JM, Winter K, Purdy JA, et al. Preliminary evaluation of low-grade toxicity with conformal radiation therapy for prostate cancer on RTOG 9406 dose levels I and II. *Int J Radiat Oncol Biol Phys*. May 1, 2003;56(1):192-8.

Moran B, Gurel, M, Visockis J, Geary P. Post-operative pain and prostate brachytherapy. *Int J Radiat Oncol Biol Phys*. 2003;54: 2(0).

Moran B, Stutz M, Gurel M. Is previous transurethral resection of the prostate a contraindication to prostate brachytherapy? *Int J Radiat Oncol Biol Phys*. 2003 (Article in Press).

Moran BJ, Friedman JL, Grimm PD. Preplanned brachytherapy for prostate cancer. *New Developments in Prostate Cancer Treatment*. Oncology Roundtable interviews. 1999: 17-20.

Moran BJ, Janson K, Raslowsky MP. The role of TURP/TUIP for chronic urinary obstruction after 125I/103Pd prostate brachytherapy. *RSNA 2000*. Supplement.

Nag S. Brachytherapy for prostate cancer : Summary of American Brachytherapy Society recommendations. *Semin Urol Oncol*. 2000;18:133-136.

Nag S, Beyer D, Friedland J, Grimm P, Nath R. ABS recommendations for transperineal permanent brachytherapy of prostate cancer. *Int J Radiat Oncol Biol Phys*. 1999;44:789-799.

Patel, RR, Orton, N, Tome, WA, et al. Rectal dose sparing with a balloon catheter and ultrasound localization in conformal radiation therapy for prostate cancer. *Radiother Oncol*. June 2003;67(3):285-94.

Pollack A, Zagars GK, Smith LG, et al. Preliminary results of a randomized radiotherapy dose-escalation study comparing 70 Gy with 78 Gy for prostate cancer. *J Clin Oncol*. 2000;18:3904-3911.

Potters L, Torre T, Feam PA, et al. Potency after permanent prostate brachytherapy for localized prostate cancer. *Int J Radiat Oncol Biol Phys*. 2001;50: 1235-1242.

Shanahan TG, Nanavati PJ, Mueller PW, Maxey RB. A comparison of permanent prostate brachytherapy techniques: preplan vs. hybrid interactive planning with postimplant analysis. *Int J Radiat Oncol Biol Phys*. 2002;53:490-496.

Stokes SH. Comparison of biochemical disease-free survival of patients with localized carcinoma of the prostate undergoing radical prostatectomy, transperineal ultrasound-guided radioactive seed implantation, or definitive external beam irradiation. *Int J Radiat Oncol Biol Phys*. 2000;47: 129-136.

Stutz MA, Gurel MH, Moran BJ. Potency preservation after prostate brachytherapy. *Int J Radiat Oncol Biol Phys*. 2003;54:2(0).

Tapen E, Blasko J, Grimm P, et al. Reduction of radioactive seed embolization to the lung following prostate brachytherapy. *Int J Radiat Oncol Biol Phys*. 1998;42:1063-1067.

Teh BS, Mai WY, Uhl BM, et al. Intensity-modulated radiation therapy (IMRT) for prostate cancer with the use of a rectal balloon for prostate immobilization: acute toxicity and dose-volume analysis. *Int J Radiat Oncol Biol Phys*. 2001;49:705-712.

Wallner K, Lee H, Wasserman S, Dattoli M. Low risk of urinary incontinence following prostate brachytherapy in patients with a prior transurethral prostate resection. *Int J Radiat Oncol Biol Phys*. 1997;37:565-569.

Whitmore WF Jr, Hilaris BS, Grabstald H. Retropubic implantation of Iodine-125 in the treatment of prostatic cancer. *J Urol*. 1972;108: 9180-9200.

Zelefsky MJ, Fuks Z, Hunt M, et al. High dose radiation delivered by intensity modulated conformal radiotherapy improves the outcome of localized prostate cancer. *J Urol.* 2001;166:876-881.

Zelefsky MJ, Ginor RX, Fuks Z, Leibel SA. Efficacy of selective alpha-1 blocker therapy in the treatment of acute urinary symptoms during radiotherapy for localized prostate cancer. *Int J Radiat Oncol Biol Phys.* 1999;45:567-570.

Zelefsky MJ, Leibel SA, Kutcher GJ, et al. The feasibility of dose escalation with three-dimensional conformal radiotherapy in patients with prostatic carcinoma. *Cancer J Sci Am.* 1995;1:42-50.

Zelefsky MJ, McKee AB, Lee H, Leibel SA. Efficacy of oral sildenafil in patients with erectile dysfunction after radiotherapy for carcinoma of the prostate. *Urology.* 1999;53:775-778.

CHAPTER 22

American Cancer Society. Detailed guide: prostate cancer. Available at: http://www.cancer.org/docroot/CRI/CRI_2_3x.asp?rnav=cridg&dt=36. Accessed March, 2004.

American Cancer Society. Do I have testicular cancer? Available at: http://www.cancer.org/docroot/PED/content/PED_2_3X_Do_I_Have_Testicular_Cancer.asp?sitearea=PED. Accessed October, 2003.

American Cancer Society. Sexuality for men and their partners. Available at: http://www.cancer.org/docroot/MIT/MIT_7_1x_SexualityforMenand TheirPartners.asp?sitearea=&level=. Accessed October, 2003.

Barqawi AB, Moul JW, Ziada A, Handel L, Crawford ED. Combination of low-dose flutamide and finasteride for PSA-only recurrent prostate cancer after primary therapy. *Urology.* November 2003;62(5):872-6.

Koff SG, Connelly RR, Bauer JJ, McLeod DG, Moul JW. Primary hormonal therapy for prostate cancer: experience with 135 consecutive PSA-ERA patients from a tertiary care military medical center. *Prostate Cancer Prostatic Dis.* 2002;5(2):152-8.

Moul JW. Contemporary hormonal management of advanced prostate cancer. *Oncology.* 1998 April;12(4):499-505.

Moul JW, Civitelli K. Managing advanced prostate cancer with Viadur (leuprolide acetate implant). *Urol Nurs.* December 2001;21(6):385-8, 393-4.

Moul JW, Fowler JE Jr. Evolution of therapeutic approaches with luteinizing hormone-releasing hormone agonists in 2003. *Urology.* December 2003;22;62 (6 Suppl 1):20-8.

Moul JW, Wu H, Sun L, et al. Early versus delayed hormonal therapy for prostate specific antigen only recurrence of prostate cancer after radical prostatectomy. *J Urol.* March 2004;171(3):1141-7.

Schroder FH. Hormonal therapy of prostate cancer. In: Walsh PC, Retik AB, Vaughan ED, Wein AJ, eds. *Campbell's Urology.* 8th ed. Philadelphia, PA: W.B. Saunders; 2002:3182-3208.

CHAPTER 23

American Cancer Society. Detailed guide: prostate cancer. Available at: http://www.cancer.org/docroot/CRI/CRI_2_3x.asp?rnav=cridg&dt=36. Accessed January 21, 2004.

Carter CA, Donahue T, Sun L, et al. Temporarily deferred therapy (watchful waiting) for men younger than 70 years and with low-risk localized prostate cancer in the prostate-specific antigen era. *J Clin Oncol.* November 2003;1;21(21):4001-8.

Holmberg L, Bill-Axelson A, Helgesen F, et al. Scandinavian Prostatic Cancer Group Study Number 4. A randomized trial comparing radical prostatectomy with watchful waiting in early prostate cancer. *N Engl J Med.* September 2002;12;347(11):781-9.

Kattan MW, Eastham JA, Wheeler TM, et al. Counseling men with prostate cancer: a nomogram for predicting the presence of small, moderately differentiated, confined tumors. *J Urol.* November 2003;170(5):1792-7.

Steineck G, Helgesen F, Adolfsson J, et al. Scandinavian Prostatic Cancer Group Study Number 4. Quality of life after radical prostatectomy or watchful waiting. *N Engl J Med.* September 2002;12;347(11):790-6.

CHAPTER 24

American Cancer Society. Detailed guide: prostate cancer. Available at: http://www.cancer.org/docroot/CRI/CRI_2_3x.asp?rnav=cridg&dt=36. Accessed March, 2004.

American Urological Association. Cryoablation for prostate cancer. Available at: http://www.urology-health.org/search/index.cfm?topic=42&search=cryotherapy&searchtype=and. Accessed March, 2004.

Anscher MS, Samulski TV, Dodge R, Prosnitz LR, Dewhirst MW. Combined external beam irradiation and external regional hyperthermia for locally advanced adenocarcinoma of the prostate. *Int J Radiat Oncol Biol Phys.* 1997;37(5):1059-65.

Bahn DK, Lee F, Badalament R, Kumar A, Greski J, Chernick M. Targeted cryoablation of the prostate: 7-year outcomes in the primary treatment of prostate cancer. *Urology.* 2002;60(Supp 2A):3-11.

Deger S, Boehmer D, Turk I, Roigas J, Budach V, Loening SA. Interstitial hyperthermia using self-regulating thermoseeds combined with conformal radiation therapy. *European Urology*. 2002;42(2):147-53.

Donnelly BJ, Saliken JC, Ernst DS, et al. Prospective trial of cryosurgical ablation of the prostate: five-year results. *Urology*. October 2002;60(4):645-9.

Ellis DS. Cryosurgery as primary treatment of localized prostate cancer: a community hospital experience. *Urology*. August 2002;60(2 Suppl 1):34-9.

Food and Drug Administration. FDA approves new indication for taxotere—prostate cancer. FDA News. May 19, 2004. Available at: http://www.fda.gov/bbs/topics/news/2004/NEW0 1068.html.

Hoffmann NE, Bischof JC. The cryobiology of cryosurgical injury. *Urology*. August 2002;60(2 Suppl 1):40-9.

Hurwitz MD, Kaplan ID, Svensson GK, Hynynen K, Hansen MS. Feasibility and patient tolerance of a novel transrectal ultrasound hyperthermia system for treatment of prostate cancer. *Int J Hyperthermia*. 2001;17(1):31-7.

Katz AE. Selection of salvage cryotherapy patients. *Rev Urol*. 2002;(suppl 2):S18-S23.

Kong G, Anyarambhatla G, Petros WP, et al. Efficacy of liposomes and hyperthermia in a human tumor xenograft model: importance of triggered drug release. *Cancer Res*. 2000;60(24):6950-7.

Petrylak, DP. Chemotherapy for androgen-independent prostate cancer. *Semin Urol Oncol*. August 2002;20(3 Suppl 1):31-5.

Ryu S, Brown SL, Kim SH, Khil MS, Kim JH. Preferential radiosensitization of human prostatic carcinoma cells by mild hyperthermia. *Int J Radiat Oncol Biol Phys*. 1996;34(1):133-8.

van der Zee J, Gonzalez Gonzalez D, van Rhoon GC, van Dijk JD, van Putten WL, Hart AA. Comparison of radiotherapy alone with radiotherapy plus hyperthermia in locally advanced pelvic tumours: a prospective, randomised, multicentre trial. Dutch Deep Hyperthermia Group. *Lancet*. 2000;355(9210):1119-25.

van Vulpen M, De Leeuw AA, Van De Kamer JB, et al. Comparison of intra-luminal versus intra-tumoural temperature measurements in patients with locally advanced prostate cancer treated with the coaxial TEM system: Report of a feasibility study. *Int J Hyperthermia*. 2003;19(5):481-97.

van Vulpen M, Raaymakers BW, Lagendijk JJ, et al. Three-dimensional controlled interstitial hyper-thermia combined with radiotherapy for locally advanced prostate carcinoma—a feasibility study. *Int J Radiat Oncol Biol Phys*. 2002;53(1):116-26.

Yagoda A, Petrylak D. Cytotoxic chemotherapy for advanced hormone-resistant prostate cancer. *Cancer*. February 1 1993;71(3):1098-109. Review.

CHAPTER 25

American Cancer Society. Detailed guide: prostate cancer. Available at: http://www.cancer.org/docroot/CRI/CRI_2_3x.asp?rnav=cridg&dt=36. Accessed March, 2004.

Chaussy C, Thüroff S. The status of high-intensity focused ultrasound in the treatment of localized prostate cancer and the impact of a combined resection. Curr Urol Rep. 2003 Jun;4(3):248-52.

Gelet A, Chapelon JY, Bouvier R, Rouviere O, Lyonnet D, Dubernard JM. Transrectal high intensity focused ultrasound for the treatment of localized prostate cancer: factors influencing the outcome. Eur Urol. 2001 Aug;40(2):124-9.

Gelet A, Chapelon JY, Poissonnier L, Bouvier R, Rouviere O, Bah-clozel I, Lyonnet D, Dubernard JM. Prostate Cancer Control with Transrectal HIFU in 245 Consecutive Patients. World Congress of Endourology, Montréal. 2003.

Thuroff S, Chaussy C, Vallancien G, Wieland W, Kiel HJ, Le Duc A, Desgrandchamps F, De La Rosette JJ, Gelet A. High-intensity focused ultrasound and localized prostate cancer: efficacy results from the European multicentric study. *J Endourol*. 2003 Oct;17(8):673-7.

CHAPTER 26

American Cancer Society. *A Breast Cancer Journey: Your Personal Guidebook*. 2nd ed. Atlanta, GA: American Cancer Society; 2004.

American Cancer Society. Clinical trials: what you need to know. Available at: http://www.cancer.org/docroot/ETO/content/ETO_6_3_Clinical_Trials_-_Patient_Participation.asp. Accessed January 22, 2004.

Bennett C, Adams J, Knox K, et al. Clinical trials: Are they a good buy? J Clin Oncol. 2001;19:4330-4339.

ECRI: *Should I Enter a Clinical Trial? A Patient Reference Guide for Adults with a Serious or Life-Threatening Illness*. ECRI;February 2002. Available at: http://www.ecri.org/Patient_Information/Patient_Reference_Guide/Patient_Reference_Guide_Detail.aspx?File=Clinical%20Trial.htm. Accessed April 6, 2004.

Getz K, Borfitz D. *Informed Consent: The Consumer's Guide to the Risks and Benefits of Volunteering for Clinical Trials*. Boston, MA: CenterWatch; 2002.

National Cancer Institute. *Cancer Clinical Trials: The Basic Workbook*. National Cancer Institute; October 2001. NIH Publication No. 02-5050. Available at: http://www.cancer.gov/clinicaltrials/resources/basicworkbook. Accessed April 6, 2004.

Pharmaceutical Research and Manufacturers of America. New medicines in development for cancer, 2004. Available at: http://www.phrma.org/newmedicines/newmedsdb/drugs.cfm. Accessed April 6, 2004.

CHAPTER 27

Agency for Healthcare Research and Quality. *Garlic: Effects on Cardiovascular Risks and Disease, Protective Effects Against Cancer, and Clinical Adverse Effects.* Summary, Evidence Report/Technology Assessment: Number 20. AHRQ Publication No. 01-E022, October 2000. Agency for Healthcare Research and Quality, Rockville, MD. Available at: http://www.ahrq.gov/clinic/epcsums/garlicsum.htm.

American Cancer Society. DHEA. Available at: http://www.cancer.org/docroot/ETO/content/ETO_5_3X_Dhea.asp?sitearea=ETO . Accessed May 20, 2004.

American Cancer Society. *Eating Well, Staying Well During and After Cancer*. Atlanta, GA: American Cancer Society; 2003.

American Cancer Society. Flaxseed and low-fat diet may prevent prostate cancer. ACS News Center. August 20, 2001. Available at: http://www.cancer.org/docroot/NWS/content/NWS_2_1x_Flaxseed_and_Low-Fat_Diet_May_Prevent_Prostate_Cancer.asp.

American Cancer Society. Frequently asked questions about nutrition and physical activity. Available at: http://www.cancer.org/docroot/mbc/content/MBC_6_2x_FAQ_Nutrition_and_Physical_Activity.asp?sitearea=MH. Accessed May 21, 2004.

American Cancer Society. Laetrile. Available at: http://www.cancer.org/docroot/ETO/content/ETO_5_3X_Laetrile.asp?sitearea=ETO. Accessed May 21, 2004.

American Cancer Society. Licorice. Available at: http://www.cancer.org/docroot/ETO/content/ETO_5_3X_Licorice.asp?sitearea=ETO. Accessed May 21, 2004.

American Cancer Society. PC-SPES taken off the market. ACS News Center. April 25, 2002. Available at: http://www.cancer.org/docroot/NWS/content/NWS_1_1x_Herbal_Prostate_Cancer_Treatment_PC-SPES_Not_All_Natural.asp.

American Cancer Society. Prostate cancer prevention studies underway. ACS News Center. April 11, 2002. Available at: http://www.cancer.org/docroot/NWS/content/NWS_1_1x_Prostate_Cancer_Prevention_Studies_Underway.asp.

American Cancer Society. Saw palmetto. Available at: http://www.cancer.org/docroot/ETO/content/ETO_5_3X_Saw_Palmetto.asp?sitearea=ETO. Accessed May 21, 2004.

MD Anderson. Herbal/Plant Therapies: PC-SPES. Complementary/Integrative Medicine: Reviews of Therapies. Available at: http://www.mdanderson.org/departments/cimer/display.cfm?id=66d17404-09ad-443e-b865bcfc6b635507&method=displayfull&pn=6eb86a59-ebd9-11d4-810100508b603a14. Accessed May 20, 2004.

Memorial Sloan Kettering Cancer Center. Black cohosh. About Herbs. Available at: http://www.mskcc.org/mskcc/html/11571.cfm?TAB=CON&RecordID=405. Accessed May 20, 2004.

Memorial Sloan Kettering Cancer Center. Dehydroepiandrosterone. About Herbs. Available at: http://www.mskcc.org/mskcc/html/11571.cfm?RecordID=625&tab=CON. Accessed May 20, 2004.

Memorial Sloan Kettering Cancer Center. Flaxseed. About Herbs. Available at: http://www.mskcc.org/mskcc/html/11571.cfm?TAB=CON&RecordID=690. Accessed May 20, 2004.

Memorial Sloan Kettering Cancer Center. Garlic. About Herbs. Available at: http://www.mskcc.org/mskcc/html/11571.cfm?TAB=CON&RecordID=412. Accessed May 21, 2004.

Memorial Sloan Kettering Cancer Center. Licorice. About Herbs. Available at: http://www.mskcc.org/mskcc/html/11571.cfm?RecordID=416&tab=CON. Accessed May 22, 2004.

Memorial Sloan Kettering Cancer Center. PC-SPES. About Herbs. Available at: http://www.mskcc.org/mskcc/html/11571.cfm?TAB=CON&RecordID=487. Accessed January 29, 2004.

Memorial Sloan Kettering Cancer Center. Shiitake mushrooms. About Herbs. Available at: http://www.mskcc.org/mskcc/html/11571.cfm?TAB=CON&RecordID=402. Accessed May 21, 2004.

National Cancer Institute. Cartilage (bovine and shark). Physician Data Query. http://www.cancer.gov/cancerinfo/pdq/cam/cartilage. Accessed May 21, 2004.

National Center for Complementary and Alternative Medicine. St. John's Wort and the Treatment of Depression. National Institutes of Health. Available at: http://nccam.nih.gov/health/stjohnswort/. Accessed May 21, 2004.

CHAPTER 28

National Cancer Institute. Questions and answers about the prostate-specific antigen (PSA) test. Available at: http://cis.nci.nih.gov/fact/5_29.htm. Accessed March 12, 2004.

Pound CR, Partin AW, Eisenberger MA, Chan DW, Pearson JD, Walsh PC. Natural history of progression after PSA elevation following radical prostatectomy. *JAMA*. 1999;281(17):1591-1597.

CHAPTER 29

Aaron A. The management of cancer metastatic to bone. *JAMA*. 1994;272:1206-1209.

American Cancer Society. *A Breast Cancer Journey: Your Personal Guidebook.* 2nd ed. Atlanta, GA: American Cancer Society; 2004.

American Cancer Society. *American Cancer Society's Guide to Pain Control.* 2nd ed. Atlanta, Georgia: American Cancer Society; 2004.

American Cancer Society. Recurrent prostate cancer: cryosurgery offers "curative" treatment. June 21, 2001. Available at: http://www.cancer.org/docroot/NWS/content/NWS_1_1x_Recurrent_Prostate_Cancer_Cryosurgery_Offers_Curative_Treatment.asp.

Amling CL, Lerner SE, Martin SK, Slezak JM, Blute ML, Zincke H. Deoxyribonucleic acid ploidy and serum prostate specific antigen predict outcome following salvage prostatectomy for radiation refractory prostate cancer. *J Urol*. 1999;161;857-862.

Baker L, Goodman S, Perkash I, et al. Benign versus pathologic compression fractures of vertebral bodies: Assessment with conventional spin-echo, chemical-shift, and STIR MR imaging. *Musculoskeletal Radiology*. 1990;174:495-502.

Beyer DC. Brachytherapy for recurrent prostate cancer after radiation therapy. *Sem Radiation Oncol*. 2003;13:158-163.

Bilsky M, Shannon F, Sheppard S, et al. Diagnosis and management of a metastatic tumor in the atlantoaxial spine. *Spine*. 2002;27:1062-1069.

Black P, Nair S, Giannakopoulos G, et al. Spinal Epidural Tumors. In: Wilkins RH and Setti S, eds. *Neurosurgery*. 2nd ed. Vol III. New York: McGraw-Hill Health Professions Division; 1996:1791.

Bolla M, Collette L, Blank L, et al. Long-term results with immediate androgen suppression and external irradiation in patients with locally advanced prostate cancer (an EORTC study): a phase III randomized trial. *Lancet*. 2002;360:103-106.

Brown JK, Byers T, Doyle C, et al. Nutrition and Physical Activity During and After Cancer Treatment: An American Cancer Society Guide for Informed Choices. *CA Cancer J Clin* 2003;53:268-291. Available at: http://caonline.amcancersoc.org/cgi/content/full/53/5/268.

Byers K, Axelrod P, Michael S, et al. Infections complicating tunneled intraspinal catheter systems used to treat chronic pain. *Clin Infect Dis*. 1995;21:403-408.

Caldwell JR, Rapoport RJ, Davis JC, et. al. Efficacy and safety of a once-daily morphine formulation in chronic, moderate-to-severe osteoarthritis pain: Results from a randomized, placebo-controlled, double-blind trial and an open label extension trial. *J Pain Sympt Manage*. 2002;23:4:278-291.

Cox JD, Gallagher MJ, Hammond EH, Kaplan RS, Schellhammer PF. Consensus statements on radiation therapy of prostate cancer: guidelines for prostate re-biopsy after radiation and for radiation therapy with rising prostate-specific antigen levels after radical prostatectomy. *J Clin Oncol*. 1999;17:1155.

Dawson NA. Therapeutic benefit of bisphosphonates in the management of prostate cancer-related bone disease. *Expert Opinion on Pharmacotherapy*. 2003;4:705-716.

Dehlen B, Szczeklik A, Murray JJ. Celecoxib in patients with asthma and aspirin intolerance. *NEJM*. 2001;344:142.

Food and Drug Administration. FDA approves new indication for taxotere—prostate cancer. FDA News. May 19, 2004. Available at: http://www.fda.gov/bbs/topics/news/2004/NEW01068.html.

Ghafar M, Johnson C, De La Taille A, et al. Salvage cryotherapy using an argon based system for locally recurrent prostate cancer after radiation therapy: The Columbia experience. *J Urology*. 2001;166:1333-1338.

Kahn D, Williams RD, Haseman MK, Reed N, Miller SJ, Gerstbrein J. Radioimmunoscintigraphy with In-111-labeled capromab pendetide predicts prostate cancer response to salvage radiotherapy after failed prostatectomy. *J Clin Oncol*. 1998;16:284-269.

Leventis AK, Shariat SF, Kattan MW, Butler EB, Wheeler TM, Slawin KM. Prediction of response to salvage radiation therapy in patients with prostate cancer recurrence after radical prostatectomy. *J Clin Oncol*. 2001;19:1030-1039.

Messing EM, Manola J, Sarosdy M, Wilding G, Crawford ED, Trump D. Immediate hormonal therapy compared with observation after radical prostatectomy and pelvic lymphadenectomy in men with node-positive prostate cancer. *N Engl J Med*. 1999;341:1781-1788.

Miguel R. Interventional treatment of cancer pain: the fourth step in the World Health Organization analgesic ladder? *Cancer Control*. March-April 2000;7(2):149-56.

Moyad M. The use of complementary/preventive medicine to prevent prostate cancer recurrence/progression following definitive therapy; parts I and II. *Curr Opin Urol.* 2003;13:137-151.

National Cancer Institute. What you need to know about prostate cancer. Available at: http://www.cancer.gov/cancerinfo/wyntk/prostate#19. Accessed May 21, 2004.

Pisters L. Salvage radical prostatectomy; refinement of an effective procedure. *Sem Radiat Oncol.* 2003;13:166-174.

Pound CR, Partin AW. Eisenberger MA, Chan DW, Pearson JD, Walsh PC. Natural history of progression after PSA elevation following radical prostatectomy. *JAMA.* 1999;28:1591-1597.

Saad F, Gleason DM, Murray R, et al. A randomized, placebo-controlled trial of zoledronic acid in patients with hormone-refractory metastatic prostate carcinoma. *J Natl Cancer Inst.* 2002;94:1458-1468.

Saad F, Schulman C. Role of bisphosphonates in prostate cancer. *European Urology.* 2004;45:26-34.

See WA, Wirth MP, McLeod DG, et al. Bicalutamide as immediate therapy either alone or as adjuvant to standard care of patients with localized or locally advanced prostate cancer: first analysis of the early prostate cancer program. *J Urol.* 2002;168:429-435.

Siddall PJ, Molloy AR, Walker S, et al. The efficacy of intrathecal morphine and clonidine in the treatment of pain after spinal cord injury. *Anesth Analg.* 2000;91:1493-1498.

Smith MR. Diagnosis and management of treatment-related osteoporosis in men with prostate carcinoma. *Cancer.* 2003;97: 789-795.

Smith MR, Eastham J, Gleason DM, et al. Randomized controlled trial of zoledronic acid to prevent bone loss in men receiving androgen deprivation therapy for nonmetastatic prostate cancer. *J Urol.* 2003;169:2008-2012.

Uhle EI, Becker R, Gatscher S, et al. Continuous intrathecal clonidine administration for the treatment of neuropathic pain. *Stereotact Funct Neurosurg.* 2000;75:167-175.

Valicenti RK, Gomella LG, Perez CA. Radiation therapy after radical prostatectomy: A review of the issues and options. *Sem Radiat Oncol.* 2003;13:130-140.

Wong R, Wiffen PJ. Bisphosphonates for the relief of pain secondary to bone metastases. Cochrane Review. In: *The Cochrane Library.* Chichester, UK: John Wiley & Sons, Ltd., 2002.

CHAPTER 30

American Cancer Society. Experiencing incontinence? Available at: http://www.cancer.org/docroot/M2M/content/M2M_2_7_1x_Experiencing_Incontinence_15.asp?sitearea=. Accessed May 22, 2004.

American Cancer Society. Sexuality for men and their partners. Available at: http://www.cancer.org/docroot/MIT/MIT_7_1x_SexualityforMenandTheirPartners.asp?sitearea=&level=. Accessed October, 2003.

Dawson NA. Intermittent androgen deprivation. *Curr Oncol Rep.* 2000;2:409-416.

Dewire DM, Todd E, Meyers P. Patient satisfaction with current impotence therapy. *Wis Med J.* 1995;94:542-544.

Fossa SD, Woehre H, Kurth KH, et al. Influence of urological morbidity on quality of life in patients with prostate cancer. *Eur Urol.* 1997;31(suppl 3):S3-S8.

Heiman JR. *Becoming Orgasmic: A Sexual Growth Program for Women.* Rev and Expanded ed. New York, NY: Prentice Hall Press; 1988.

Helgason AR, Adolfsson J, Dickman P, Arver S, Fredrikson M, Steineck G. Factors associated with waning sexual function among elderly men and prostate cancer patients. *J Urol.* 1997;158:155-159.

Higano CS. Intermittent androgen suppression with leuprolide and flutamide for prostate cancer: A pilot study. *Urol.* 1996;48:800-804.

Higano CS. *Side Effects Of Androgen Deprivation: The Known and the Less Well Known.* Paper presented at the 3rd Annual Pacific Northwest Prostate Cancer Conference, Portland, OR; June 2003.

Masters WH, Johnson V. *Human Sexual Inadequacy.* Boston: Little Brown; 1970.

Masters WH, Johnson V. *Human Sexual Response.* Boston: Little Brown; 1966.

Van Kampen M, de Weerdt WD, Claes H, Feys H, De Maeyer M, Van Poppel. Treatment of erectile dysfunction by perineal exercis, electromyographic biofeedback, and electrical stimuation. *Phys Ther.* 2003;83:536-543.

CHAPTER 31

American Cancer Society. New unique protein marker for prostate cancer identified. ACS News Center. November 11, 2003. Available at: http://www.cancer.org/docroot/MED/content/MED_2_1x_New_Unique_Protein_Marker_For_Prostate_Cancer_Identified.asp.

Apakama I, Robinson MC, Walter NM, et al. bcl-2 overexpression combined with p53 protein accumulation correlates with hormone-refractory prostate cancer. *Br J Cancer.* October 1996;74(8):1258-1262.

Bansal A, Critchfield GC, Frank TS, et al. The predictive value of BRCA1 and BRCA2 mutation testing. *Genet Test.* 2000;4(1):45-48.

Brewster SF, Oxley JD, Trivella M, Abbott CD, Gillatt DA. Preoperative p53, bcl-2, CD44 and E-cadherin immunohistochemistry as predictors of biochemical relapse after radical prostatectomy. *J Urol.* April 1999;161(4):1238-1243.

Culig Z, Klocker H, Bartsch G, Steiner H, Hobisch A. Androgen receptors in prostate cancer. *J Urol.* October 2003;170(4 Pt 1):1363-1369.

Edwards J, Krishna NS, Grigor KM, Bartlett JM. Androgen receptor gene amplification and protein expression in hormone refractory prostate cancer. *Br J Cancer.* August 4 2003;89(3):552-556.

Fey MF. Microsatellite markers in leukaemia and lymphoma: comments on a timely topic. *Leuk Lymphoma.* December 1997;28(1-2):11-22.

Gardner TA, Sloan J, Raikwar SP, Kao C. Prostate cancer gene therapy: past experiences and future promise. *Cancer Metastasis Rev.* 2002;21(2):137-145.

Grignon DJ, Caplan R, Sarkar FH, et al. p53 status and prognosis of locally advanced prostatic adenocarcinoma: a study based on RTOG 8610. *J Natl Cancer Inst.* January 15 1997;89(2):158-165.

Kaminski JM, Summers JB, Ward MB, Huber MR, Minev B. Immunotherapy and prostate cancer. *Cancer Treat Rev.* June 2003;29(3):199-209.

Koivisto P, Kononen J, Palmberg C, et al. Androgen receptor gene amplification: a possible molecular mechanism for androgen deprivation therapy failure in prostate cancer. *Cancer Res.* January 15 1997;57(2):314-319.

Mabjeesh NJ, Zhong H, Simons JW. Gene therapy of prostate cancer: current and future directions. *Endocr Relat Cancer.* June 2002;9(2):115-139.

McDonnell TJ, Navone NM, Troncoso P, et al. Expression of bcl-2 oncoprotein and p53 protein accumulation in bone marrow metastases of androgen independent prostate cancer. *J Urol.* February 1997;157(2):569-574.

National Human Genome Research Institute. Prostate Cancer Genetic Backgrounder. National Institutes of Health. Available at: http://www.genome.gov/ 10003513.

Oxley JD, Winkler MH, Parry K, Brewster S, Abbott C, Gillatt DA. p53 and bcl-2 immunohistochemistry in preoperative biopsies as predictors of biochemical recurrence after radical prostatectomy. *BJU Int.* January 2002;89(1):27-32.

Qian J, Jenkins RB, Bostwick DG. Genetic and chromosomal alterations in prostatic intraepithelial neoplasia and carcinoma detected by fluorescence in situ hybridization. *Eur Urol.* 1999;35(5-6):479-483.

Ruijter E, van de Kaa C, Aalders T, et al. Heterogeneous expression of E-cadherin and p53 in prostate cancer: clinical implications. BIOMED-II Markers for Prostate Cancer Study Group. *Mod Pathol.* March 1998;11(3):276-281.

CHAPTER 32

American Cancer Society. Detailed guide: prostate cancer. Available at: http://www.cancer.org/ docroot/CRI/CRI_2_3x.asp?rnav=cridg&dt=36. Accessed May 26, 2004.

Bolla M, Collette L, Blank L, et al. Long-term results with immediate androgen suppression and external irradiation in patients with locally advanced prostate cancer (an EORTC study): a phase III randomised trial. *Lancet.* July 13, 2002;360(9327):103-6.

Gohagan JK, Prorok PC, Hayes RB, Kramer BS. Prostate, Lung, Colorectal and Ovarian Cancer Screening Trial Project Team. The Prostate, Lung, Colorectal and Ovarian (PLCO) Cancer Screening Trial of the National Cancer Institute: history, organization, and status. *Control Clin Trials.* December 2000;21(6 Suppl):251S-272S.

Holmberg L, Bill-Axelson A, Helgesen F, et al. A randomized trial comparing radical prostatectomy with watchful waiting in early prostate cancer. *N Engl J Med.* 2002;347 :781-9.

Klein EA, Lippman SM, Thompson IM, et al. The selenium and vitamin E cancer prevention trial. *World J Urol.* May 2003;21(1):21-7.

Lawton CA, Winter K, Murray K, et al. Updated results of the phase III Radiation Therapy Oncology Group (RTOG) trial 85-31 evaluating the potential benefit of androgen suppression following standard radiation therapy for unfavorable prognosis carcinoma of the prostate. *Int J Radiat Oncol Biol Phys.* March 15, 2001;49(4):937-46.

Logothetis CJ. Docetaxel in the integrated management of prostate cancer. Current applications and future promise. *Oncology* (Huntingt). June 2002;16(6 Suppl 6):63-72.

National Cancer Institute. NCI High Priority Clinical Trial—Phase III Randomized Study of Prostatectomy Versus Expectant Management With Palliative Therapy in Patients With Clinically Localized Prostate Cancer (PIVOT). Clinical Trials: Physician Data Query. Available at: http://www.cancer.gov/ templates/view_clinicaltrials.aspx?version= healthprofessional&cdrid=63882. Accessed May 22, 2004.

National Cancer Institute. Prostate cancer prevention trial (PCPT): questions and answers. June 24, 2003. Available at: http://www.cancer.gov/newscenter/pressreleases/PCPTQandA.

Schellhammer P. Clinical trials in prostate cancer. *BJU Int*. August 2003;92(3):186-7.

Syed S, Petrylak DP, Thompson IM. Management of high-risk localized prostate cancer: the integration of local and systemic therapy approaches. *Urol Oncol*. May-June 2003;21(3):235-43.

Thompson IM, Goodman PJ, Tangen CM, et al. The influence of finasteride on the development of prostate cancer. *N Engl J Med*. July 17, 2003;349(3):215-24.

Verma M, Srivastava S. New cancer biomarkers deriving from NCI early detection research. Recent Results. *Cancer Res*. 2003;163:72-84; discussion 264-6.

Wilt TJ, Brawer MK. The Prostate Cancer Intervention Versus Observation Trial (PIVOT). *Oncology* (Huntingt). August 1997;11(8):1133-9;discussion 1139-40, 1143

INDEX

Sphincter implants, 298
SPIRIT study, 332
Spread, tumor, 70–72
  imaging studies to determine, 137–142
  lymph nodes and, 143
Squamous cell carcinoma, 6
St. John's wort, 267
Staging
  definition of, 133
  and Gleason grades, 69, 70–71f, 136
  improved through molecular biology research, 324–325
  M categories, 135
  N categories, 135
  and stage grouping, 136
  T categories, 134–135
  TNM system of, 133–136
State risk pools, 121
Statistical models of outcomes, 151–152
Steroids, 291
Stress, 86
Supplemental Security Income (SSI), 124
Supplements, prostate-healthy, 264
Support networks
  assembling, 110–111
  after diagnosis, 8, 84
Surgery. See also Prostatectomy
  advantages of different types of, 180, 184
  anesthesia complications, 190
  blood loss, 187–188
  cardiovascular complications, 190
  catheters after, 177–180, 189
  conversion during, 188
  ejaculation effects of, 195
  expected outcomes, 181, 185, 189
  impotence after, 31, 40–41, 58, 193–194
  incontinence after, 185, 189, 192–193
  infections after, 189, 191–192
  laparoscopic radical prostatectomy (LRP), 186–189
  nerve-sparing prostatectomy, 178–179, 183, 193–194
  orchiectomy, 216, 219t, 224–229
  organ injury due to, 195
  pain, 184, 187, 189, 190
  potential consequences of, 180, 185, 188–195
  questions to ask about, 166–167
  radical perineal prostatectomy, 181–185
  radical retropubic prostatectomy, 175–181
  recovery from, 178–180, 184, 188
  scarring after, 184, 190
  side effects, 169, 180, 185, 188–189, 192–195, 227
Survival rates, 152, 293–294
Symptoms
  abdominal pain or digestive, 31
  back or pelvic pain, 32
  blood in semen, 31, 58
  blood in urine, 29, 58
  clotting disorder, 32
  describing, 42
  erectile dysfunction, 31
  follow-up plans after treatment, 272
  inability to urinate, 29

kidney failure, 29
leg pain, numbness, or weakness, 32
painful or frequent urination, 29
score index, 30t
sexual, 31, 40–41, 42, 58
sudden, 31
urinary, 29–31, 40–41, 42
weak urination, 29
weight loss, fatigue, or generalized weakness, 31
what may be indicated by, 27–28
in young men, 30

T
T categories of staging, 134–135
Tadalafil, 302–303
Tamsulosin, 303
Targeted therapies, 326
Taxol, 242t, 288
Taxotere, 242t, 243, 288
Testes, 4, 216
  orchiectomy, 216, 219t, 224–227
Testosterone, 13, 215–216, 227
  replacement therapy, 14
Thalidomide, 335
Thalomid, 335
Three-dimensional conformal radiation therapy
      (3DCRT), 198
TNM staging system, 133–136
Tofranil, 297
Tofu, consumption of, 19, 20, 24
Tolterodine, 297
Tomato products, consumption of, 19, 20
Transitional cell carcinoma, 6
Transrectal biopsies, 55, 56, 60
Transrectal ultrasound (TRUS), 41, 45, 49, 55, 59–62,
      140–142, 205, 238
  delivering treatment for cancer, 62, 246f
  Doppler flow machine, 62
  -guided biopsy, 55, 56, 60, 61f
Transurethral resection of the prostate (TURP), 196, 210
Treatments. See also Surgery
  adjuvant therapy, 165, 218
  alternative, 263–267
  assistance programs, 126
  brachytherapy, 167, 169, 204–214, 273, 300t, 332
  caregiver support for decisions about, 114
  chemotherapy, 241–244, 287–288, 300t, 334–335
  choosing centers for, 95–98
  clinical trial, 253–262
  common guidelines for, 157–160, 161t
  consulting with the health care team about, 164–165
  cryotherapy, 169, 175, 237–241, 287
  delivered via transrectal ultrasound (TRUS), 62, 246f
  designating a personal advocate during, 99
  expected outcomes of, 150, 153, 181, 185, 189, 204,
      214, 222, 227
  external beam radiation therapy (EBRT), 167, 169,
      197–204, 287
  factors that help determine the most appropriate, 159t
  follow-up plans, 167, 272–276

We Care About Your Opinions.

Please take a moment to complete this survey and fax it to *Books/Product Marketing Specialist* at **404-325-9341**, or email your comments and suggestions to us at **trade.sales@cancer.org**. *Thank you!*

PLEASE PRINT.

First Name _____

Last Name _____

Address _____

City _____ State _____ Zip _____

Email _____

1. Gender: ☐ Female   ☐ Male

2. Age: ☐ 20–39   ☐ 40–59   ☐ 60+

3. How many health books have you bought or read in last 12 months? _____

4. How did you find out about this book? (Please choose one.)
   ☐ Recommendation   ☐ Store Display   ☐ Online
   ☐ Advertisement   ☐ Catalog/Mailing ☐ TV/Radio

5. Is there a topic you feel should appear in the next edition of this book?
   _____

6. What attracts you most to a book? (Please rank 1–4 in order of preference; 1 being most important.)
   ____ Title ____ Content ____ Cover Design ____ Author

7. If you would you like more information about other books published by the American Cancer Society, please tell us how you prefer to be contacted:
   ☐ Email   ☐ Mail